Bioethical Dilemmas
A Jewish Perspective

Other Books by the Same Author

Providence in the Philosophy of Gersonides
Contemporary Halakhic Problems, Vols. I–IV
Jewish Bioethics: A Reader (ed. with Fred Rosner)
Judaism and Healing
Bircas ha-Chammah
With Perfect Faith: Foundations of Jewish Belief (ed.)
Time of Death in Jewish Law
Be-Netivot ha-Halakhah, Vols. I–III

Bioethical Dilemmas
A Jewish Perspective

J. David Bleich

KTAV Publishing House, Inc.
Hoboken, NJ

Library of Congress Cataloging-in-Publication Data

Bleich, David J.
Bioethical dilemmas: a Jewish perspective / David J. Bleich.
p. cm.
"...consists of a variety of less technical lectures and papers presented before diverse forums over period of several decades"-—Pref.
Includes indexes.
ISBN 0-88125-473-8
1. Bioethics—Religious aspects—Judaism. 2. Medicine—Religious aspects—Judaism. 3. Medical laws and legislation (Jewish law) 4. Ethics, Jewish. I. Title.
BM538.H43B54 1998
296.3' 64957—dc21 98-28595
CIP

Manufactured in the United States of America

ועל דא אצטריך לאסיא חכים לאשתדלא עליה אי יכיל למיתב ליה אסוותא מן גופא יאות ואי לאו יתן ליה אסוותא לנשמתיה, ודא הוא אסיא דקב"ה ישתדל עליה בהאי עלמא ובעלמא דאתי.

זהר, דברים דף רצ"ט.

A person needs a wise physician to endeavor on his behalf. If he can prescribe a remedy for the body, good! If not, he should provide a remedy for his soul. It is on behalf of such a physician that the Holy One, blessed be He, endeavors in this world and in the world to come.

Zohar, Deuteronomy 299a.

Contents

Preface

Analyses of many of the issues discussed in this work have been presented in the various volumes of my *Contemporary Halakhic Problems* and in *Judaism and Healing* as well as in essays published in *Jewish Bioethics*. The material included in the present volume consists of a variety of less technical lectures and papers presented before diverse forums over a period of several decades. Some were addressed to general audiences and readers and designed simply to convey the broad ethical teachings of Judaism. As such, they are exercises in consciousness-raising and are directed to Jews and non-Jews alike. Others were designed to express a nuanced formulation of Jewish teaching and are addressed to Jews for whom the minutiae of Halakhah taken collectively represent the ultimate source of moral authority. Thus, the reader should not be surprised at the absence of a uniform style in the various selections.

Portions of this work served as the subject matter of *shi'urim* and seminars on behalf of the students of the Rabbi Isaac Elchanan Theological Seminary and the Benjamin N. Cardozo School of Law. The ongoing support of the Leonard and Bea Diener Institute of Jewish Law in facilitating my investigation of the application of Jewish law to contemporary legal and moral issues is gratefully acknowledged.

I wish to express my thanks to my brother-in-law, Rabbi Mordecai Ochs, for his painstaking reading of the manuscript; to my son, Rabbi Moshe Bleich, for drawing my attention to sources that otherwise would have eluded me and for his many valuable insights; to Dr. Joel Wolowelsky, associate editor of *Tradition*, both for his patience and for his many welcome suggestions; to Rabbi Jacob B. Mandelbaum of the Mendel Gottesman Library of Yeshiva University, whose encyclopedic bibliographic knowledge has been of immeasurable aid; to Mr. Zalman Alpert, Mr. Zvi Erenyi, Mrs. Chaya Gordin and Mr. Tuvia Lasdun of the Mendel Gottesman Library for their constant helpfulness and assistance; to Mrs. Racheline Habousha of the library of the Albert Einstein College of Medicine for her unfailing graciousness in expediting my many requests; and to Dr. Fred Rosner, Dr. Edward Reichman and Dr. Richard Weiss for assisting me in obtaining pertinent medical sources.

My thanks also to the publisher of this volume, Mr. Bernard Scharfstein, for his unfailing indulgence and patience and his warm friendship; to Dr. Yaakov Elman for making his technical and scholarly expertise available at all times; and to Dr. Richard White for his painstaking efforts, tirelessness and good humor in shepherding the manuscript through the various stages of publication.

Above all, I am grateful to the Almighty for my cherished collaborators—the members of my family. It is our fervent prayer that this endeavor, as our earlier efforts, serve to promote Torah study and to enhance the moral climate in which we live.

Introduction

The second half of the twentieth century has witnessed triumph after triumph in the development of medical science and technology. Diseases such as smallpox have been eradicated; others such as tuberculosis and poliomyelitis have become rare or have been geographically contained. Many chronic diseases are no longer debilitating. Disabled persons who in days gone by would have been confined to bed or home are now productive and self-fulfilled members of society. The biblical era excluded, longevity anticipation is more favorable than at any time since the dawn of civilization.

These advances are universally acclaimed. But other achievements are just as widely perceived as a mixed blessing. The life of a comatose patient can be extended by placing him or her on a ventilator but only with dedicated efforts of often overburdened care-givers and anguish on the part of family members. Malignant diseases can be treated, generally with no guarantee of success but with the assurance of discomfort. Life-saving transplantation of vital organs is quite feasible but only with attendant risk of failure followed by the imminent demise of the recipient, not to speak of the dilemma involved in assuring that the organ is harvested without causing the death of the donor.

Not only can modern medicine prolong life in ways that were unimaginable barely a few decades ago, medical technology can also enable man to generate life in highly novel ways. Assisted reproduction has brought joy to many couples who would otherwise have remained childless. But assistance in the form of artificial insemination has also spawned moral dilemmas centering upon family values and the sanctity of marital bonds. Surrogate motherhood and ovum donation have given rise to previously unexplored questions regarding maternal identity. Confidentiality surrounding many fertility programs has resulted in realistic concern regarding potential consanguineous relationships. In vitro procedures may yield a higher than normal incidence of neonatal defects. And, of course, the specter of human cloning presents issues we have only begun to define.

These problems and many others are novel in the sense that in past generations they would have been theoretical rather than actual. The science fiction of yesteryear has become the reality of today. Only in the past two or three decades have philosophers, ethicists, theologians and legal scholars been forced to address such matters. In grappling with these problems our society seeks not only practical guidance but also formulation of a value system in which the solutions are morally coherent. Accordingly, even secular theoreticians find themselves looking to religious traditions—of which Judaism is by far the oldest—not always for definitive answers, but for insights that may inform their own decision making. Jewish medical practitioners and patients committed to a Jewish lifestyle must perforce look both to Halakhah for a determination of normative rules and to Jewish tradition for the values against which any contemplated procedure must be examined. With increasing frequency halakhic scholars are called upon to plumb the depths of rabbinic literature for sources and precedents applicable to novel bioethical dilemmas.

Jews have seldom endeavored to impose Jewish teaching

upon society at large. Judaism regards most areas of Jewish law as being relevant only to Jews. To the extent that some bioethical issues involve matters of Noahide law it is necessary to examine those issues from the perspective of the provisions of the Noahide Code itself. Of equal concern is the impact of public policy and the prevailing moral climate upon Jews themselves and upon their need to adhere steadfastly to the values and principles of Judaism while living in a pluralistic society. To that end, Jews must be aware of the duties incumbent upon them and non-Jews must be sensitized to Jewish values, needs and concerns. It is to that purpose that this endeavor has been undertaken.

One must also be mindful of the comment made by R. Judah ha-Levi in his *Kuzari*, Part II, sec. 36: "As the heart is to the body, so is Israel among the nations." The role and function of the heart and its the importance to, and influence upon, the human organism is vastly disproportionate to its modest size. Likewise, the potential moral influence of Israel upon the nations of the world is far greater than demographic figures would suggest. And just as a healthy heart fulfills its crucial biological function without conscious effort, or even awareness, either on its own part or on the part of the organism it serves so can ethically committed, spiritually healthy Jews exercise moral influence over the dominant society simply by the example provided in adherence to their own code of conduct, a code that has governed Jewish behavior since it was received at Sinai.

1

Medical and Life Insurance: A Halakhic Mandate

I. EARLY RESPONSA

Psalms 37:3, rendered by the classic commentaries as "Trust in the Lord and do good; dwell in the land and seek sustenance[1] in faith," is cited by both Ramban[2] and R. Baḥya ben Asher[3] as the locus of Jewish teaching regarding man's need to trust in the Deity for satisfaction of his needs. To be sure, both philosophers understand the phrase "dwell in the land" as negating man's right to rely solely upon divine beneficence in abjuring any attempt to seek sustenenance by means of human endeavor. Nevertheless, the concept of reliance, or *bitaḥon*, might readily be understood as precluding concern for possible reversal of fortune and certainty as excluding reliance upon other mortals, as distinct from one's own labor and industry to restore economic well-being. Indeed, the Gemara, *Sotah* 48b, quotes R. Eliezer the Great as declaring, "One who has bread in his basket but says 'What will I eat tomorrow?' is but of those who have little faith." R. Baḥya ibn Pekuda asserts that failure to place one's trust in God results, not merely in failure to achieve benefit commensurate with such faith, but has deleterious effects as well: "For if a person does not put his trust in God, he places his trust elsewhere. If he puts his trust elsewhere than in the Eternal, God withdraws His providential care from that individual and leaves him in the power of the one in whom he trusted, so that he will be in the condition of the one concerning whom it was said, 'For my people have committed two evils: Me they have forsaken, the fountain of living waters to hew them out cisterns, broken cisterns . . .' (Jeremiah 2:13)."[4]

Insurance of all sorts including life, medical, accident, fire, theft, flood, etc., is designed to mitigate adverse circumstances that may arise at some future time as a result of natural events as well as from human negligence. or malfeasance. Insurance, by its very nature, reflects a lack of reliance on divine protection against misfortune.[5] Moreover, insurance coverage represents an attempt by policyholders to provide for a need that does not yet exist and that, in the case of many forms of insurance, may never exist. In addition, arguably, insurance represents tangible reliance upon mortals, rather than upon the Deity, to satisfy those needs when they do arise. Furthermore, the Gemara, *Gittin* 75b, records that Samuel decreed that a person lying on his death-bed who seeks to execute a conditional divorce in order to exempt his wife from the obligation of levirate marriage should declare, "If I do not die, it shall not be a *get*, but if I die, it shall be a *get*" rather than "If I die, it shall be a *get;* but if I do not die, it shall not be a *get*" because a person ought not anticipate and render primary his own misfortune *(lo makdim inish puranuta le-nafshei).* That, in turn is a reflection of the notion enunciated by the Gemara, *Mo'ed Katan* 18a and *Sanhedrin* 102a, to the effect that "a covenant is entered into with the lips." Similarly, the Gemara, *Berakhot* 19a, admonishes, "A person should not open Satan's mouth." The concern reflected in that statement is that verbalizing an untoward contingency may serve to cause its occurrence. The mere mention of misfortune may be the mother of the event since it may prompt examination by heaven of whether the misfortune is indeed deserved. Thus, there is *prima facie* reason to fear that execution of an insurance policy designed to alleviate the effects of a catastrophe may itself trigger that untoward event.

The foregoing notwithstanding, examination of discussions of insurance in the responsa literature dating from the medieval period fails to reveal the slightest hint of censure of insurance against financial loss. The earliest form of insurance devised by man was probably maritime insurance designed to protect a merchant from the loss of what might represent his entire fortune in the event that a ship carrying his merchandise to market sinks at sea or is abducted by pirates. The earliest discussion in halakhic sources of what is analagous to a rudimentary insurance contract involves a maritime transaction. R. Isaac ben Sheshet (1326–1408), known as Rivash, was consulted with regard to an arrangement involving a loan of twenty *dinars* to be secured by a ship about to embark upon a sea voyage. Repayment in the amount of twenty-four *dinars* was to be contingent upon return of the ship "in peace" to the port of embarkation. Repayment of a sum greater than that extended in the form of a loan is, of course, prohibited by Jewish law. However, this transaction was unlike an ordinary loan agreement in that it provided for forfeit of capital in the event of misadventure. In effect, a transaction of this nature is a hybrid in that it represents a loan coupled with a contract for indemnification against loss of the ship.[6] The additional four *dinars* might be construed either as interest on the loan,[7] a premium for insurance coverage, or both.[8] In his reply, *Teshuvot Rivash,* no. 308, Rivash forbids the arrangement on two grounds: (1) based upon a discussion recorded in *Bava Meẓi'a* 69b, Rivash argues that, since the recipient would not return the coins entrusted to him but would expend the funds on his own behalf, the funds represent a loan despite the fact that the recipient was not to be released from repayment in the event of misadventure and, accordingly, the additional payment constitutes illicit interest; (2) since the merchant accepted absolute liability for all forms of misadventure that might occur before the ship sails as well as for misadventure that might occur subsequent to safe return of the ship but prior to repayment, the funds constitute a loan and hence any additional payment represents interest.[9] Nevertheless, Rivash maintains that since, due to exoneration in the event of misadventure, even return of the principal is not certain, the violation is rabbinic, rather than biblical, in nature.

The identical question was later addressed by R. David ibn Zimra (1479–1589), *Teshuvot Radvaz,* I, no. 497. Radvaz adopts an even more stringent position in ruling that the repayment of twenty-four *dinars* represents a biblically prohibited form of interest. Radvaz argues that the merchant is liable, at least "at the hands of heaven,"[10] for repayment of the principal under all circumstances. He maintains that, according to rabbinic edict, the release conditioned upon misadventure is not binding because the financier does not really envisage that such a contingency will actually occur and hence the transfer of funds is not accompanied by the state of mind required to effect transfer of title. Radvaz rules that, by virtue of rabbinic decree, delivery of funds in the absence of such mental determination constitutes an ineffective *asmakhta* and hence the insurance contract is not enforceable in Jewish law.[11] Accordingly, the recipient, not having received valid title, must return the funds even in the case of misadventure. Thus, those funds have the character of a loan that must be repaid. As a result, even voluntary repayment of any additional funds constitutes payment of interest.

The novelty of Radvaz' position lies in the fact that the transfer of title to the funds is biblically valid and, moreover, despite being rendered invalid by rabbinic decree, return of the funds cannot be enforced by a *Bet Din.* Yet, maintains Radvaz, even an unenforceable rabbinic obligation to return the funds is sufficient to endow the transfer with the guise of a loan so that any additional payment constitutes biblically prohibited interest.[12]

In the earlier cited responsum Rivash discusses a conventional form of maritime insurance which he describes as a common practice and with which he finds no fault. That arrangement is described as indemnity coverage of merchandise transported by ship in return for a fee or premium of ten percent of the amount guaranteed. Rivash does entertain the objection that, if the premium is paid in advance, indemnification in the event of accident in excess of the premium originally paid might represent a return in the form of interest. Rivash dismisses that contention on the grounds that title to the premium vests in the insurer immediately upon delivery of the payment without vesting a simultaneous concommitant obligation for repayment. Unlike Radvaz, he finds no problem of *ashmakhta* in such an arrangement since the insured events are both foreseeable and not within the power of the parties to prevent. Rivash's opinion with regard to contracts of that nature is codified in *Shulḥan Arukh, Yoreh De'ah* 173:19. There are, to be sure, numerous later responsa dealing with maritime arrangements.[13] For most part they concern themselves with problems of interest.[14] Entirely absent in those discussions is any hint of censure of the concept of insurance as a means of indemnification against loss.

Little can be inferred from the early literature concerning maritime insurance that is applicable to more common types of insurance. Talmudic sources temper the principle of reliance with emphasis upon prudence. Thus the Gemara, *Berakhot* 35b, stresses that one dare not go to the extreme in trusting that God will provide to the extent of renouncing any attempt to seek sustenance by means of gainful employment. It is in this context that the Gemara presents the oft-cited dictum of R. Ishmael: "'And you shall gather in your corn' (Deuteronomy 11:14). Conduct yourself in the manner of the world." Likewise, not only did the Sages issue a general admonition warning that one dare not tempt fate by placing oneself in danger,[15] they also formally promulgated a series of ordinances prohibiting conduct that might lead to untoward results.[16] They further declared that providential guardianship extended to persons engaged in fulfilling divine commands does not encompass situations in which harm may be anticipated.[17] In days gone by, sea voyages were fraught with danger as amply evidenced by the halakhic requirement for recitation of a blessing of thanksgiving upon safe return. Insurance against pecuniary loss under such circumstances could hardly be categorized as a reflection of imperfect faith.

There are, at the very minimum, two sources that, in at least limited circumstances, go beyond ideological neutrality to positive advocacy of insurance coverage. At the time of the Portuguese expulsion of Jews, a certain person died leaving his fortune in the hands of a younger brother who had made his way to Franconia. The children of the deceased resided in Turkey. The younger brother wished to relocate to Turkey as well. He turned to R. Samuel de Medina (1505–1589) with an inquiry concerning the property that had been entrusted to him. Should he leave the property of his orphaned nephew in the custody of the *Bet Din* of Franconia or, despite the substantial risk of loss in transport, should he bring his nephew's fortune with him and deliver it to his nephew in Turkey? R. Samuel de Medina, *Teshuvot Maharashdam, Ḥoshen Mishpat,* no. 46,[18] counseled that the valuables be transported, but only on the condition that they be insured in the most extensive and reliable manner possible "even if the expense is somewhat more than customary" and that the costs of coverage be charged to the heirs as a legitimate expenditure on their behalf.[19]

A closely related question was presented to R. Moshe Alshikh (1508–1600). The whereabouts of a certain Turkish Jew was unknown and, since there was reason to believe that he had been killed, a guardian was appointed to safeguard that gentleman's property on behalf of his young son. The man's wife sought to relocate to *Ereẓ Yisra'el* together with her son and wished to take with her the movable property that remained in her husband's estate. The guardian and relatives of the husband sought to prevent her from doing so. R. Moshe Alshikh, *Teshuvot Maharam Alshikh,* no. 38,[20] ruled that she was entitled to custody of the child and was free to choose a place of domicile. However, Alshikh further ruled that she could be prevented from placing the child's inheritance at risk unless insurance was provided or she herself guaranteed to indemnify the estate for any loss.

Again, the positive attitude toward insurance evidenced in these responsa cannot be construed as encouragement of general coverage. Apart from the relatively high risk of loss in those cases, they both involved potential loss that would be borne by another party and, moreover, they involved a potential loss that the guardian had a fiduciary obligation to prevent. Man has no right to rely upon God to discharge obligations he has assumed vis-à-vis others. Thus, insistence upon insurance coverage in such cases does not reflect an ideological endorsement of insurance *per se*; rather, it reflects the broad responsibility of a guardian.

However, there are also a number of responsa whose focal point is that insurance costs represent a customary and usual business expense. Such a holding certainly suggests the absence of any ideological odium. R. Shimon ben Ẓemaḥ Duran (1364–1444) was queried with regard to payment of a *ketubah* executed in Majorca. The sum to which the husband had obligated himself was expressed in the local currency, i.e., in gold reals. At the time of payment the parties resided in a locale, apparently Algeria, in which the coins of the realm were gold dinars. Gold, we are informed, was exported from *Tashbaẓ'* locale to "the land of the Christians" and hence was more valuable in Europe than in North Africa. In *Teshuvot Tashbaẓ,* III, no. 74, he replies that, for purposes of Halakhah, gold is treated as a commodity. *Tashbaẓ* asserts that a person who, for example, obligates himself to deliver a quantity of wax in a locale in which wax is expensive but who finds himself in a place in which wax is less expensive is obligated to pay the value of wax in the locale in which the obligation was assumed. *Tashbaẓ* rules that the same principle applies to payment of the value of the gold stipulated in the *ketubah*. He adds, however, that the payor may deduct the fee that would have been paid "to one who assumes liability for danger of the sea." *Tashbaẓ'* ruling apparently reflects the theory that, had the buyer received the reals in Majorca, the insurance premium would have been incurred by the buyer as a necessary cost of shipping the gold to North Africa.

In a much more recent responsum, dated 5643, a nineteenth-century authority, R. Shlomoh Drimer, *Teshuvot Bet Shlomoh, Ḥoshen Mishpat,* no. 48, writes that, since insurance is now customary, one partner who pays the premium for fire insurance may recover half the cost from the second partner.[21] *Bet Shlomoh* declares that such costs are of the same category as expenditures for securing a city by means of walls and fortifications. The costs of such fortifications are apportioned among all the townspeople and no one may claim that he does not desire such protection. *Bet Shlomoh*'s analogy of insurance to erection of fortifications for the defence of a city certainly indicates that seeking protection against financial loss is ideologically no different from seeking protection against marauders.

II. THE IDEOLOGICAL PROBLEM

In Jewish sources, the first rabbinic authority directly to address the issue of insurance as antithetical to *bitaḥon* or placing one's trust in the Deity, is R. Eliezer Deutsch, *Teshuvot Pri ha-Sadeh,* II, no. 44.[22] Actually, the arrangement brought to his attention was not a conventional form of insurance against loss but was more akin to a savings plan involving periodic deposits with the guarantee of the return of a specified sum after a certain number of years. Such policies were typically bought on behalf of infants or young children and were designed to provide funds for wedding expenses or, in more recent times, for college tuition. Although such policies were certainly not designed to provide a hedge against adversity attributable to Providence, they were apparently regarded by some as problematic because seeking assurance that funds will be available for such cases purportedly reflects a lack of confidence that God will provide "sufficient for his lack that is lacking to him" (Deuteronomy 15:8).

It is indeed quite difficult to grasp the nature of the problem since the arrangement, in actuality, is no more than a pooled investment with a stipulated return. The lump sum payment represented return of capital plus a portion of accrued profits. The funds received by the insurance company were typically invested in interest-bearing loans. The guarantee of the return of a specified sum was meaningful only so long as the insurance company remained solvent and its investments profitable. One searches in vain for any hint in rabbinic literature that interest-bearing loans (to non-Jews) or commercial investments offend *bitaḥon*. Quite to the contrary, only Providence can guarantee that such endeavors realize a profit. Pooling investment funds in a mutual or cooperative venture in order to spread risk and to realize the benefits of expertise and economy in the management of the investment cannot be other than salutary. Nevertheless, the response of *Pri ha-Sadeh,* authored in 1907, is instructive.

Pri ha-Sadeh's interlocutor cites the comments of *Tosafot, Kiddushin* 41a, in support of his thesis that, during the period of our exile, reliance upon God is mitigated, at least to some degree, as a norm of conduct. The Gemara declares that, despite the biblical provision granting a father the authority to give a minor daughter in marriage, rabbinic law forbids such practice until such time as the child "becomes mature and declares 'I wish so-and-so.'" *Tosafot* take notice of the fact that, despite the seeming halakhic impropriety, betrothal of minors was a relatively frequent and customary phenomenon in their day. *Tosafot* defend the practice on the grounds that "each day the exile becomes more severe" with the result that, although a person may presently possess sufficient resources to defray wedding expenses and to provide a dowry, at some future time he may find himself unable to do so with the result that his daughter may remain a spinster. *Tosafot* did not find the father's failure to trust that God will provide to constitute a lack of faith, at least during the period of Israel's exile.

Pri ha-Sadeh cites a further comment of *Tosafot* that serves to establish the same point. The Gemara, *Bava Meẓi'a* 70b, records a view positing a rabbinic prohibition against lending money to a non-Jew at interest despite explicit biblical sanction for the practice as reflected in Deuteronomy 23:21. The policy consideration prompting promulgation of this edict was a desire to minimize fraternization between Jews and non-Jews lest the Jew "learn from (the non-Jew's) actions." The Gemara does, however, permit such moneylending on the part of scholars who are unlikely to be influenced by the deportment of non-Jews and also permits any other person to engage in such enterprises to the limited extent necessary for that person's sustenance. Here, too, *Tosafot* take notice of the fact that during the medieval period moneylending was a common Jewish occupation. *Tosafot* justify the practice on two separate grounds: (1) the oppresive taxes imposed by "kings and princes" create a situation such that whatever is earned in this manner is no more than is necessary for our sustenance; (2) since, in exile, Jews live among the nations of the world it is impossible to engage in any means of earning a livelihood other than by entering into commercial relations with non-Jews. Accordingly, there is no reason to prohibit moneylending more so than any other activity. Again, there is no intimation that one ought to refrain from such commercial intercourse and place one's trust in God.

Pri ha-Sadeh adds one incisive comment. The prophet declares, "Cursed is the man who trusts in man and makes flesh his arm and turns his heart from God" (Jeremiah 17:5). The phrases of that verse are presented as a conjunction; the prophet does not declaim against human endeavor or against seeking the aid of a fellow-man, but only against doing so while failing to recognize that all assistance ultimately comes from God who is the "Cause of all causes." Insurance, asserts *Pri ha-Sadeh*, is also of divine origin for it is the Deity who prompted the founders of insurance companies to gather together in order to create such an enterprise for the benefit of mankind.

The issue of whether life insurance in particular evidences a lack of reliance upon Providence is addressed by R. Moshe Feinstein, *Iggerot Mosheh, Oraḥ Ḥayyim*, II, no. 111. *Iggerot Mosheh*, in effect, dismisses the problem out of hand. For Rabbi Feinstein, life insurance is in the nature of "business" or "commerce" (*misḥar*), as are fire, theft and automobile insurance. No man, he declares, has a right to refrain from engaging in business or labor in order to secure a livelihood on the plea that God will provide.[23] Such reliance reflects unwarranted hubris born of a conviction that the person conducting himself in such a manner has earned sufficient merit entitling him to an inordinate level of divine guardianship. Moreover, total failure to seek a livelihood is tantamount to reliance upon a form of providential guardianship that must be equated with the miraculous. No individual, even one who is deserving of such guardianship, has a right to rely upon a miracle.

A person is entitled to engage in commercial activity in order to provide for his needs and for the needs of his family. He is also entitled to engage in such activity throughout his lifetime in order to provide for his old age and for the needs of his heirs after his demise. *Iggerot Mosheh* regards insurance as no different from any other investment or mercantile activity. Indeed, he finds it a highly appropriate means of providing for the needs of heirs since adequate coverage means that the insured will not need to labor as arduously as otherwise in order to satisfy those needs.

As did *Pri ha-Sadeh* before him, *Iggerot Mosheh* also sees insurance as the manifestation of divine Providence. Unlike *Pri ha-Sadeh* who sees establishment of insurance companies as the product of Providence, *Iggerot Mosheh* focuses upon the insured's desire for coverage as being the result of providential guardianship. *Iggerot Mosheh* cites Onkelos' rendition of Deuteronomy 8:18 in establishing that point. The cited phrase is conventionally translated "for it is He who gives you power to generate wealth." Onkelos, however, renders the phrase as "for it is He who gives you counsel to acquire possessions," i.e., intellectual acumen to consummate a profitable transaction is a gift from God. Since, in recent generations, God has granted man wisdom to formulate and comprehend the concept of insurance it is entirely proper for even the most God-fearing to purchase such coverage for "it is God who counsels the purchase of insurance." *Iggerot Mosheh* appends a pithy final comment in which he seeks to identify the nature of reliance upon God for which one should strive. *Iggerot Mosheh* remarks that reliance upon God "that one will be able to pay [the premium] when the time arrives each year—that is the *bitaḥon* to which we are obligated."

To these considerations one further observation may be added. The verse included in the *tokhaḥah*, i.e. the list of misfortunes destined to befall transgressors, "and you shall have no assurance of your life" (Deuteronomy 28:66) is interpreted by the Gemara, *Menaḥot* 103b, as referring to a person who "relies upon a baker." Reflected in that interpretation is the concept that self-sufficiency is a blessing while reliance upon others is a curse. A person who bakes his own bread has no worry with regard to his daily nourishment; a person who must buy bread is dependent upon the availability and good will of others. The *bitaḥon* of the God-fearing does not include reliance upon God to employ other mortals as instruments of His guardianship. No one may dare to presume that he will be spared from sickness and death or even that he will be spared the ill effects of a natural disaster. *Bitaḥon* is meaningful only in the sense that, even in such circumstances, God will exercise compassionate care in ameliorating the consequences of such events. However, a serious financial burden generated by a major catastrophe can ordinarily be mitigated only through the generosity of others. Reliance upon charity is not integral to trust in God. Quite the contrary, the need for such reliance is depicted as a curse to be avoided.

A similar view is expressed by R. Ovadiah Yosef, *Yeḥaveh Da'at,* III, no. 85, who, *inter alia,* cites both *Iggerot Mosheh* and *Pri ha-Sadeh.* In particular, he cites the argument of *Pri ha-Sadeh* with approbation but somewhat inaccurately describes that responsum as addressing the issue of life insurance.

The issue of preparing for one's own misfortune and possible violation of the warning against "opening Satan's mouth" was apparently first raised by R. Mordecai Ze'ev ha-Kohen of Baden in a query concerning the propriety of acquiring life insurance. The identical question seems to have been presented by the rabbi of Baden to a number of authorities whose responses are published in their own responsa collections. Among them are R. Chaim Zevi Ehrenreich, *Teshuvot Kav Ḥayyim*, no. 26, and his brother R. Shlomoh Zalman Ehrenreich, *Teshuvot Leḥem Shlomoh, Yoreh De'ah*, II, no. 67.[24] *Teshuvot Kav Ḥayyim* notes that *Teshuvot Rivash*, no. 114, declares that it is entirely proper for a person to prepare shrouds during his lifetime.[25] By the same token, as noted by a third author consulted by the rabbi of Baden at approximately the same time,[26] execution of a last will and testament has long been regarded as an accepted practice. Rivash explains that death is a contingency that must be anticipated by all and that the Sages encouraged reflection upon human mortality as an expedient prompting repentance. Rabbi Ehrenreich also notes that life insurance policies typically provide for payment to the insured, rather than to the beneficiary, upon the attainment of a specified advanced age. Accordingly, the policy may be categorized as no less anticipatory of a ripe old age than of death.

R. Yechezkel Halberstam, known as the *Shiniver Rebbe* and renowned as the author of *Divrei Yeḥezkel,* is quoted as remarking that purchase of life insurance does not represent anticipation of misfortune; on the contrary, it is a means of enhancing one's prospect of longevity. It is evident that insurance companies are highly profitable and that the owners of those companies are blessed with success and wealth. Their continued good fortune is predicated upon ongoing collection of periodic premiums and upon not being called upon to make early payment of the sums specified in the policies they issue. Accordingly, the providential guardianship that provides for their good fortune must perforce preserve the life of the insured.[27]

Other objections to life insurance expressed in non-Jewish sources are not mirrored in rabbinic literature. In the early years of life insurance, many Christian theologians considered it irresponsible not to insure property but decried life insurance because it diminished an individual's need to plan for the future and thereby, they contended, "paralyzes a man's effort" and contributes to lack of industry and laziness.[28] For such reasons, most European countries enacted laws during the sixteenth and seventeenth centuries banning life insurance.[29] In a similar vein, life insurance was decried by the *New York Times* in an editorial published in 1853 on the grounds that life insurance "is calculated to encourage reliance upon something besides economy and industry and to lead accordingly to the relaxation and decay of those cardinal virtues of society."[30] Judaism, in contrast, regards "by the sweat of your face shall you eat bread" (Genesis 3:19) as a curse but not a command and never decried attempts to mitigate expenditure of human energy. Quite to the contrary, Judaism encourages husbanding of both time and energy so they may be devoted to study of Torah and worship of God.[31]

Objections to life insurance have also been advanced on the grounds that such coverage may be construed as turning human life into "an article of merchandise."[32] This is undoubtedly a reflection of the Roman law principle *Liberum corpus nullem recipit aestimationem* (The life of a freeman can have no monetary assessment). Accordingly, successorial contracts were nullified because they surround death with financial consideration. At one time, French courts declared all contracts on the lives of persons, including successorial contracts, trusts and life insurance to be illegal.[33] Again, there is no hint of such concern in halakhic sources. Indeed, in certain limited circumstances, Jewish law does recognize that the value of a lifetime of labor can be capitalized. Even more significantly, Jewish law would surely recognize that since insurance contracts may be written for amounts either greater than or less than the pecuniary value of the life of the insured, and since beneficiaries are not required to demonstrate a pecuniary loss to themselves as a result of the decease of the insured as a condition of collecting the insurance, life insurance does not represent compensation for loss of life. Unlike insurance against fire or theft, life insurance is not a contract of indemnity. The principal is paid upon occurence of a contingency that is universal and certain, i.e., death. Uncertainty exists only with regard to the time at which payment must be made. That uncertainty endows the insurance contract with the aura of an actuarial gamble rather than an undertaking for indemnification in case of a loss.

III. IMPLEMENTING THE MANDATE

The plethora of mail solicitations and the frequent appearance of notices in various publications pleading for funds to defray medical expenses of uninsured members of the Jewish community bear testimony to the consequences of inadequate health care coverage. An organized *kehillah* would not only have the ability to arrange group coverage for its members but would also have halakhic power to compel each of it members to enroll in a medical insurance plan.

There is no gainsaying the fact that patients bereft of insurance coverage are frequently deprived of access to quality medical care.[34] Disparity in the quality of care is directly reflected in survival rates.[35] Although any particular individual may never experience catastrophic illness requiring treatment that is beyond his financial ability, it is a virtual certainty that some members of a community will suffer such illness. The essence of insurance is the spreading of losses or costs among a large pool of insured persons so that an onerous financial burden does not fall upon a single person. In the case of health coverage, insurance also serves to provide access to life-saving care and treatment. It is that aspect of medical insurance that opens the door to enforcing enrollment of all members of the community.

The Mishnah, *Bava Batra* 7b, declares that townspeople may compel one another to contribute to the cost of erecting a wall around the town and to the construction of fortifications as protection against marauders and military asssault. Financial cooperation can be compelled even though there exists no imminent threat. The mere possibility of future need is sufficient substantiation of a demand for protection on the part of any inhabitant. No resident may avoid payment of the assessment levied for this purpose on the plea that he is willing to forego protection and assume the resultant risk. Although the danger is neither imminent nor certain, with the result that erection of fortifications is not encompassed within the fundamental personal obligation of *pikuaḥ nefesh*, satisfaction of a need of that nature is no less a social amenity that residents may demand of one another than is digging a well or purchase of religious works for purposes of study. *Shulḥan Arukh, Ḥoshen Mishpat* and Rema 163:1–2, rule that even a minority of the residents may insist that a levy be imposed upon all townspeople in order to raise funds for such purposes.

All members of a community are at risk for illness and disease even though only a small number may actually become ill. Quite obviously, no individual resident may decline to assume his share of the financial burden upon renouncing his perogative to avail himself of the benefit to be made available. Moreover Rema, *Ḥoshen Mishpat* 163:3, rules that even inhabitants who demonstrably have no need for a particular amenity, e.g., a ritualarium or a wedding hall, must contribute to the levies assessed for such purposes. In addition, Rema, *Ḥoshen Mishpat* 163:1, specifically rules that townspeople may compel one another to contribute to a fund to provide for the needs of strangers in their midst and to provide alms for the needy. The community clearly has an obligation to provide for the medical needs of the indigent and a person lacking medical insurance who suffers serious illness will perforce rapidly become indigent. Thus, establishment of a fund to defray medical expenses represents both a needed social amenity as well as a charitable obligation and the community is fully empowered to levy a tax for either purpose.

Establishment of a communal fund for such anticipated needs is, in reality, a form of self-insurance. Practicality and economic efficiency would augur against establishment of such a fund; rather, they would be strong factors in favor of using the funds to purchase commercial insurance coverage for the entire community. The community would presumably be in a position to negotiate a favorable rate for group coverage as a fraternal organization. Although an argument might be made on behalf of compelling all members of the community to participate in such insurance and to disallow the substitution of other coverage, such a policy would be economically wasteful and would undoubtedly meet with disfavor. The community might simply levy a "tax" equal to the insurance premium and allow that obligation to be satisfied either by payment directly to the community or by evidence of remittance either of that premium to the insurance carrier or of a premium for comparable coverage to a reputable insurance company. The most obvious benefit of such an arrangement is that persons who receive medical insurance as an employment benefit would not be required to pay for redundant coverage.

In this writer's opinion, a member of a community is also fully entitled to demand that the community subscribe to group coverage in the form of an indemnity plan as opposed to subscription to a managed care program. The crucial consideration is that the insured must be accorded the opportunity to be treated by a practitioner of his choice at a cost that is affordable by him.

The Palestinian Talmud, *Nedarim* 4:3 and *Ketubot* 13:2, declares, "Not by every person is an individual privileged to be cured." The consideration reflected in that dictum may well be naturalistic. Medical diagnosis and treatment constitute an art in that the personal dynamic between doctor and patient may play a crucial role in the treatment of any given malady. The confidence that a patient has in his physician may itself be a crucial element in therapeutic efficacy. A somewhat analogous statement recorded by the Gemara, *Avodah Zarah* 55a, "At the time afflictions are sent upon a person they are sworn not to depart other than on a specified day, at a specified hour and at the hands of a specified individual," certainly conveys a message with regard to the operation of Providence. Regardless of the nature of their consideration, the Sages certainly recognized that even equally competent physicians may not achieve identical results in treating any given patient. Hence a patient is entitled to untrammeled freedom of choice with regard to medical services.

Indemnity plans that provide for the costs of coverage of services rendered typically require some form of copayment. That arrangement is designed to prevent frivolous utilization of medical services and may also serve as a prophylactic against hypochondria. Such a requirement also reduces the required premium and is perfectly acceptable provided that, as is generally the case, there is also a cap on copayment so that the cost of treatment never becomes too burdensome for the patient. Nor can there be a serious objection to a group plan that provides treatment at no cost, or for a nominal fee, if the patient chooses a participating physician but requires copayment up to a reasonable limit when the patient chooses a non-participating physician. A form of coverage, typical of an HMO, that requires the patient to select a primary-care physician who serves as a gatekeeper whose permission must be sought before visiting a specialist or before seeking the services of a non-participating physician represents a form of economic duress that effectively deprives the patient of the freedom of choice that the Sages recognized as a crucial factor in the therapeutic process.

A quite similar argument might be made for a communal policy requiring mandatory life insurance coverage. Sadly, there have been cases in which a young breadwinner has died at an early age leaving a widow and minor children destitute. The support of the widow and orphans then becomes a communal burden. The community certainly has a charitable obligation with regard to their support and an organized community enjoys the authority to impose a tax for that purpose. It also has the authority to impose a tax in order to establish a charitable fund in anticipation of such needs, an arrangement that is, in effect, a form of self-insurance. It would appear that the community would also have the right to use those funds to defray the cost of a group life insurance policy for each of its members if for no other reason than on the grounds that such an arrangement is cheaper, more efficient and more dignified than simple charity. Again, since the premium is a charity "tax," it may be levied even upon the wealthy whose families are unlikely to become beneficiaries of charity. But with regard to life insurance as well, it would be both wise and equitable to accept evidence of payment for alternative life insurance coverage as satisfaction of the communal levy.

Unfortunately, to our detriment in many social and religious matters, the Jewish community in most countries is no longer organized in a *kehillah* structure. The resultant inability to assure universal insurance coverage for members of the community is one such detriment. Nevertheless, in relatively small and cohesive geographic areas, establishment of a *kehillah* is quite feasible even as a short-term goal. A more limited and more practicable goal in any area is establishment of a *kehillah* in which membership and participation would be voluntary.

NOTES

1. See commentaries of Rashi, *Meẓudat David* and Ibn Ezra. Cf., Ramban, *Ha-Emunah ve-ha-Bitaḥon*, chap. 1, *Kitvei Ramban*, ed. R. Bernard Chavel (Jerusalem, 5724), II, 357, who renders the verse "and cleave to faith as to a friend."
2. *Ha-Emunah ve-ha-Bitaḥon,* chap. 1, (Chavel, pp. 355–357).
3. "Bitaḥon," *Kad ha-Kemaḥ*, in *Kitvei Rabbenu Baḥya,* ed. R. Bernard Chavel (Jerusalem, 5730), p. 170.
4. *Ḥovot ha-Levavot, Sha'ar ha-Bitaḥon,* trans. Moses Hyamson (Jerusalem, 1965), I, 281.
5. In Ibsen's *Ghosts* one of the characters criticizes insurance as ungodly. Manlus, a parish clergyman, argues that insuring an orphanage would scandalize the community because it would symbolize a lack of "proper reliance upon divine protection." See *Four Great Plays* (New York: Bantam Books, 1971), pp. 81–82.
6. A transaction in the forrn of a loan on bottomry was well-

known in the ancient world and consisted of an advance upon a ship for the period of the voyage. If the ship came safely to port the loan was repaid together with a premium commensurate with the risk, but if the ship was lost or suffered misadventure the borrower was free from making any payment of either capital or interest. The ship was hypothecated for payment of the debt and hence a real right was created rather than a personal one. The term "bottomry" is derived from the pledge of the ship (i.e., the keel or "bottom" of the ship) as security. See *Black's Law Dictionary,* 6th ed. (St. Paul, 1990), p. 186. The term "respondentia" was used to denote hypothecation of the cargo or goods on board a ship as security for repayment of the loan. See *Black's Law Dictionary,* p. 1312. For a discussion of bottomry see Harold E. Raynes, *A History of British Insurance* (New York, 1983), p. 5. See also W.S. Holdsworth, *History of English Law,* 3rd ed. (London, 1922), VIII, 274, and Frederic R. Sanborn, *Origins of the Early English Maritime and Commercial Law* (New York, 1930), pp. 236–239. There is some evidence that a contract similar to bottomry was known in antiquity to merchants of Babylon and was given legal force in the Code of Hammurabi (2250 B.C.E.). See C.F. Trennery, *The Orgin and Early History of Insurance Including the Contract of Bottomry* (London, 1926), pp. 5ff. It is well established that such contracts were in use in Greece as early as the fourth century B.C.E. From the Greeks the contract passed to the Romans and from them to the maritime nations of Europe during the Middle Ages. In the year 533, an edict of the Roman Emperor Justinian restricted interest on money advanced on bottomry (which was previously unregulated in the Roman Empire) to 12 percent, as opposed to 20 percent in the Code of Hammurabi, as compared with 6 percent for other advances. See Victor Dover, *A Handbook to Marine Insurance,* 8th ed. (London, 1975), pp. 4–5, and John H. Magee, *General Insurance*, 6th ed. (Homerwood, Ill., 1961), p. 2.

7. The *Corpus Juris Canonici* prohibited the taking of interest but allowed for some exceptions. One such exception included bottomry loans in which the lender assumed the risk of the venture. However, in 1243, Pope Gregory IX promulgated a decree that was presumed to declare such loans to be usurious as well. It has been speculated that the maritime contract of insurance was invented for the specific purpose of evading that prohibition, i.e., the loan was extended without interest but a

separate contract was entered into for assumption of risk in return for which a fee was charged. See Magee, *General Insurance,* p. 6, note 27. Other writers have credited Jews as being the prime movers in the emergence of insurance in the medieval period. For a review of those sources see Magee, *General Insurance*, p. 6, note 27, and Stephen M. Passamaneck, *Insurance in Rabbinic Law* (Edinburgh, 1974), p. 2.

8. If, as may well have been the case, the loan was entered into in order to defray the cost of acquiring merchandise transported by the ship, an expedient in the form of a variation of the standard *hetter iska* would have been readily available and would have accomplished the desired result. Instead of advancing the funds as a loan, the financier might have engaged the merchant as his commercial agent with instructions to buy and sell the merchandise on the former's account. The agreement might have readily stipulated that the financier's profit, if any, be limited to four dinars with the balance accruing to the merchant as compensation for his services. This may have been the intent of *Teshuvot Maharashdam, Yoreh De'ah,* no. 220, who writes that "there are forms of *cambios* that are entirely permissible." At that time, however, merchants were apparently often unaware of the nuances of structure necessary to make such transactions permissible. For a survey of responsa discussing usury problems involved in *cambio* arrangements see Jacob Bazak, "Heskemei Bituaḥ Yami (Cambium) be-Sifrut ha-She'elot ve-Teshuvot shel ha-Me'ah ha-Tet-Zayin," *Sinai* (Nisan–Iyar 5734), pp. 40–60. Later *hetter iska* arrangements, which provide that as soon as the stipulated return is realized the funds convert to an interest-free loan, probably did not become common among Jews until the time of Maharam Avigdors in the sixteenth century. An instrument reflecting a precursor of a *hetter iska* arrangement is examined by J.D. Goitein, *A Mediterranean Society* (Berkeley, 1967), I, 175–176. For a comprehensive discussion of such arrangements among non-Jews to avoid prohibitions against usury and the ensuing debate among canon law theorists see John T. Norman, Jr., *The Scholastic Analysis of Usury* (Cambridge, 1987) and the review of that material by Passamaneck, *Insurance in Rabbinic Law*, pp. 181–190.

9. Cf., *Shulḥan Arukh, Yoreh De'ah* 173:18.

10. Radvaz cites, and refutes, a much earlier authority who permitted such an arrangement on the grounds that no prohibition against usury pertains to any situation in which the lender's cap-

ital is at risk. See *Gittin* 30a but cf., *Tosafot, ad locum,* s.v. *kivan.* The source cited is R. Estori ha-Farḥi, *Kaftor va-Feraḥ*, chap. 24 (Jerusalem, 5659), II, 576. *Kaftor va-Ferah,* in turn, attributes this view to one of his forebears, a twelfth-century French authority, R. Meir ben Yitzchak.

11. Later responsa discussing the *asmakhta* problem and enforceability of insurance contracts are cited by R. Menachem Slae, *Ha-Bituaḥ be-Halakhah* (Tel Aviv, 5740), pp. 79–82
12. Radvaz suggests that the parties enter into an alternative arrangement: Instead of extending a loan the financier might sell the merchandise at any agreed price with payment conditional upon safe return of the ship. Since title to the merchandise passes immediately and is absolute there is no problem of *asmakhta.*
13. For a survey of those responsa see R. Menachem Slae, *Ha-Bituaḥ be-Halakhah,* particularly pp. 21–48.
14. See also sources cited in *Ha-Bituaḥ be-Halakhah*, pp. 82–91.
15. *Shabbat* 32a.
16. See *Yoreh De'ah* 116.
17. *Pesaḥim* 8b.
18. This responsum, as well as many of the sources discussed below, are cited in *Ha-Bituaḥ be-Halakhah,* chap. 18, pp. 136–142.
19. Mahrashdam cites the statement of *Maggid Mishneh, Hilkhot Naḥalot* 11:3, to the effect that guardians should not transport property of orphans by sea, or even by land when there is danger of loss, but apparently had reason to assume that that consideration did not apply because conditions were such that the property was not secure in Turkey. In a later responsum, *Ḥoshen Mishpat,* no. 434, Mahrashdam cites the argument of an executor who wished to transport property of an orphan from France to Salonika. The executor contended that *Maggid Mishneh's* ruling should not prevent him from doing so because "he has found someone who will insure the property." Maharashdam comments that adducement of that argument is superfluous since transportation was necessary in order too assemble all of the orphan's property in one locale.
20. In the immediately following responsum, *Teshuvot Maharam Alshikh,* no. 39, R. Moshe Alshikh quotes and analyzes the earlier cited responsum of Rivash with whom he concurs. A translation of that responsum is presented by Passamaneck, *Insurance in Rabbinic Law,* pp. 51–66.
21. A similar point is made by *Teshuvot Mahari'az*, no. 72. See also R. Samuel Engel, *Teshuvot Maharash*, VI, no. 103, sec. 3. Cf.

also, R. Shlomoh Kluger, *Ḥokhmat Shlomoh, Ḥoshen Mishpat* 176, who rules that if civil law permits purchase of insurance without, or in excess of, a pecuniary interest, the partner who paid the premium is entitled to the proceeds in their entirety. See also, the opposing view of R. Mordecai ha-Levi Solovey, *Yad Ramah*, no. 20, as well as sources cited by R. Isaac Sternhal, *Kokhvei Yiẓḥak* (Brooklyn, 5729), I, no. 22, secs. 7–8, regarding the respective rights of the payor of the premium and the owner of the property. Cf. *Teshuvot Maharash*, VI, no. 103.

22. This responsum as well as many of the sources discussed below are cited by R. Ovadiah Yosef, *Yeḥaveh Da'at*, III, no. 85.
23. A similar point is made by R. Chaim David Halevy, *Aseh Lekha Rav*, VI, part 2, no. 92, on the basis of a comment of *Sifrei* on Deuteronomy 15:18. *Sifrei* interprets the verse "and the Lord your God shall bless you in all that you shall do" as indicating that divine blessing is predicated upon human endeavor.

    In response to the argument that idemnity insurance serves no significant purpose since a divine decree mandating financial loss will be fulfilled in some other way, Rabbi Halevy avers that not every loss is to be attributed to divine decree since many losses are the result of human foolishness, negligence and the like. In addition, it should be noted that many medieval philosophers maintain that, at times, misfortune may simply be the result of natural causes. For discussion of some of those views see J. David Bleich, *Providence in the Philosophy of Gersonides* (New York, 1973), part 1, chapters 1 and 2 and *idem, With Perfect Faith* (New York, 1983), pp. 498–500.
24. This source is cited both by *Yeḥaveh Da'at* and by Rabbi Slae. However, I have been unable to find the cited responsum in the works of R. Shlomoh Zalman Ehrenreich.
25. See also *Bet Yosef, Yoreh De'ah* 339.
26. See R. Shalom Yitzchak Levitan, originally of Lithuania and later rabbi of Oslo, Norway, in his *Kuntres Sukkat Shalom*, no. 11, appended to R. Shlomoh of Pintshok, *Bet Shlomoh* (Pietrkow, 5687).
27. See *Kokhvei Yiẓḥak*, I, no. 22, sec. 1. Rabbi Sternhal cites an anonymous scholar who suggests that life insurance may not be in the best interest of the insured. The consideration advanced is that a person's life may be prolonged, not on the basis of his own merit, but because he is the instrument of Providence to provide sustenance for his wife and family. Providing for their welfare by means of an insurance policy, goes the argument, re-

moves the need to preserve their breadwinner. That argument, however, seems incorrect. A significant principle with regard to the operation of Providence is that performance of a *mizvah* cannot be the cause of negative consequences that would otherwise not befall an individual. That principle is expressed in the verse "He who observes a commandment shall not know an evil thing" (Ecclesiastes 8:5) and in the talmudic dictum "Those engaged in the performance of a commandment meet no harm" (*Pesaḥim* 8b). Support of one's family constitutes a *mizvah* as declared by the Gemara, *Ketubot* 50a: "'Happy are . . . they that perform charity at all times' (Psalms 106:3). Is it then possible to perform charity at all times? . . . [The reference is to] one who supports his sons and daughters when they are minors." Accordingly, assuring that one's family will be provided for after one's death will not result in an early demise.

28. See Freeman Hunt, *Worth and Health: A Collection of Maxims, Morals and Miscellannies for Merchants and Men of Business* (New York, 1856), pp. 38, 346 and 386.
29. Viviana A. Rotman Zelizer, *Morals and Markets: The Development of Life Insurance in the United States* (New York, 1979), p. 33.
30. *New York Times,* February 23, 1953, p. 4.
31. Islamic law forbids life insurance because it prohibits all speculation on human life. For that reason life insurance presently remains unrecognized in Saudi Arabia and Libya. See Zelizer, *Morals and Markets,* p. 33.
32. George Albree, *The Evils of Life Insurance* (Pittsburgh, 1870), p. 18.
33. See Zelizer, *Morals and Markets,* p. 44.
34. Even in the same medical facility patients lacking medical insurance are not only deprived of the services of physicians of their choice but were shown in one study to be 29 percent to 70 percent less likely too undergo each of five high-cost or high-discretion procedures. They were also 50 percent less likely to have normal results on tissue pathology reports for biopsies performed during a variety of endoscopic procedures. See Jack Hedley, Earl Steinberg and Judith Feder, "Comparison of Uninsured and Privately Insured Hospital Patients," *Journal of the American Medical Association,* vol. 265, no. 3 (January 16, 1991), pp. 374–379.
35. See, for example, John Z. Ayanian, Betsy A. Kohler, Toshi Abe and Arnold M. Epstein, "The Relation Between Health Insurance Coverage and Clinical Outcomes Among Women With Breast Cancer," *New England Journal of Medicine,* vol. 329, no. 5

(July 29, 1993), pp. 326–331. That study reported a 49 percent higher risk of death for uninsured patients during the interval between 54 and 89 months after diagnosis. The risk for medical patients during the same period was 40 percent higher than for privately insured patients

2

Disclosure of Information

My task is to describe the halakhic view regarding the disclosure of information to a patient, apprising him of the terminal nature of his illness. In fact, I am prepared to make two statements on the topic. The first will be very, very brief. In fact, it will be no more than three words. But let me preface those words with a somewhat longer story. This story concerns a rather modern congregation that had established a number of standing committees. Every year, at the annual dinner, the chairman of each of the various committees was called upon to deliver a report. One of the committees was the ritual committee. The chairman was a gentleman of the old school and each year he got up and delivered the same report. The report consisted of two words: "*Men davent.*" Finally, one year he got up and delivered a three-word speech: "*Men davent nisht*!"

My first statement with regard to disclosing information

This paper was originally delivered at the First International Physicians' Conference on Medicine and Halachah sponsored by the Raphael Society of the Association of Orthodox Jewish Scientists in New York City, January 1989, and is presented, with minor revisions, as published in the conference proceedings, *Medicine and Jewish Law*, I, Fred Rosner, ed. (Northvale, N.J., 1990), pp. 31–63.

regarding the terminal nature of an illness is extremely simple: "*Men tor nisht*"—It is prohibited! In the second statement I will attempt to elaborate upon the sources from which that conclusion is drawn, and also to modify that statement in some small way.

I. RABBINIC DISCUSSIONS OF THE PROHIBITION

1. *Contemporary Sources*

Let me begin with several contemporary sources that ostensibly deal with somewhat different issues but nevertheless serve to illustrate the focal point of this discussion. The first source is in the last volume of Rabbi Moshe Feinstein's responsa collection published during his lifetime.[1] The responsum deals with a situation involving a patient occupying an intensive care unit (ICU) bed. The question addressed to Rabbi Feinstein is whether the patient may be moved to another room because there is now another patient who can derive more benefit from the type of comprehensive and constant care that is available only in an ICU. In addition to discussing a number of other considerations, Rabbi Feinstein remarks that, if in the process of moving the patient from the ICU to another unit the patient may develop anxiety or emotional distress because he recognizes that he is being relegated to less than intensive care due to the fact that his condition has been judged to be terminal, it is prohibited to move the patient from the ICU. Rabbi Feinstein states very clearly that it is forbidden to reveal the terminal nature of an illness to the patient by either word or deed and that this prohibition is grounded in considerations of *tiruf ha-da'at*—a concern that the emotional distress or anguish produced by such a disclosure might foreshorten the brief period of life that is still available to the patient.

A second responsum in the same volume[2] makes the same point, but in somewhat different language. There the question is "How does one treat a terminally ill patient?" The responsum is addressed to a specific situation in which no efficacious therapy is available; the physician has nothing to offer that might be of benefit to the patient. Nevertheless, Rabbi Feinstein counsels that that patient be given a placebo, some innocuous substance that serves no medical purpose. Rabbi Feinstein reasons that, in order to prevent the patient from becoming despondent, he must be led to believe that he is being medicated. The physician is obligated to occupy himself with the patient, to spend time with him, to give him attention, and to prescribe medication because despondency is detrimental to the patient's welfare. In the course of formulating this position, Rabbi Feinstein uses an expression somewhat different from that employed in his earlier responsum. Here the concern is not the fear of emotional shock in the form of *tiruf ha-da'at* that is associated with the revelation of a particular item of information that the patient cannot assimilate. Rather, the concern is that slowly, over a period of time, the patient will become aware of the fact that no one is attempting to treat him, that no one is taking him seriously as a patient, and that he has, in effect, been medically abandoned. The result will be a form of despondency or melancholy and that state, in and of itself, is described by Rabbi Feinstein as "the most detrimental harm to the patient."

Evidence demonstrating the existence of the latter phenomenon, one that is far more widespread than situations usually associated with the concept of *tiruf ha-da'at*, can be found in the Torah in a verse that otherwise defies comprehension. Moses was told to return to Egypt but before returning he took leave of his father-in-law Jethro: "And he said, I will go and return to my brothers in Egypt to see whether they are still alive" (Exodus 4:18). Moses went to Jethro and told him that he must go back to Egypt. Interpreted literally, this verse tells us that Moses wished to see his brethren in Egypt because he wanted to determine whether they were still alive; it had been such a long time since he had seen them that he was unsure of what may have happened to them in the interim. However, if one endeavors to understand this verse literally, it is simply incomprehensible. The Lord had already told Moses to go to Pharaoh in order to redeem the Israelites and to take them out of Egypt (Exodus 3:12). If the purpose of Moses' return to Egypt was to facilitate the redemption of the Jews, then of course they must still have been alive. One cannot redeem people unless they are among the living. And yet Moses went to Jethro saying that he was not sure whether his brethren in Egypt were indeed still alive. Moses' statement seems to constitute an obvious falsehood. Nevertheless, among the classical commentaries, only the *Or ha-Ḥayyim*, Exodus 4:18, draws attention to this apparent falsehood.

Rabbi Ben-Zion Firer[3] explains this passage in a very simple manner. Moses was directed to return to Egypt to deliver the divine command to Pharaoh and ultimately to lead the Jews out of Egypt. But Moses was concerned that the Jews would neither believe him nor listen to him (Exodus 4:1). He was afraid that, even if he were to transmit God's instructions, people would not accept them. Scripture confirms that this is what, in fact, did occur. The Jews did not listen to Moses because of their oppression and hard labor (Exodus 6:9). They did not accept his message with alacrity because they believed that redemption was impossible. Their slavery, oppression and persecution had been so intense and had continued for such a long time that they were in a state of severe despondency. A person who is despondent and melancholic has no desire to live; chronic depression is itself a form of mental illness. For a person in such a condition, life is not really life. When Moses went to Jethro and told him that he must determine whether the Jews in Egypt were still alive, he meant it quite literally. Was there anyone to rescue? Was there anyone to redeem? Did they still desire to live? If Moses' brethren had no desire to live, then redemption would have been an impossibility.

Rabbinic sources emphasize one basic and fundamental point that is crucial to understanding the Jewish approach to the practice of medicine. Insofar as Judaism and Jewish tradition are concerned, not only is every human life of infinite and inestimable value, but every moment of life is of infinite value as well. There is absolutely no hint within Jewish tradition of a notion of a period of life-anticipation that is so brief or so ephemeral as to be morally meaningless. That concept comes from an entirely different system of ethics. It has no place within an ideological or ethical framework predicated upon the teachings of Judaism.

2. *Early Sources*

The moral imperative mandating preservation of every possible moment of human life is spelled out in clear detail in a number of sources. The first and perhaps the most obvious is the statement of the Gemara, *Mo'ed Katan* 26b, to the effect that an ill person is not to be informed of the death of a relative or close friend lest he become emotionally upset upon receiving the news. The patient is not to be informed because he might experience *tiruf ha-da'at*. Note that the Sages of the Talmud did not say that every terminally ill patient is subject to *tiruf ha-da'at*. They did not say that every patient will die as a result of the shock of receiving this information. They *did* say that there is a cogent and rational fear that disclosure of such information constitutes at least *safek pikuaḥ nefesh* (possible danger to life). For that reason one must refrain from conveying information of this nature.

There is another provision in an entirely different area of Jewish law that, it seems to me, is also predicated upon a concern for avoiding *tiruf ha-da'at*. The concern embodied in the principle "The words of a dying person (*shekhiv mera*) are as if written and delivered," as formulated by the Gemara, *Gittin* 13a, is based upon the fear that if one fails to fulfill the desire of a dying person he may die sooner, even momentarily sooner, than he would have died otherwise. Ordinarily, one cannot transfer ownership of property other than by employing one of the formal modes of conveyance (*kinyan*). Judaism does not recognize disposition of property by means of testament. Hence, if a person wishes to avoid distribution of his property by operation of the laws of inheritance, he must effect some form of *inter vivos* gift. In order to accomplish that end, there must be some form of *kinyan*. However, the Sages carved out an exception to that rule that prevails in certain limited circumstances. In the case of a person suffering from a serious and possibly terminal illness, the Sages declared that the requirement of *kinyan* is to be completely waived. For a *shekhiv mera*, a mere oral declaration is sufficient to effect a transfer of property; the oral declaration in and of itself serves as the conveyance. The Sages were afraid that, on his deathbed, a person might realize that he lacks the capacity to dispose of his estate in the manner in which he chooses, and that this realization could result in mental anguish that might foreshorten his life.

Concern for mental anguish or distress was recognized by early rabbinic authorities (*rishonim*) in a remarkable situation. Rabbi Asher ben Yeḥiel, known as Rosh, states in his commentary on *Bava Batra* 9:18 that a person who is being led out in chains to his execution is also categorized as a *shekhiv mera*, and if a person wishes to divest himself of his property under such circumstances, the provision for *kinyan* is to be dispensed with. Rosh cites the position of Rabbi Isaac Alfasi, known as Rif, who declares that dispensation with the provision for *kinyan* applies not only to a patient who is terminally ill and to a person about to be executed, but even to someone who is about to embark upon a sea voyage or a caravan journey. Rosh disagrees with Rif with regard to the latter two cases—that is, with regard to the dispensation applied in the case of a person who is about to embark upon a sea voyage or a caravan trip. Although danger may arise in the course of travel, argues

Rosh, nevertheless such travelers cannot be regarded as being in danger at the time they embark upon their journey. Certainly, the concept of mental anguish (*tiruf ha-da'at*) has no meaningful application in such cases since individuals setting out on a journey are not in a debilitated state such that emotional anguish might hasten their death. However, Rosh agrees that these provisions of Jewish law are fully applicable in the case of a person who is about to be executed. Rosh regards the person being led to his execution as being included in the same category as the terminally ill patient.[4]

Let us analyze the implications of Rosh's position. In the case of a person about to be executed, we are not confronted with a situation involving a person suffering from a terminal illness. The condemned prisoner does not suffer from any debilitating malady. Nevertheless, according to Rosh, since he is about to be executed, rabbinic legislation places him in the same category as a person who is dying of a terminal and debilitating illness. What can the concern possibly be? The person being led to his execution, although he may be shackled in chains, is, as yet, entirely healthy. Once the executioner begins discharging the duties of his office, however, this individual has no chance whatsoever of surviving. The concern must be that, even in instances of death by execution, the process of dying may be completed speedily or it may be prolonged over a somewhat protracted period of time. Apparently, Rosh reasons that if the condemned prisoner were to become emotionally upset, agitation might hasten his death, even though death occurs by means of execution. For that reason, the condemned prisoner is regarded as being within the parameters of the category of *shekhiv mera*—that is, a person whom one dare not excite or cause to become agitated because his death may thereby be hastened.

There is another source that employs somewhat different nomenclature in expressing an identical concern. The Gemara, *Horayot* 12a, describes the case of a person who is about to embark on a journey and wishes to know whether he will return safely or whether early demise will prevent his return. The Gemara suggests that the would-be traveler retire to a dark place and observe whether or not his shadow casts a second shadow. If his shadow also casts a shadow, he may be assured that he will return; but if his shadow does not cast its own shadow, he has reason to fear that he will not return. The Gemara immediately qualifies this by remarking that the procedure is not to be recommended because the person attempting this form of divination may become upset, and as a result his "luck" (*mazal*) may be spoiled. Rashi explains that the Gemara's concern is that the shadow test is not foolproof; it is possible that a person may not cast a double shadow but yet return from his journey in perfect safety. Nevertheless, since the traveler fails to observe a double shadow he may become disturbed or upset, and the resultant agitation may itself lead to disastrous consequences. Quite obviously, the concern is to avoid a situation in which a person may become overly apprehensive because that type of mental stress can only have a deleterious effect upon a person's general health and well-being.

There is also a talmudic source that speaks of despondency in comparable terms. The Gemara, *Nedarim* 40a, states that one should not visit a sick person either in the first three hours of the day or in the last three. If one wishes to visit a sick friend or relative, one should do so during the mid-portion of the day. Why should one not pay a sick call during the early morning or late afternoon hours? Because during the first three hours of the day the patient appears to be fresh and relatively healthy. As a result, the visitor will not be prompted to pray for a speedy and complete recovery on behalf of the patient because he will think that prayer is unnecessary. During the last three hours of the day the patient seems weaker and his medical condition appears to have deteriorated. As a result, the visitor may be led to think that there is no hope and hence he will not pray on behalf of the patient. Clearly, then, the concern of the Sages extended beyond disclosing negative information to the patient himself. They counseled even against creating a situation in which negative information is imparted to someone other than the patient because they recognized that despondency, even of friends and relatives, can have a negative effect upon the patient. Even if despondency is not contagious, which may well be the case, it has a negative effect in that it causes relatives and friends to despair of divine mercy and hence to abandon hope and abjure prayer.

There are at least two sources that explicitly discuss divulging the diagnosis of a terminal condition to the patient. The Midrash, *Kohelet Rabbah* 5:6, comments upon the biblical narrative that tells of the visit of the prophet Isaiah to King Hezekiah when the latter was ill. God instructed Isaiah to inform Hezekiah that the latter was terminally ill and would not live. The prophet dutifully discharged his mission. Isaiah visited Hezekiah and delivered the message as charged by God and also admonished Hezekiah to give his family final instructions because death was imminent. The Midrash informs us that Hezekiah reproved the prophet saying, "Customarily, when one visits the sick, he says, 'May Heaven have mercy upon you.' A physician who visits [a patient] tells him, 'This you may eat and that you may not eat. This you may drink and that you may not drink.' Even if [the physician] sees that [the patient] is about to die he does not say to him, 'Leave a testament to your household' lest the [patient's] mind faint." One is supposed to pray for the patient and give him a blessing. A visitor tells the patient that God will help, and gives advice with regard to diet: This food you may eat, but do not eat other foods. Drink this liquid, but not some other beverage. And even if the physician sees that the patient is about to die, he does not tell him, "Write your last will and testament because you are about to die." "Why, then," queries Hezekiah of Isaiah, "did you instruct me to put my affairs in order because I will not live?" Had God not specifically commanded Isaiah to deliver that message, Isaiah would indeed have been remiss in informing Hezekiah that he was about to die. The concern embodied in that rebuke, the Midrash tells us, is a concern for *tiruf ha-da'at*, "lest the mind faint"; i.e., if a patient suffers distress and anguish, that emotional state may itself cause the foreshortening of his life.

Another incident recorded in the Bible is understood by some commentaries in precisely the same way. As recorded in II Kings 8:7–10, Ben-Haddad, the King of Aram, became sick and sent a messenger, Azael, to Elisha. The messenger was to pose one question: Would Ben-Haddad recover from this illness? Elisha informed the messenger Azael that, in fact, Ben-Haddad would die, but he instructed Azael to tell the king, "You shall surely recover." R. Levi ben Gershon, known as Ralbag, commenting on this verse, indicates that Elisha's concern was precisely a concern for *tiruf ha-da'at*, or mental anguish. Elisha's concern was based upon the very real possibility that the shock of receiving a true response—namely, a prediction of impending death—might, in and of itself, serve to trigger termination of the life of the patient.

II. ARGUMENTS FOR FULL DISCLOSURE

Both the Sages of the talmudic period and the early talmudic commentators were extremely clear in formulating their position against divulging the diagnosis of a terminal illness. In contemporary times, four arguments have been presented in support of a policy that is diametrically opposed to the negative view regarding full disclosure that is reflected in rabbinic sources. Two of those arguments arc medical or scientific in nature and two can be categorized as ethical or moral in nature. I will first list those arguments and then discuss them each in turn.

The first argument consists of a simple denial of the phenomenon of emotional distress as a life-shortening factor. The concern of *Ḥazal* for *tiruf ha-da'at*, runs the argument, is entirely misplaced. Scientifically speaking, *tiruf ha-da'at* is a nullity; it does not exist. Emotional pain and psychological anguish do not really shorten anybody's life. The second argument is based upon a claim that truthful information regarding the condition of the patient, even if the patient is terminally ill, is actually beneficial in a variety of ways. Hence, it is in the patient's best interest to be given full and complete information concerning his condition. Thirdly, the patient has a right to know: How can anyone take it upon himself to deny another human being such basic information—information he is rightfully entitled to receive? The fourth argument is that information can be withheld only by means of some type of subterfuge. Usually, an outright lie of one type or another is required. But a lie cannot be sanctioned because lying is absolutely immoral. Lying is a sin; one has no right to lie even if one believes that the lie is designed to achieve a good purpose.

These are the arguments in favor of full disclosure to the patient that have appeared in the medical and psychological literature. Let me deal with them *seriatim*.

1. *Psychological and medical considerations*

As noted, the first argument is that *tiruf ha-da'at*, or emotional trauma that might foreshorten life, simply does not exist. The most prominent, but by no means the only, exponent of that position is Elizabeth Kübler-Ross in her books *On Death and Dying*[5] and *Questions and Answers on Death and Dying*.[6] Kübler-Ross has developed an extremely complex theory regarding the psychology of dying and claims to have identified five distinct psychological stages of dying. She argues that ultimately the patient comes to accept death and does so without adverse effect. Kübler-Ross' scientific objectivity and the validity of her conclusions have been challenged by a number of her colleagues,[7] and other researchers have reported markedly different findings.[8] Nevertheless, *arguendo*, I am perfectly willing to accept as absolutely true everything that Kübler-Ross has said, but not more than she has said. Dr. Kübler-Ross conducted experiments involving some 200 subjects. I am perfectly willing to grant her the benefit of any possible doubt, and to concede that the five stages she has identified and labeled constitute an accurate report of the phenomena observed in every one of her 200 subjects. I am also willing to concede that there were no adverse physical effects in any one of those 200 patients. Having done so, I nevertheless find no contradiction in her reports to anything found in rabbinic literature. In examining the words of the Gemara, *Mo'ed Katan* 26b, one should note that the Sages expressed concern "*lest* the patient suffer mental anguish"; in other words, they were concerned about the *possibility* of inducing mental anguish by disclosure of information. They did not contend that this result would obtain in all cases, or even in the majority of cases. They contended only that it may occur in some cases; they did not even hint at how small that minority of cases might be. All forms of inductive reasoning fall short of ultimate proof and demonstration because one cannot examine every possible case. Kübler-Ross has shown, at best, that there were no adverse effects in two hundred patients. Who knows what might happen in the case of the two-hundred-and-first patient?

At least one contemporary study does record and confirm the phenomenon of emotional trauma associated with being informed of an unfavorable diagnosis. It is noteworthy that this fact is conceded by physicians who nevertheless argue for divulging such information to the patient. In an article entitled "Should the Doctor Tell the Patient that the Disease is Cancer? Surgeon's Recommendation,"[9] Victor Gilbertsen and Owen Wangensteen advocate full disclosure. They specifically discuss the question of whether or not one should disclose a diagnosis of cancer to the patient and they cite statistics that, in their opinion, augur in favor of disclosure. Four percent of surgical patients who received such information became emotionally upset upon learning the nature of their affliction and remained so throughout the course of their illness. Only four percent suffered emotional distress and manifested that emotional distress during the entire course of the illness. How many more suffered emotional distress but did not manifest symptoms of distress during the entire course of the illness is not stated. But at least four percent *did* manifest emotional distress—and did so until they died! I submit that, if the life of every individual is precious, and if every moment of that life is of infinite and inestimable value, four percent is a very, very high rate of incidence. If we are dealing only with even four percent who experienced the phenomenon of *tiruf ha-da'at*, statistically, that phenomenon is extremely significant; and our Sages certainly had ample reason to make their concern known to us and to make that concern an integral consideration in determining how one is to relate to a terminally ill patient.

At least one source advances the view that full disclosure of information may actually be beneficial to the patient. In an article published in the *British Medical Journal*,[10] Jean Aitken-Swan and E. C. Easson claim that, at least for some patients, disclosure of even the bleakest prognosis serves either to eliminate fear and anxiety or at least to significantly reduce these feelings. The same authors indicate that other benefits are attendant upon this type of disclosure. Presumably this means that, in the case of some patients, the result of full disclosure is a lesser degree of danger of *tiruf ha-da'at*. As will be shown later, the exceptions that these authors have reported are paralleled in at least one rabbinic source. Such observations in no way negate the concern for *tiruf ha-da'at* as a phenomenon that must be anticipated. At the very most, those studies show that there are some people who may actually benefit from having such information revealed to them. The argument developed in explaining the reaction of these patients is that knowledge, even knowledge of the worst, is easier for them to handle than doubt and uncertainty. Even if this thesis is correct, it does not negate or contradict rabbinic teachings regarding disclosure. Even taking that consideration into account, rabbinic authorities regarded the consequences of *tiruf ha-da'at*, in the cases in which it does occur, as too serious to be disregarded. Any benefit attendant upon disclosure that may be enjoyed by some patients must be weighed against the serious harm such disclosure may cause others. Therefore, "do not disclose" is the recommended course of action. Since the potential harm of full disclosure involves the foreshortening of human life, the harm outweighs any possible benefit that may result.

I will cite two examples of the phenomenon that evoked our Sages' concern which I have personally observed in my own "clinical practice" as a pulpit rabbi. Many years ago, a middle-aged attorney was hospitalized and told that he was suffering from diverticulitis, an inflammation in small outpouchings from the large bowel. One day, I walked into the patient's room to find that this individual, whose spirits had been fine up to that point, was in tears; he was broken and shattered, an emotional basket-case. If ever there was a case of *tiruf ha-da'at*, there it was, in front of my eyes! I asked him what happened; why was he so upset? By mistake, a nurse had left his chart in the room. The patient had glanced at the chart and seen the dreaded word: *carcinoma*. I brazenly told him that I was sure there was some mistake: "I know your condition. I spoke with your doctor. You don't have cancer; you have diverticulitis. Wait a minute. I'll go outside and have a look at your chart." I walked outside and paced back and forth in the hall for ten minutes, doing absolutely nothing. I came back into the room and said, "I saw your chart. The word carcinoma does not appear there." The patient's reaction was, "Rabbi, are you sure? Are you absolutely positive that you checked the chart carefully? I'm so glad!"

That is not the end of the story. The man lingered on for six or seven weeks, and on subsequent visits I saw a patient with widely fluctuating moods. On some days he was perfectly cheerful and happy. Those were the days on which he believed the lie I had told him. On other days he was extremely depressed. Those were the days on which he told me, "Rabbi, I know that you were lying. I know that you were not telling me the truth." For the psychologist, here was a perfect case of denial and counterdenial. For the student of Jewish law, here was a perfect example of *tiruf ha-da'at*. While one cannot state with certainty that the patient's death was actually hastened by the knowledge he had inadvertently obtained, that knowledge certainly was not beneficial to him. It assuredly caused emotional trauma, and it is not at all far-fetched to suspect that it may have hastened his demise. As one contemporary writer has succinctly stated: "Not only can deception cure, but truth can kill."[11]

Another example is presented by a situation that did not involve so serious a condition and that fortunately had a different outcome. An elderly gentleman experienced back pain while walking home from *shul* on *Shabbat*, broke out in a cold sweat, and became extremely pale. No one would have challenged the diagnosis of a possible "heart attack." I assume all physicians would agree that a person manifesting such symptoms ought to be sent to a hospital, put into a coronary care unit, and carefully monitored. This man was in fact sent to the hospital. When I visited him there, he told me that his doctor had informed him that "On a scale of 1 to 10, you had a heart attack that is 0.5." Some heart attacks are more severe than others, but, by definition, a "heart attack" means that there has been some damage to the cardiac muscle. The patient's cardiologist had commendably told the patient the truth but had couched the message in language designed to minimize concern. The next evening I received a telephone call from the man's wife. She had been in touch with a relative who happened to be a cardiac surgeon. The relative spoke to the patient over the telephone and told him, "You will probably need bypass surgery." He then proceeded to spell out in great detail the procedures and risks involved in bypass surgery. At that time, when bypass surgery was in its infancy, the dangers were significant. When I visited the patient the next day, he was in a terrible state; he was clearly in a state of *tiruf ha-da'at* and for no real reason. Fortunately, the man came home after several days and recovered fully and uneventfully without surgery.

This clearly is a situation in which it was irresponsible for the patient's relative to furnish him with a definitive diagnosis and prognosis. The diagnosis happened to be inaccurate, and the patient was alarmed needlessly. But even if the information had been correct, it should not have been conveyed in so insensitive a manner. This is certainly a very dramatic example of disclosure that did not do the patient any good at all. It is an instance in which one may clearly see the phenomenon of *tiruf ha-da'at*.

This phenomenon also finds scientific confirmation in the medical literature. A famous surgeon, J. M. T. Finney, who for many years served as a professor of surgery at the Johns Hopkins Medical School, publicly testified that his years of experience had taught him to be selective in accepting patients. The mortality rate among his patients was very, very low. Dr. Finney refused to perform major surgery on any patient who expressed fear with regard to the potential success of the contemplated procedure. Dr. Finney's clinical experience had led him to conclude that fear contributes to a high mortality rate, and he managed to keep the mortality rate among his patients artificially low by accepting only patients who were not afraid.[12]

There is also a report in the psychological literature that serves to demonstrate that hopelessness can be a cause of death in animals. A series of experiments was performed with wild rats that were first confined in a metal cage. They were then forced into a black opaque bag in which they could not move. Later they were removed from the bag and their whiskers were cut off in order to cause loss of stimulation. Finally, the rats were dropped into a water-filled glass jar in which they might swim until they were overcome by exhaustion, but from which there was no escape. The procedure was designed to eliminate all hope of escape and to cause the rats to feel threatened.

A significant number of rats died as soon as they were taken out of the bag even before they were dropped into the water; others died immediately upon being placed in the water. None of the rats survived in the water for any significant period of time. In a control group, however, when hopelessness was eliminated, the rats did not die. The elimination of hopelessness was achieved by repeatedly holding the rats briefly and then freeing them, and by immersing the rats in water for only a few moments on several occasions and immediately removing them from the water. The rats quickly learned that the situation was not hopeless. They became aggressive, tried to escape and swam for much longer periods of time. Many rats in this control group swam for a period of between 40 and 60 hours. Clinical tests indicated a slowing of the heartbeat and respiratory rate and lowering of body temperature among the rats that died. Autopsies revealed enlarged hearts distended with blood. Researchers who conducted this experiment attributed the early death of the experimental rats to the overstimulation of the parasympathetic nervous system.[13]

Apparently, the rats in the control group, at least on an instinctive level, still had hope; they anticipated salvation in one form or another. Be that as it may, one is clearly confronted here with a situation in which anticipation of survival, even among animals, contributes to survival, whereas anticipation of death contributes to death. In many cases, such anticipations become self-fulfilling prophecies.

There are other psychological studies that serve to confirm that phenomenon. During World War II a considerable number of unaccountable deaths were reported among soldiers in the armed forces. Those deaths occurred among men who were apparently in good health. In autopsies, no pathology was observed. Deaths occurred not as a result of wounds, but of some other unexplained cause. Deaths are also regularly reported among individuals who imbibe small, definitely sublethal doses of poison and among persons who inflict minor, nonlethal wounds upon themselves. In those cases it is assumed that the sole cause of death is simply the victims' belief in their impending doom.[14]

In a well-known investigation of "voodoo death," Dr. Walter Cannon demonstrated that such deaths are readily explainable and have absolutely nothing to do with black magic. The hex is pronounced, and, as a result, the individual is overcome by profound misery, refuses food and drink, and literally "pines away." The explanation offered is that death occurs as a result of persistent excessive activity of the sympathetic adrenal system. Continuous injection of adrenaline produces a constriction of the blood vessels. The resultant decrease in blood pressure causes blood volume to be reduced until it becomes insufficient for maintenance of adequate circulation. Thereupon, deterioration occurs in the heart and nerve centers. As a result of the damage to the organs necessary for adequate circulation, they become less and less able to maintain effective blood circulation. The result is death.[15] Death occurs even though there is no significant reason for such dysfunctions to have occurred in the first place. Death occurs simply because the patient experiences the fear that he is going to die and this fear itself sets into motion physiological processes that ultimately cause death to occur.

A most eloquent formulation of this phenomenon, written by Louis Thomas, appears in the first volume of the *Journal of Medicine and Philosophy*:

> It is not unlikely that there is a pivotal moment at some stage in the body's reaction to injury or disease, maybe in aging as well, when the organism concedes that it is finished and the time for dying is at hand, and at this moment the events that lead to death are launched, as a coordinated mechanism. Functions are then shut off, in sequence, irreversibly, and while this is going on, a neural mechanism held ready for this occasion, is switched on. . . .[16]

Although the article from which this excerpt is quoted appeared in the *Journal of Medicine and Philosophy*, it certainly is not philosophy, and I doubt that it is medicine. But it is certainly poetically moving and serves eloquently to describe the phenomenon of *tiruf ha-da'at.*[17]

2. *Ethical Considerations*

Enough has been said in rebutting the medical counterarguments to the halakhic concern regarding *tiruf ha-da'at.* Let me turn to the ethical arguments, the first of which is based upon the putative right to know. That right, in turn, flows from the concept of personal autonomy—that is, the notion that a person enjoys the right to absolute freedom with regard to himself and to his destiny; hence he is entitled to any and all information with regard to himself that he wishes to obtain. The response to that argument is quite simple: No such right is recognized by Judaism. To the extent that liberty and personal autonomy constitute a value, such value consists of freedom *from*, not freedom to. For Judaism, freedom as a moral value is freedom from external constraint. The God-given right to develop one's potential to serve the Lord does not include the right to dispose of one's life and one's body in a manner of one's own choosing.

This concept is expressed most beautifully in the language of Halakhah in two sources. One is a responsum of Rabbi

Betzalel Stern[18] and the other is to be found in a compendium edited by Rabbi Shlomoh Zalman Braun.[19] In both sources, the specific question involves a father who demands of his son that the latter tell him explicitly and unequivocally the nature of his illness. Both authorities rule in no uncertain terms that, even when confronted with a possible infraction of the commandment to honor one's father, there is absolutely no obligation to disclose this type of information. The responsum authored by Rabbi Stern consists of a lengthy dissertation devoted to a delineation of the parameters of the commandment concerning the honor due one's father and mother. Insofar as the specific question itself is concerned, it might have been addressed in a very brief sentence. The request for disclosure of information is tantamount to the father's demanding of his son that the latter do something in violation of a commandment of the Torah; under the circumstances, there is no obligation whatsoever to "honor" one's father. A virtually identical and equally brief statement to that effect appears in the work of Rabbi Braun.

Let me turn to the fourth argument in favor of disclosure—namely, that in failing to provide information, one becomes involved in either a subterfuge or an outright lie. The author who formulates that argument most clearly is Sissela Bok, in her book *Lying: Moral Choice in Public and Private Life*.[20] This argument reflects great concern with regard to the grave sin of "lying." After all, Scripture unequivocally declares, "Keep thee far from a false matter" (Exodus 23:7).

At least two of the early rabbinic authorities who enumerate the 613 biblical commandments—Rabbi Moses of Coucy, *Semak*, no. 104, and Rabbi Isaac of Corbeil, *Semag*, no. 226—do indeed list this admonition as one of the 613 commandments. However, other eminent authorities, including some of the most prominent of those who have compiled listings of the commandments (e.g., Rambam, Ramban, *Ba'al Halakhot Gedolot* and *Sefer ha-Ḥinnukh*), do not enumerate this scriptural admonition among the 613 biblical commandments. For them, this verse must undoubtedly be understood as interpreted by Abraham Ibn Ezra in his biblical commentary—namely, as an exhortation to the *Bet Din*. According to Ibn Ezra, the cognitive import of this verse parallels the commandment "In righteousness shalt thou judge thy neighbor" (Leviticus 19:15). Indeed, the concluding phrase of the scriptural verse exhorting against falsehood is "and do not slay the innocent and the righteous" (Exodus 23:7), an admonition that is clearly addressed to the judicial authorities. Talmudic exegesis of this verse interprets the first part of the verse as also dealing with matters pertaining to a *Bet Din*. The Gemara, *Shevu'ot* 31a, declares, "From where is it derived that the *Bet Din* dares not listen to one of the litigants before the other litigant appears? From the verse 'Keep thee far from a false matter.'" Failure to observe that procedure would result in a "false matter"—that is, an erroneous decision. Similarly, the Gemara, *Shevu'ot* 30b, queries, "From where is it derived that a judge should not allow an ignoramus to sit before him? From the verse 'Keep thee far from a false matter.'" An ignoramus who participates in the deliberations of the court is likely to utter nonsense, but in doing so he may sway the judges and cause a false decision to be issued. The rabbinic applications of the verse clearly show that the verse is associated with a commandment to the *Bet Din*. Rabbi Sa'adia Ga'on, *Sefer ha-Mizvot*, no. 22, adduces additional evidence in support of the position that there is no biblical prohibition against uttering a falsehood.

Let me be very precise. I do not wish it to be said that I have made a blanket statement to the effect that lying is permissible. There are other prohibitions associated with various forms of falsehood. There is a prohibition against perjury: "Thou shalt not utter a false report" (Exodus 23:1). There is a prohibition against a *Bet Din* issuing a false judgment: "Thou shalt not wrest the judgment" (Exodus 23:6). There is a prohibition against lying for purposes of illicit monetary gain:

"Neither shall ye deal falsely, nor lie one to the other" (Leviticus 19:11). There is a prohibition against various forms of deception. If one is about to go to the mailbox and another person is in the process of leaving the house, one dare not say, "Wait, I will accompany you." One dare not deceive by pretending to perform an act on behalf of another person when that act is actually being performed on behalf of oneself. Such conduct is a prohibited form of *geneivat da'at*, "stealing another person's mind."

Telling a lie for the purpose of causing pain or anguish to another person is prohibited: "Ye shall not wrong one another" (Leviticus 25:14). The statement that, for some authorities, uttering a falsehood is not forbidden is limited solely to a perfectly innocuous lie that harms no person—in other words, a "white lie" from which no one will suffer financially, physically, or even emotionally. Thus, the area of possibly permissible falsehood is extremely limited.

It seems to me that this controversy regarding the permissibility of an innocuous lie is really the substance of a dispute between *Bet Shammai* and *Bet Hillel* as recorded in the Gemara, *Ketubot* 16b-17a. *Bet Hillel* declare that, under any and all circumstances, one should praise a bride's pulchritude as well as her good qualities and traits by lauding her as beautiful and gracious. *Bet Shammai* in effect ask: What if she is a little bit lame or is blind in one eye? Does one still call her beautiful and gracious? Is it not written "Keep thee far from a false matter"? The Torah commands us not to lie! Elsewhere, in *Kallah*, chapter 10, the Gemara clarifies the position of *Bet Hillel*. *Bet Hillel* is reported as having responded that when the Torah commands "Keep thee far from a false matter," it is in the context of the concluding phrase of the verse, "Do not slay the innocent and the righteous" (Exodus 23:7). Thus it is quite evident that *Bet Hillel* espouse an interpretation identical to that of Ibn Ezra and regard the admonition as being addressed to a court of law commanding them to abjure any form of falsehood that may result in the death of the innocent and the righteous. However, when undertaken for a laudable purpose, such as to avoid causing distress to another, lying is entirely permissible.

Why is it necessary to belabor that point, particularly since there are other circumstances with regard to which *Bet Shammai*—as well as the authorities who maintain that "Keep thee far from a false matter" is one of the 613 biblical commandments binding upon all Jews—would certainly concede that lying is permissible? There is no question that all would agree that lying is permissible for purposes of preserving or prolonging a human life. The point that requires emphasis is this: The majority of early rabbinic authorities maintain that distortion in order to preserve the well-being of another is not a matter of choosing the lesser of two evils. It does not constitute a situation in which the law against lying is set aside or waived because of a higher cause, such as one in which the act is intrinsically a transgression but is sanctioned because of an overriding consideration. Failure to tell the truth for the purpose of preventing distress, or even for the purpose of promoting a sense of well-being, is not at all a transgression and hence does not engender a situation with regard to which a person should suffer any remorse whatsoever.

This statement may be very unconvincing, at least to some. Sissela Bok, for example, would be totally unswayed by this analysis of "Keep thee far from a false matter." It would not impress her at all, and I understand her point of view. I understand her perspective very well because it is endemic to the American mentality. I have many shortcomings; one of them is that, despite my white beard and black hat, I am very much a product of American culture. An American can understand and forgive virtually anything and everything, with one exception: he cannot forgive a lie. If you lie to him, even if it is an innocuous lie, he will never forgive you. He will no longer look you in the eye, and he will not willingly continue to have dealings with you. I know because I suffer from that mentality. I react that way. Moreover, I also believe that there is support in Jewish tradition for such a reaction. King David reacted that way when he said, "He that speaketh falsehood shall not be established before mine eyes" (Psalms 101:7). Even in circumstances in which telling a lie is not an outright transgression, it is certainly distasteful and odious and hence lying should be eschewed unless there are serious considerations warranting communitcation of an untruth. But when there is sufficient reason for doing so, there is no reason to harbor feelings of guilt.

Even more significantly, in the situation that we are addressing, the physician's statement denying the terminal nature of an illness is not necessarily a lie. It is not a lie for two reasons. In his commentary on the Bible, Deuteronomy 11:13, Rabbi Baḥya ben Asher of Saragossa remarks that the power of prayer is so great that it can even nullify a divine decree and cause a change in the operation of the laws of nature. To tell a patient that he is not terminally ill does not constitute a lie. Insofar as Judaism is concerned, there is no irreversible malady: *Al titya'esh min ha-puraniyot*—Do not become despondent because of misfortune"; it is always possible to effect a cure. Rabbi Yechezkel Abramsky, of blessed memory, once put it to me in a very beautiful way. He remarked that, in the blessings preceding *keri'at shema*, we speak of God as a *bore refu'ot*, a Creator of cures. Creation connotes the generation of *yesh me-ayin*, something out of nothing. If God is the Creator of cures, then a cure can surely be created literally "out of nothing." Hence one has no right to assume that a cure is impossible.

There is yet another reason why telling a patient that he is not terminally ill should not be regarded as a lie. The Dutch scholar Hugo Grotius argued that lying is always forbidden.[21] However, there are many situations in which everybody concedes that a person ought to lie. An obvious example is a case in which someone solicits information that he will use for some nefarious purpose. For example, a burglar breaks into a house and asks, "Where can I find the rifle so that I can use it to threaten your life?" Clearly, only a fool would disclose that information. Grotius argues that, under such circumstances, dissemblance is not a lie. Since the would-be malefactor is not entitled to such information in the first place, denial of that information is not a lie. There is a rabbinic source for that position, a little book by Rabbi Ya'akov Yecheskel Fisch that was published not long ago entitled *Titen Emet le-Ya'akov* (literally, *Give Truth to Jacob*).[22] The work is devoted to the explication of the virtues of truth-telling, but also contains a series of some seventy-five responsa that should properly be titled *Titen Sheker le-Ya'akov* (literally, *Give Falsehood to Jacob*), since these responsa enumerate a series of leniencies with regard to falsehood. One of the considerations cited in this work in permitting certain forms of falsehood is very similar to that advanced by Grotius, but with one important variation. To take a slightly different example from that of Grotius:

Suppose someone calls me on the telephone and asks, "What are you doing?" I happen to be counting my money, but I do not wish to tell the caller what I am doing. May I lie or may I not lie? The author of *Titen Emet le-Ya'akov* argues that this is information to which the caller is not entitled. I have no obligation to disclose the truth. But if I were to answer truthfully, "I don't want to tell you. It's none of your business," the caller would be offended. Accordingly, runs the argument, this is a situation in which it is permissible to withhold the truth "for the sake of peace." This consideration allows falsification even when the truth is innocuous, simply because the interlocutor has no claim to the information that he seeks. *A fortiori*, if a patient is not entitled to certain information because the patient has no claim to information that may lead to *tiruf ha-da'at*, and, for obvious reasons, one cannot very well tell him, "I do not wish to answer," the license to lie is clear and unequivocal. Under those circumstances the "lie" is certainly not to be defined as a falsehood within the parameters of the prohibition of "Keep thee far from a false matter."

Does this mean that there are no exceptions to the principle that a patient should not be informed that he is suffering from a terminal illness? On the basis of this discussion it would seem that there are none. It sounds very much as if this entire presentation is in the form of what, in legal circles, would be termed a general denial. The jocular example of a general denial is portrayed in the situation of an attorney representing a chicken thief. The defendant is accused of having stolen chickens. The attorney goes to court and says, "Your honor, my client is innocent. First of all, he did not steal the chickens; secondly, he returned the chickens; and finally, the chickens were not worth very much anyway." It sounds as if what I have been saying is: First of all, it is not a lie; second, if it is a lie it is a permissible lie; and finally, the truth is not worth knowing in the first place. Since the truth will do more harm than good, what is the point of telling the truth?

Nevertheless, in the real world there certainly are exceptions. First, an exception must be admitted in a situation in which disclosure is necessary in order to secure the cooperation of the patient in his treatment. Second, there are situations in which the patient is bound to discover the truth and he may learn the nature of his illness in circumstances that will cause greater harm than would result from disclosure by the physician. In some cases, early, sensitive disclosure may constitute the better part of valor.

These exceptions are formulated in a somewhat different manner by Dr. Abraham S. Abraham in *Nishmat Avraham, Yoreh De'ah* 338:3. The author distinguishes between diagnosis in the early stages of an illness and discovery of a terminal condition in the final stages of the illness. He remarks that, in the early stages of the illness, one should inform the family *and* the patient, both in order to secure the patient's cooperation and to assuage the patient's fears. Of course, one must be very supportive and stress the fact that therapy is available and that there is great hope. However, when the malady is discovered at an advanced stage and only palliative treatment is available, Dr. Abraham sees no point in informing the patient. I can accept that recommendation up to a point. I can conceive of the case, for example, of a very independent middle-aged person to whom the physician has already lied. The patient's tumor was surgically removed and, at the time, there was no reason to disclose the malignancy. Later, the patient develops such symptoms as weight loss, blood in the stool, lack of appetite and nausea. At this point no cure is available. The physician wishes to administer radiation therapy for palliative purposes, but the patient does not know what is wrong with him. After making a recitation of the symptoms and a review of laboratory reports, the physician informs the patient that he must undergo radiation therapy. The patient may say, "Doctor, why are you worried about my loss of weight? For years you have been telling me to lose weight. Are you concerned about the blood in my stool? I have hemorrhoids, you know that. I don't have any appetite because my wife is not cooking as well as she used to. Occasional nausea—for that you want me to take radiation? Doctor, you know that radiation can cause leukemia! Do you want me to expose myself to that risk just because of a little nausea?" Under those circumstances, the physician will certainly find it necessary to reveal the diagnosis to the patient in order to obtain his cooperation even for palliative treatment. Of course, the physician must be careful not to inform the patient of the severity of his condition and of the fact that the treatment is merely palliative in nature.

Not all patients are alike. There are some clinical symptoms that one cannot mask, disguise or "misinterpret" if one is treating, for example, a patient who happens to be a physician or a professor of pharmacology. Indeed, in the present-day world, it is difficult to conceal the import of such symptoms from any educated and sophisticated patient. This is even more likely to be the case in the advanced stages of a malady than in early stages. Under these circumstances, one has no choice; one must confirm to the patient what the patient already knows. However, at any stage of illness, the patient should be given unfavorable information only to the extent that it is necessary for his physical and psychic well-being.[23] And, even more significantly, his condition and prognosis should be portrayed in the most favorable light possible under the circumstances.[24]

Simply for purposes of intellectual honesty, let me also cite the statement of Rabbi Judah the Pious, *Sefer Ḥasidim*, no. 154. Rabbi Judah writes of a physician who is reported to have had the remarkable capability of being able to determine whether or not a patient would die simply by examining his urine. I marvel at this doctor who, without laboratory facilities, was able to examine a specimen of urine and determine that the patient was afflicted with a terminal illness. Be that as it may, Rabbi Judah declares that, under such circumstances, if the patient tells the physician, "Do not hide anything from me. I know you doctors. You do not tell the truth because you are afraid of causing *tiruf ha-da'at*. But I would be happier and more at peace if I knew the truth," the rule is as follows: If the patient does not wish to live and if he is also experiencing excruciating pain, one may tell him the truth. Rabbi Abraham Price, in his commentary on *Sefer Ḥasidim, Nishmat Avraham*, advances what seems to me to be a cogent analysis of the approach outlined there. The exception posited by *Sefer Ḥasidim*, he states, is limited to a case in which the patient is suffering great pain and, as a result, is already in a state of *tiruf ha-da'at*. Although it is forbidden to hasten the death of any patient, nevertheless—since this patient is already experiencing a type of *tiruf ha-da'at* in that he is already in a state of mental anguish and he truly wishes to die in order to be spared further agony—any information he will receive about his condition will serve only to calm him. It is only in this type of situation, in which *tiruf ha-da'at* is already present, that disclosure does no harm and may do some good. I cannot say that the approach of *Sefer Ḥasidim* is necessarily normative Jewish law. In instances in which rulings of *Sefer Ḥasidim* are incorporated in the writings of the early talmudic commentators and codes of Jewish law, they become accepted practice by virtue of that incorporation. In instances such as this, in which *Sefer Ḥasidim* is not cited by early authorities, its comments are not necessarily to be regarded as normative Halakhah.

III. PRACTICAL APPLICATIONS

What should be done when one is confronted with a patient who is suffering from a serious disease or a patient who is suffering from a terminal illness? Clearly, the concerns that point in the direction of disclosure are cogent. They include the concern that the individual have the opportunity for recitation of *viduy*, or final confession before God, and repentance. He should have the opportunity to put his affairs in order and to make provisions for his family. Those are concerns that were recognized by rabbinic authorities as well. They counsel that the patient be told, "Confess and do not be fearful, for many people have confessed and did not die, and many who did not confess have died. Some people survive in the merit of having repented and confessed." That is the traditional manner in which one recites *viduy* with a terminally ill patient. On several occasions I have taken the liberty of shortening and paraphrasing this statement by telling the patient, "*Viduy* is a *segulah* for longevity; the merit of *viduy* can lead to a long life." Recitation of *viduy* can indeed reverse the heavenly edict and cause a favorable decree to be issued.

Rabbi Abraham Danzig, *Ḥokhmat Adam* 151:11, reports a practice that certainly constitutes an appropriate paradigm. He reports that the practice of the Jewish community of Berlin was that, if a person did not attend synagogue for three consecutive days, officers of the *Bikkur Ḥolim* society would pay a visit to that person at his home. The *Bikkur Ḥolim* society did not make house calls for every case of sniffles. In eighteenth-century Berlin, a Jew was absent from the synagogue for three consecutive days only if seriously ill; one did not miss communal worship because of mere discomfort. Accordingly, if a person did not appear in the synagogue for three days, it was assumed that he was seriously ill. The *Bikkur Ḥolim* society visited the patient and informed him that they had come to recite *viduy* with him. But the patients did not become afraid because they knew that the society habitually visited everyone who was absent from the synagogue for three days. Many such patients experienced a complete recovery and resumed their normal practice of attending synagogue services three times a day.

It seems to me that this constitutes a model for how the modern-day physician should comport himself. Long before a definitive diagnosis is possible, the physician should be able to say to the patient, "Look, I tell all my patients the same thing: We are going to do laboratory tests. We may even put you in the hospital for observation. I hope that it will turn out to be nothing, but I give every patient the same advice anyway." The physician should then proceed to tell the patient that any medical condition may become serious and that one should order one's affairs accordingly. Most significantly, this information should be conveyed long before the situation is known to be serious. Moreover, the emphasis must be not so much on what is said, because in some situations there is no way to avoid the truth, but on how it is said. The tone of voice, the facial expression, and the demeanor of the physician are tremendously significant, and even more important than the spoken words.

The physician has absolutely no right whatsoever to tell any patient that there is nothing that can be done for him. He has absolutely no right whatsoever to tell the patient that there is no hope. Even if the nature of the disease has to be identified and even if the severity of the illness must be spelled out, it should always be in a context and in a manner that is supportive, hopeful and assuring, and that conveys the message that everything that can be done on behalf of the patient will be done.

I am well aware of the fact that there is great resistance to the policy that I have outlined. But since the teachings and values of Judaism are often unpopular, that is not surprising. I will conclude with a brief story. Years ago, when I was a young student, I remember someone returning to the yeshiva after having spent a *Shabbat* in Lakewood, New Jersey. Rabbi Aaron Kotler, of blessed memory, used to deliver his weekly *shi'ur* on Saturday evening after the conclusion of the Sabbath. Lakewood, at the time, was a popular resort area, and many Jews went there for weekends. Many visitors would go to the yeshiva on Saturday evenings to hear Rabbi Kotler's discourse and occasionally one would ask a question during the course of the *shi'ur*. The story that was brought back was that, on the previous Saturday evening, a gentleman had interrupted Rabbi Kotler and asked him a question. Rabbi Kotler answered. The man proceeded to argue with Rabbi Kotler. Rabbi Kotler answered a second time. The man continued to argue until finally Rabbi Kotler exclaimed, "If you disagree with me, it must be a sign that I am right because the views of *ba'alei battim* are opposite to the views of Torah. So it is written in the *Sema, Ḥoshen Mishpat* 3:23." The actual comment of *Sema* is not quite as strong as the words quoted in his name. However, *Sema*—citing a responsum of Maharil—does state that what is accepted as normative by the general public and what is regarded as normative by Torah scholars are unfortunately, more often than not, not one and the same. Often they are diametrically opposed. Moral dilemmas should not be resolved on the basis of intuition. *Vox populi* is not always intuitively reflective of *vox Dei* and it is to the latter that our ears must be attuned.

NOTES

1. *Iggerot Mosheh, Ḥoshen Mishpat*, II, no. 73, sec. 2.
2. *Ibid.*, II, no. 75, sec. 6.
3. *Panim Mazbirot ba-Torah*, II (Tel Aviv, n. d.), pp. 24–26.
4. Of course, it might be argued that Rosh asserts only that all persons experiencing imminent danger are to be treated in an identical manner; the concept of *lo plug* [no exceptions] might be invoked in justifying such a rule—i.e., many rabbinic edicts are universal in nature and do not admit of exceptions even when cogent grounds exist for not including all situations within the ambit of an edict. Accordingly, it might be argued that a rabbinic law designed to ameliorate a specific concern may well apply in all similar cases even though the concern may be entirely absent in those cases. If so, provisions with regard to those facing imminent death may apply not only to the terminally ill but to those facing execution as well. Nevertheless, the case of a condemned prisoner is readily distinguishable from that of a terminally ill patient and there is no talmudic evidence indicating that the Sages sought to treat both cases in an identical manner because of considerations of *lo plug*. The class of the terminally ill is quite different and much narrower than the broader class of persons facing imminent death, and talmudic references are to the former rather than to the latter. Since Rosh extends this principle to the condemned prisoner despite the absence of substantiating talmudic evidence and without explicit reference to the principle of *lo plug*, it certainly appears that he regarded that case to be entirely analogous to that of the terminally ill person, i.e., he presumably regarded *tiruf ha-da'at* to be a cogent concern even in the case of the condemned prisoner.
5. New York, 1970.
6. New York, 1974.
7. See R. Schultz and D. Aderman, "Clinical Research and the Stages of Dying," *Omega*, vol. 5 (1974), pp. 137–143, and R. Branson, "Is Acceptance a Denial of Death? Another Look at Kübler-Ross," *Christian Century* (May 7, 1975), pp. 464–468. See also *Time* (Nov. 12, 1979), p. 81.
8. See J. M. Hinton, "The Physical and Mental Distress of Dying," *Quarterly Journal of Medicine*, vol. 32 (1963), pp. 1–21; and K. A. Achte and M. L. Vaukkonen, "Cancer and the Psyche," *Omega*, vol. 2 (1971), pp. 46–56.

9. In *The Physician and the Total Care of the Cancer Patient* (New York, 1962), pp. 80–85, a collection of papers presented at a symposium sponsored by the American Cancer Society.
10. March 21, 1959, pp. 779–783.
11. Bradford Wixen, "Therapeutic Deception: A Comparison of Halacha and American Law," *Journal of Legal Medicine*, vol. 13, no. 1 (March 1992), p. 78.
12. See W. B. Cannon, "'Voodoo' Death," *American Anthropologist*, vol. 44 (1942) no. 2; reprinted in *Psychosomatic Medicine*, vol. 19 (1957), p. 189.
13. See C. P. Richter, "On the Phenomenon of Sudden Death in Animals and Man," *Psychosomatic Medicine*, vol. 19 (1957), pp. 191–198.
14. *Ibid.*, p. 197.
15. Cannon, pp. 182–190.
16. L. Thomas, "A Meliorist View of Disease and Dying," *Journal of Medicine and Philosophy*, vol. 1 (September 1976), p. 219.
17. For a report of a study demonstrating that positive expectations can have a salutary clinical effect and of a number of other studies demonstrating that negative expectations can have deleterious effects, see Wixen, "Therapeutic Deception," pp. 77–78.
18. *Teshuvot be-Ẓel he-Ḥokhmah,* II, no. 55.
19. *She'arim Meẓuyanim be-Halakhah* 193:2.
20. New York, 1978.
21. *On the Law of War and Peace*, trans. F. M. Kelsey *et al.* (Indianapolis, 1925), Book III, chapter 1.
22. Jerusalem, 1982.
23. See Wixen, "Therapeutic Deception," p. 93.
24. A sensitive discussion by a physician of how to communicate such information to a patient is presented by Shimon Glick, *Assia*, no. 42–43 (Nisan 5747), pp. 8–15, reprinted in *Sefer Assia*, VII (5754), 15–24 and in "Telling the Truth to a Patient," *B'Or Ha'Torah*, no. 9 (1995), pp. 51–59.

3

Treatment of the Terminally Ill

I. PRESERVATION OF LIFE

1. *The Dilemma*

Medicine has long subscribed to the adage "Thou shalt not kill; but needs't not strive officiously to keep alive."[1] Nevertheless, until relatively recent times, medical science was able to offer either all or nothing in its treatment of virtually all illnesses and diseases. Either the patient responded to treatment, when treatment was available, and was cured or else he or she succumbed to the ravages of the malady. These dichotomous possibilities generated few moral dilemmas for the medical practitioner. Patients, by and large, sought treatment and physicians strained to do all in their power in order to effect a cure. To be sure, theologians and ethicists agonized over such questions as the moral legitimacy of euthanasia for patients who found continued existence too painful to bear and the extent to which the patient was obliged to seek extraordinary means in effecting a cure; but the number of people with regard to whom such perplexities were germane was not nearly as great as in our day.

In recent years medical science and technology have made tremendous strides. Some diseases have been virtually eradicated; for others, effective remedies have been found. Concomitantly, ways and means have been developed which enable physicians to sustain life even when known cures do not exist. As a result, issues concerning prolonging the life of the terminally ill now arise with heretofore unprecedented frequency. Economic considerations coupled with the stark reality of patients suffering from debilitating illnesses, often incapable of engaging in meaningful or satisfying activities, have combined to create a milieu in which the focus of concern is upon quality of life.

The physician's practical dilemma can be stated in simple terms: to treat or not to treat. In deciding whether or not to initiate or to continue treatment, the physician is called upon to make, not only medical, but also moral determinations. There are at least two distinguishable components which present themselves in all such quandaries. The first is a value judgment: Is it desirable that the patient be treated? Should value judgments be made with regard to the quality of life to be preserved? The second question pertains to the personal responsibilities of the physician and of the patient: Under what circumstances, and to what extent, is the physician morally obligated to persist in rendering aggressive professional care? Is the patient always obliged to seek treatment designed to prolong life even though a cure is not anticipated?

Jewish teaching with regard to these questions is shaped by the principle that, not only is human life in general of infinite and inestimable value, but that every moment of life is of infinite value as well.[2] Accordingly, obligations with regard to treatment and cure are one and the same regardless of whether the person's life is likely to be prolonged for a matter of years or merely for a few seconds. Thus, on the Sabbath, no less so than on a weekday, efforts to free a victim buried under a collapsed building must be continued even if the victim is found in circumstances such that he cannot survive for longer than a brief period of time.[3]

Life with suffering is regarded as being, in many cases, preferable to cessation of life and with it elimination of suffering. The Gemara, *Sotah* 22a, followed by Rambam, *Hilkhot Sotah* 3:20, indicates that the woman who was required to drink "the bitter waters" (Numbers 6:11–31) did not always die immediately. If she possessed other merit, though guilty of the offense with which she was charged, rather than causing her to perish immediately, the waters produced a debilitating and degenerative state which led to a protracted termination of life. The added longevity, although accompanied by pain and suffering, is deemed a privilege bestowed in recognition of meritorious actions. Life accompanied by pain is thus viewed as preferable to death.[4] It is this sentiment which is reflected in the words of the Psalmist, "The Lord has indeed chastened me, but He has not left me to die" (Psalms 188:18).

The practice of euthanasia—whether active or passive—is contrary to the teachings of Judaism. Any positive act designed to hasten the death of the patient is equated with murder in Jewish law, even if death is hastened by only a matter of moments. No matter how laudable the intentions of the person performing an act of mercy killing may be, the deed constitutes an act of homicide.

One nineteenth-century commentator finds this principle reflected in the verse "But your blood of your lives will I require; from the hand of every beast will I require it; and from the hand of man, from the hand of a person's brother, will I require the life of man" (Genesis 9:5). Fratricide is certainly no less heinous a crime than ordinary homicide. Why then, having already prohibited homicide, is it necessary for Scripture to prohibit fratricide as well? R. Jacob Zevi Mecklenburg, in his commentary on the Pentateuch, *Ha-Ketav ve-ha-Kabbalah*, astutely comments that, while murder is the antithesis of brotherly love, in some circumstances the taking of the life of one's fellow man may be perceived as indeed being an act of love par excellence. Euthanasia, designed to put an end to unbearable suffering, is born not of hatred or anger, but of concern and compassion. It is precisely the taking of life in circumstances in which it is manifestly obvious that the perpetrator is motivated by feelings of love and brotherly compassion that the Torah finds necessary to brand as murder, pure and simple. Despite the noble intent which prompts such an action, mercy killing is proscribed as an unwarranted intervention in an area which must be governed by God alone. The life of man may be reclaimed only by the Author of life. So long as man is yet endowed with a spark of life—as defined by God's eternal law—man dare not presume to hasten death, no matter how hopeless or meaningless continued existence may appear to be in the eyes of a mortal perceiver.

2. *Personal Autonomy*

In stark contrast to the value system posited by Judaism, decisions in a series of cases handed down by American courts in recent years have upheld the right of a mentally competent adult to decline any and all forms of medical intervention even in instances in which it is clear that death will ensue.[5] The sole recognized exceptions involve situations in which the adult is the parent of a minor child or in which intervention is necessary to preserve the life of a fetus. In such situations earlier decisions have recognized the State's "compelling interest" in not allowing a situation to develop in which the child might become a ward of the State[6] and a number of decisions have recognized the State's interest in safeguarding the life and health of an unborn child.[7]

The touchstone of a democratic society is the concept of individual freedom and personal autonomy. Democratic societies are quite properly dedicated to the maximization of personal freedom and find it necessary to justify any violation of personal privacy and any intrusion into the personal affairs of their citizens. These democratic traditions stand diametrically opposed to the absolutism which is the hallmark of the autocratic systems of government whose excesses cause so much human suffering.

No one will dispute the claim that personal freedom and individual autonomy are religious values as well. Yet it is readily apparent that, in a hierarchical ranking of values, the values of personal freedom and autonomy do not occupy a position within a religiously oriented ethical system identical to that which they occupy in a secular system of values. That certainly is the case insofar as Jewish tradition is concerned and serves to explain why a patient dare not refuse treatment that is clearly required to preserve life.

Judaism teaches that man has no proprietary interest either in his life or in his body. Man's body and his life are not his to give away. The proprietor of all human life is none other than God Himself. As Radvaz, *Hilkhot Sanhedrin* 18:6, so eloquently phrases it: "Man's life is not his property, but the property of the Holy One, blessed be He."[8]

According to Jewish teaching, personal privilege as well as personal responsibility as extended to the human body and to human life are similar to the privilege and responsibility of a bailee with regard to a bailment with which he has been entrusted. It is the duty of a bailee who has accepted an object of value for safekeeping to safeguard the bailment and to return it to its rightful owner upon demand. With regard to the human body, man is but a steward charged with preservation of this most precious of bailments and must abide by the limitations placed upon his rights of use and enjoyment. Hence, any claim to absolute autonomy is specious.

This moral stance is reflected in the mores of society at large, although not to the same degree. Despite contemporary society's commitment to individual liberty as an ideal, it recognizes that this liberty is not entirely sacrosanct. Although there are those who wish it to be so, self-determination is not universally recognized as the paramount human value. There is a long judicial history of recognition of the State's "compelling" interest in the preservation of the life of each and every one of its citizens, an "interest" which carries with it the right to curb personal freedom. What the jurist calls a "compelling state interest" the theologian terms "sanctity of life." It is precisely this concept of the sanctity of life which, as a transcendental value, supersedes considerations of personal freedom. This is implicitly recognized even in the provisions of the Natural Death Act enacted in various jurisdictions; otherwise such legislation would grant its citizens unequivocal authority to terminate life by any means and in all circumstances. Were autonomy recognized as the paramount value, society would not shrink from sanctioning suicide, mercy killing, or indeed consensual homicide, under any or all conditions.

Jewish tradition certainly recognizes liberty as a value but defines freedom and liberty in a very particular way. The Mishnaic dictum "*ve-lo atah ben ḥorin le-hibatel mimenah*" (*Ethics of the Fathers* 2:16) is rendered by the fifteenth century commentator R. Isaac Abarbanel, not in the usual manner as "nor are you free to desist from it," i.e., from obedience to the law, but as "nor in desisting from it are you a free man." Freedom is the absence of constraint which would interfere with realization of man's potential. The laws of the Torah are designed to facilitate man's endeavors in fulfilling the Divine plan inherent in creation. Hence casting off the yoke of law is not an act of freedom but its antithesis. This concept is very similar to what the British philosopher T. H. Green called "positive freedom."

Liberty, as the term is conventionally understood, is a paramount value only when it does not conflict with other divinely established values. In secular terms, personal autonomy must give way to preservation of the social fabric. The state has an interest, which is entirely secular in nature, in the preservation of life of each of its citizens. In the absence of other competing interests, it may assert its authority in compelling the preservation of a life against the wishes of a citizen in spite of the deprivation of liberty which is entailed thereby because public policy accepts the moral thesis that the preservation of life must be regarded as a superior value, taking precedence over the right to privacy and the value of personal autonomy.

Yet as reflected in Jewish law, Judaism bestows a privileged position upon preservation of human life as a moral value in a manner that is unparalleled in other value systems. As a moral desideratum, it takes precedence over virtually all other values. Exceptions to the general rule that preservation of life takes precedence over all other considerations are transgression of the three cardinal sins for purposes of preserving life. These are murder (hardly an exception), idolatry, and sexual offenses such as incest and adultery. All other laws are suspended for purposes of conservation of life. Even the mere possibility of preserving life mandates suspension of biblical restrictions, however remote the likelihood of success in saving human life may be.

3. *Prayer for Death*

The aggressiveness with which Judaism teaches that life must be preserved is not at all incompatible with awareness that the human condition is such that there are circumstances in which man would prefer death to life. The Gemara, *Ketubot* 104a, reports that Rabbi Judah the Prince, redactor of the Mishnah, was afflicted by what appears to have been an incurable and debilitating gastrointestinal disorder. Rabbi Judah had a female servant who is depicted in rabbinic writings as a woman of exemplary piety and moral character. This servant is reported to have prayed for his death. On the basis of this narrative, the thirteenth-century authority, Rabbenu Nissim of Gerondi, in his commentary on *Nedarim* 40a, states that it is permissible, and even praiseworthy, to pray for the death of a patient who is gravely ill and in extreme pain. Rabbenu Nissim chides those who are remiss in discharging the obligation of visiting the sick, remarking of such an individual, ". . . not only does he not aid [the patient] in living but even when [the patient] would [derive] benefit from death, even that small benefit [prayer for his demise] he does not bestow upon him."

Although man must persist in his efforts to prolong life, he may, nevertheless, express human needs and concerns through the medium of prayer. There is no contradiction whatsoever between acting upon an existing obligation and pleading to be relieved of further responsibility.[9] Man may beseech God to relieve him from divinely imposed obligations when they appear to exceed human endurance. In the context of suffering associated with a debilitating illness, the patient, even while discharging his obligations as a bailee, is fully entitled to beseech God to terminate those responsibilities by reclaiming His bailment, i.e., the life entrusted to man. Thus, in appropriate circumstances, a patient while dutifully swallowing his prescribed medication need not utter the prayer recorded in *Shulḥan Arukh, Oraḥ Ḥayyim* 230:4, "May it be Your will, O Lord, my God, that this endeavor be a cure for me,"[10] but may actually pray that the medication not prolong his life. The ultimate decision, however, is God's, and God's alone. There are times when God's answer to prayer is in the negative. But that, too, is an answer.

Contemporary rabbinic writers point out that even after Rabbi Judah's servant expressed her feelings and conveyed information regarding her master's pain and discomfort to his disciples, they not only declined to join her in prayer for his decease but did not desist from praying for prolongation of his life.[11]

There is one responsum which deals with the particular question of prayer for termination of suffering through death, but which has important implications for decision-making in general. R. Chaim Palaggi, *Ḥikekei Lev*, I, *Yoreh De'ah*, no. 50, accepts the view of Rabbenu Nissim but adds an important caveat. *Ḥikekei Lev* asserts that only totally disinterested parties may, by even so innocuous a method as prayer, take any action that may lead to a premature termination of life. Husband, children, family, and those charged with the care of the patient, according to R. Chaim Palaggi, may not pray for death. The considerations underlying this reservation are twofold in nature: (1) Those who are emotionally involved, if they are permitted even such non-physical methods of intervention as prayer, may be prompted to perform an overt act which would have the effect of shortening life and thus be tantamount to euthanasia. (2) Precisely because of their closeness to the situation, they are psychologically incapable of reaching a detached, dispassionate and objective decision in which considerations of patient benefit are the sole controlling motives. The human psyche is such that the intrusion of emotional involvement and subjective interest preclude a totally objective and disinterested decision.

II. TREATMENT OF THE TERMINALLY ILL

1. *Modes of Treatment: Natural vs. Artificial; Ordinary vs. Extraordinary*

The foregoing discussion reflects the unique position that preservation of life occupies in the hierarchy of values posited by Judaism. Judaism regards human life as being of infinite and inestimable value. The quality of life that is preserved is thus never a factor to be taken into consideration. Neither is the length of the patient's life expectancy a controlling factor.

Since Judaism regards every moment of life as sacred the patient is obliged to seek treatment[12] and religious laws are suspended for the sake of such treatment even if there is no medical guarantee of a cure. Similarly, the physician's duty does not end when he is incapable of restoring the lost health of his patient. The obligation "and you shall restore it to him" (Deuteronomy 22:2) refers, in its medical context, not simply to the restoration of health, but to the restoration of even a single moment of life. Again, Sabbath restrictions and other laws are suspended even when it is known with certainty that human medicine offers no hope of a cure or restoration to health. Ritual obligations and restrictions are suspended so long as there is the possibility that life may be prolonged even for a matter of moments.

Nevertheless, there remains considerable doubt, and perhaps even a measure of disagreement, within the Jewish community with regard to the permissibility of withholding various forms of medical treatment from the terminally ill. In Israel the matter has been exacerbated by the adoption of a statute exonerating a physician or any other person from criminal liability "for a medical action or treatment performed with lawful permission of an individual for the person's benefit." In an attempt to dispel confusion the following statement was issued recently by a group of leading Israeli rabbinic decisors:

> According to the law of the Torah it is obligatory to treat even a patient who, according to the opinion of the physicians, is a terminal, moribund patient with all medications and usual medical procedures as needed. Heaven forfend that the demise of a terminal patient be hastened by withholding nutrients or medical treatments in order to lessen his suffering. *A fortiori*, it is forbidden to hasten his demise by means of an overt act (other than if it is clear that these are his last hours in which case even movement [of the patient] is forbidden since he is a *goses*.
>
> Below is a list of medical treatments compiled by senior physicians.
>
> In accordance with what has been stated above, it is incumbent upon the families of terminally-ill patients to concern themselves and to request that the patients receive treatment in accordance with the above stated principles.
>
> (*Signed*)
>
> Joseph Shalom Eliashiv — Shlomoh Zalman Auerbach
> Shmu'el ha-Levi Woszner — S. Y. Nissim Karelitz

Appended to this statement is a list of mandatory treatments that includes intravenous or gastric feeding, IV fluid replacement, insulin injections, controlled dosages of morphine, antibiotics and blood transfusions. The Hebrew text of this statement appeared in various periodicals, including the 29 Kislev 5755 issue of the English-language edition of *Yated Ne'eman.*[13]

In addition, the following heretofore unpublished statement, dated 9 Adar 5756 (February 29, 1996), was issued by Rabbi Aaron Soloveichik:

> It is my unmitigated, convinced opinion that a doctor must do his utmost to treat terminally ill patients. This is true whether doctors believe that the patient can survive for even an extremely brief period of time, or even if they believe that the patient is brain dead. The situation of a *goses* does not even have to be considered since today very few, if any, patients manifest the symptoms of a *goses*. Even in a case where the patient has been unconscious for a year or more, pulling the plug constitutes an act of homicide. Anyone who commits such a crime violates the Biblical prohibition of *lo tirẓaḥ*.
>
> The Gemara in *Masekhet Mo'ed Katan* that tells the story of *amta de-bei Rebbi* is in no way a justification for a doctor to deny a terminally ill patient his life support. The Gemara there relates that when the maid of Rebbi saw his unbearable pain in his dying moments, she went up on the roof and prayed to *Ha-Kadosh Barukh Hu* that He should expedite his death. The maid prayed to *Ha-Kadosh Barukh Hu*. He has title to all souls and therefore He can do with them whatever He in His infinite wisdom sees fit to do. A human being, however, cannot play God and therefore he may not decide the fate of other human beings.
>
> (*Signed*) Aaron Soloveichik

Jewish law with regard to care of the dying is spelled out with care and precision. The terminal patient, even when he is a *goses*, i.e., a person who has become moribund and whose death is imminent, is regarded as a living person in every respect. One must not pry his jaw, anoint him, wash him, plug his orifices, remove the pillow from underneath him or place him on the ground.[14] It is also forbidden to close his eyes "for whoever closes the eyes with the onset of death is a shedder of blood."[15] Each of these acts is forbidden because the slightest movement of the patient may hasten death. As the Talmud puts it, "The matter may be compared to a flickering flame; as soon as one touches it, the light is extinguished."[16] Accordingly, any movement or manipulation of the dying person is forbidden. Furthermore, passive euthanasia involving the omission of a therapeutic procedure or the withholding of medication which could sustain life is also prohibited by Jewish law. The terminal nature of an illness in no way mitigates the physician's responsibilities since the physician is charged with prolonging life no less than with effecting a cure.

Although, as will be noted presently, there may well be some limitations upon the obligation to preserve life, many commonly asserted moral distinctions have no basis in Jewish teaching. Any distinction between "natural" and "artificial" means of treatment is without precedent in Jewish law. Indeed, upon examination, the distinction is fundamentally specious. Medical substances synthesized in the laboratory are certainly not "natural," yet it is unlikely that ethicists would regard such medications as "artificial." For that matter, even drugs extracted from plants and the like are hardly "natural" sources of nutrition for man but assuredly would not be classified as artificial. The obligation to revive a person from drowning is one of the paradigms of *pikuaḥ nefesh* advanced by the Gemara, *Sanhedrin* 73a. That obligation includes the duty to throw a life preserver to the potential victim. In what sense is a respirator designed to deliver oxygen to the lungs different from the casting of a life preserver? If the drowning person is too exhausted to grasp the life preserver of his own accord he must certainly be assisted in doing so. In what sense is the pumping action of the apparatus designed to facilitate absorption of the oxygen by the blood stream different from physically placing the life preserver around the waist of the drowning victim?

Rambam's remarks in his *Commentary on the Mishnah, Pesaḥim* 56a, serve to dispel any distinction that might be drawn between the "natural" and the "artificial" in such a context. The Tosefta records that King Hezekiah performed six memorable acts; three of those acts were censured by the Sages and three received their approbation. Among the latter was his suppression of a certain "book of cures." Rashi explains that Hezekiah was concerned because, upon being stricken by illness, the sick were immediately able to cure their maladies simply by consulting this manual and following its directions. As a result "their heart did not become humble," i.e., they failed to recognize sickness as a manifestation of Providence designed to induce introspection and repentance. In offering his own totally disparate explanation of Hezekiah's motives Rambam cites an anonymous interpretation quite similar to that of Rashi and dismissively comments:

> How could they attribute to Hezekiah a foolishness that it would not be proper to attribute to the meanest of the populace? . . . According to their flighty and confused opinion, a person who is starving and goes to bread and eats of it, without doubt when he is cured of that severe illness, viz., the illness of hunger, is he then forsaken and will no longer rely upon God? We say to them: O fools! Just as I give thanks to God upon eating for having made available to me the wherewithal to satiate myself and dispel my hunger in order to live and be sustained, so shall I give thanks to Him when I am cured for having made available to me a cure to heal my sickness.

In those remarks Rambam eloquently affirms the notion that the Deity provides for all of the needs of mankind. God causes man to seek bread instinctively in order to assuage hunger; in a similar manner God providentially makes medication and technology available to man so that man may cure illnesses. The "artificiality" of medications in no way diminishes their role as instruments of Providence. As such, medicaments must be attributed to God and acknowledged with gratitude. In precisely the same manner, all medical artifacts must be recognized as having been spawned by Providence and designed to serve as instruments of *pikuaḥ nefesh*.

God created food and water; we are obliged to use them in staving off hunger and thirst. God created drugs and medicaments and endowed man with the intelligence necessary to discover their medicinal properties; we are obliged to use them in warding off illness and disease. Similarly, God provided the materials and the technology which make possible catheters, intravenous infusions and respirators; we are likewise obligated to use them in order to prolong life. Medication, therefore, may not be withheld from an incurable patient.

Similarly, the commonly drawn distinction between "ordinary" versus "extraordinary" means of treatment and the exclusion of "heroic" measures in preserving life have no parallel in Jewish sources. Indeed, one is hard pressed to find appropriate terminology in rabbinic Hebrew to express such distinctions. Those distinctions have entered contemporary moral discourse through the mediation of an entirely foreign religious tradition.

In discharging his responsibility with regard to prolongation of life the physician must make use of any medical resources that are available. However, as shown elsewhere,[17] he is not obligated to employ procedures which are themselves hazardous in nature and which may potentially foreshorten the life of the patient. Nor is either the physician or the patient obligated to employ a therapy which is experimental in nature.[18]

The question of treatment in face of intractable pain will be considered in a later section.

For these same reasons, Judaism cannot sanction a "living will" or the provisions of legislation such as the various versions of the Natural Death Act which have been enacted by a number of state legislatures. Such legislation is designed to bind the physician to respect the wishes of the patient and, under certain conditions, to withhold or withdraw life-sustaining procedures in the event of a terminal malady. Judaism denies man the right to make judgments with regard to quality of life. The category of *pikuaḥ nefesh* extends to human life of every description, including the feeble-minded the mentally deranged, and even persons in a so-called vegetative state. The *mizvah* of saving a life is neither enhanced nor diminished by virtue of the quality of life preserved. Nor, in the final analysis, does the desire of the patient to have, or not to have, his or her life prolonged play a role in the halakhic obligation to initiate or maintain life-sustaining procedures.[19]

2. *Palliation of Pain*

Assuredly, elimination of pain is a legitimate and laudable goal. According to some authorities mitigation of pain is encompassed within the general obligation to heal.[20] Palliative treatment is certainly mandated by virtue of the commandment "and you shall love your neighbor as yourself" (Leviticus 19:18). Yet, when the dual goals of avoidance of pain and preservation of life come into conflict with one another, Judaism recognizes the paramount value and sanctity of life and, accordingly, assigns priority to preservation of life. Thus, a number of authorities have expressly stated that non-treatment or withdrawal of treatment in order for the patient to be released from pain by death constitutes euthanasia and is not countenanced by Judaism.[21] This remains the case even if the patient himself pleads to be permitted to die. As stated by one prominent authority, "Even if the patient himself cries out, 'Let me be and do not give me any aid because for me death is preferable' everything possible must be done on behalf of the patient."[22]

Nevertheless, every prudent effort should be made to alleviate the patient's suffering. This includes aggressive treatment of pain even to a degree which at present is not common in current medical practice. Physicians are reluctant to use morphine in high dosages because of the danger of depression of the cerebral center responsible for respiration. The effect of morphine administered in high doses is that the patient cannot control the muscles necessary for breathing. There is, however, no halakhic objection to providing such medication in order to control pain in the case of terminal patients even though palliation of pain may ultimately entail maintaining such a patient on a respirator. Similarly, there is no halakhic objection to the use of heroin in the control of pain in terminal patients. The danger of addiction under such circumstances is, of course, hardly a significant consideration. At present, the use of heroin is illegal even for medical purposes. Judaism affirms that everything in creation is designed for a purpose. Alleviation of otherwise intractable pain is a known beneficial use of heroin. Marijuana is effective in alleviating nausea that is a side-effect of some forms of chemotherapy. There is every reason to believe that these drugs were given to man for the specific purpose of controlling pain and discomfort. Jewish teaching would enthusiastically endorse legislation legalizing the use—with adequate accompanying safeguards—of those substances in treatment of terminal patients.

III. THE GOSES

1. *Definition of a Goses*

Although euthanasia in any form is forbidden, and the hastening of death, even by a matter of moments, is regarded as tantamount to murder, there is one situation in which treatment, according to some authorities,[23] may be withheld from the moribund patient in order to provide for an unimpeded death. While the death of a *goses*[24] may not be hastened, according to those authorities, there is no obligation to perform any action which will lengthen the life of a patient in this state. The distinction between an active and a passive act, as drawn by those authorities, applies to a *goses* and to a *goses* only. When a patient is, as it were, actually in the clutches of the Angel of Death and the death process has actually begun, argue these authorities, there is no obligation to heal. In support of that position, those scholars cite the words of Rema, *Yoreh De'ah* 339:1, who permits the removal of "anything which constitutes a hindrance to the departure of the soul, such as a clattering noise or salt upon his tongue. . . since such acts involve no active hastening of death, but only the removal of the impediment."

As will be shown, Rema's ruling is subject to at least three possible interpretations. The most obvious is that Rema distinguishes between an overt act that may foreshorten life and passive withholding of life-prolonging measures. It cannot be overemphasized that even those authorities who interpret Rema in this manner and sanction acts of omission do so only when the patient is in a state of *gesisah*.[25] At any earlier stage, withholding of treatment is tantamount to euthanasia. What, then, are the criteria indicative of the onset of this state? Rema, in both *Even ha-Ezer* 121:7 and *Ḥoshen Mishpat* 211:2, defines this state as being that of a patient who "brings up secretion in his throat on account of the narrowing of his chest."[26] Of course, if the condition is reversible there is an obligation to heal.[27] According to those authorities, when the condition of *gesisah* is irreversible there is no obligation to continue treatment and, according to some of those authorities, there is even a prohibition against prolonging the life of the moribund patient.

Rema's description, while a necessary criterion of *gesisah*,[28] is certainly not a sufficient one. Were the patient to present this symptom but in the opinion of medical practitioners be capable of survival, he would clearly not be considered a *goses* and all usual obligations would remain in force. Moreover, the physiological criteria of *gesisah* must be spelled out with care. It is surely clear that a patient whose life may be prolonged for weeks and even months is not yet moribund; the actual death process has not yet started to set in and hence the patient is not a *goses*. The halakhic provisions governing care of a *goses* may most emphatically not be applied to all who are terminally ill.

It appears that any patient who may reasonably be deemed capable of potential survival for a period of seventy-two hours cannot be considered a *goses*. If the patient is capable of surviving that length of time, the death process cannot be deemed to have commenced. It would appear that Halakhah assumes axiomatically that the death process or the "act of dying" cannot be longer than seventy-two hours in duration.[29] This is evidenced by the ruling recorded in *Shulḥan Arukh, Yoreh De'ah* 339:2, to the effect that one must commence to observe the laws of mourning three days after a relative has been observed in a state of *gesisah*. Some authorities even permit a wife to remarry in the absence of witnesses testifying to the actual death of the husband provided that testimony is forthcoming to the effect that her husband was observed in a state of *gesisah*.[30] These authorities maintain that the testimony of witnesses with regard to *gesisah*, *ipso facto*, constitutes legal proof of a state of widowhood commencing three days following the onset of *gesisah*.

It further appears that this state is not determined by a patient's ability to survive for this period solely by natural means unaided by drugs or medication. The implication is that a *goses* is one who cannot, under any circumstances, be maintained alive for a period of seventy-two hours.[31] Testimony with regard to the existence of a state of *gesisah* as conclusive evidence of impending death implies that the state is not only irreversible but also not prolongable even by artificial means. Otherwise, there would exist a legal suspicion that life may have been prolonged artificially by means of extraordinary medical treatment. The obvious conclusion to be drawn is that, if it is medically feasible to prolong life, the patient is indeed not a *goses* and, therefore, in such instances there is a concomitant obligation to preserve the life of the patient as long as possible.

It follows that a specific physiological condition may or may not correspond to a state of *gesisah* depending upon the state of medical knowledge of the day. When medical care is of no avail and the patient manifesting the symptoms described by Rema is expected to expire within seventy-two hours, he is deemed to be in the process of "dying." When, however, medication can prolong life, such medicine, in effect, delays the onset of the death process. Accordingly, the patient who receives medical treatment enabling him to survive for a period of three days or more is not yet in the process of "dying." It follows, therefore, that those responsible for his care are not relieved of their duty to minister to his needs and to postpone the onset of death by means of medical treatment.

References to the precise maximum duration of a state of *gesisah* are found in the works of a number of disciples of the thirteenth-century German authority, R. Meir of Rothenberg, and constitute the basis of Rema's earlier-cited ruling incorporated in the laws of mourning. *Mordekhai, Mo'ed Katen*, sec. 864, reports that the following situation was brought to the attention of R. Meir of Rothenberg: A certain woman found herself in a locale a four-day journey distant from her husband. Several Jewish travellers arriving from the husband's place of residence informed her that, at the time of their departure, her husband was a *goses*. R. Meir of Rothenberg ruled that she must immediately commence observance of the prescribed period of mourning. That ruling was predicated upon the talmudic presumption recorded in *Gittin* 28a to the effect that "the majority of *gosesin* die." R. Meir of Rothenberg amplifies that principle and indicates that the halahkic presumption is that "the majority of *gosesin* do not live two days or three."[32] A similar version of the incident is recorded by another disciple of R. Meir of Rothenberg, Rabbenu Asher, in Rosh, *Mo'ed Katan* 3:97, with the slightly varying concluding statement, ". . . the majority of *gosesin* do not live three days or four." A report of the same incident found in *Sefer ha-Agudah, Mo'ed Katan* 3:56, contains neither concluding remark but begins by indicating that the "woman was distant from her husband a journey of three or four days." The version cited by *Mordekhai* is reflected in R. Meir of Rothenberg's work *Ḥiddushei Maharam: Hilkhot Semaḥot*, edited by R. Isaac Gatineiv (Saloniki, 5555), no. 6,[33] and is the basis of the ruling recorded by *Tur Shulḥan Arukh, Yoreh De'ah* 339, as well as by *Shulḥan Arukh, Yoreh De'ah* 339:2.[34]

2. *Withdrawal of Treatment from a Goses*

Rema's ruling regarding cessation of wood chopping in order to allow a *goses* to expire is taken directly from *Sefer Ḥasidim* (Jerusalem, 5720), no. 723. Rema has been understood as drawing a distinction between performance of an overt act for the purpose of hastening death and withdrawal of an impediment so that death can occur naturally.[35] In effect, according to this understanding, Rema sanctions passive euthanasia in the case of a *goses*. That interpretation is bolstered by Rema's concluding phrase "for in this there is no act at all; rather, he removes the impediment."

Granted that Rema's ruling is limited to a *goses*, the paramount problem with regard to his ruling is why the general obligation to prolong life does not extend to a *goses* as well.[36] As noted earlier, the obligation to preserve life is not limited either by the quality of life preserved or by longevity anticipation. Moreover, Rema in his commentary on *Tur Shulḥan Arukh, Darkei Mosheh, Yoreh De'ah* 339:1, goes beyond the ruling incorporated in *Shulḥan Arukh*. In his gloss to *Shulḥan Arukh, Yoreh De'ah* 339:1, Rema rules simply that it is permitted to remove an impediment to the departure of the soul from the body whereas in his *Darkei Mosheh* he declares it to be forbidden to interfere with the departure of the soul. This understanding of Rema is reflected in *Teshuvot Bet Ya'akov*, no. 59, who accepts the comment of *Darkei Mosheh* declaring prolongation of the life of a *goses* not only to be unnecessary but actually prohibited.[37] In a manner entirely consistent with that view, *Teshuvot Bet Ya'akov* rules that it is forbidden to violate the Sabbath[38] on behalf of a *goses*.[39]

Although he does not comment upon the ruling of *Sefer Ḥasidim* and Rema, R. Jacob Reischer, *Teshuvot Shevut Ya'akov*, I, no. 13, cites *Teshuvot Bet Ya'akov* and takes sharp issue with the author of that work in stating, "His words are incomprehensible. Certainly it is forbidden for one who is not proficient in medicine to prevent the departure of the soul but it is certainly permissible for one who is proficient in medicine to ward off *gesisah* temporarily." Accordingly, *Teshuvot Shevut Ya'akov* rules that otherwise forbidden acts may be performed on *Shabbat* on behalf of a *goses* even in order to prolong his life only ephemerally.[40] In support of that position *Shevut Ya'akov* cites the advice offered by the Gemara, *Avodah Zarah* 12b: "One who swallows a wasp cannot live. Nevertheless, let him be given a *revi'it* of strong vinegar to drink. Perhaps he will live briefly, long enough to set his house in order."[41] However, in the light of Rema's definition of a *goses* as one who cannot bring up secretions from his chest, that statement of the Gemara does not necessarily substantiate *Shevut Ya'akov*'s position. Not every moribund patient is a *goses*. A *goses* is a patient whose death is imminent and who has also lost control of bodily functions as manifested by his inability to bring up secretions from the chest. Indeed the ability to swallow the prescribed *revi'it* of vinegar is inconsistent with the inability to bring up secretions beause of constriction of the chest that, for Rema, is emblematic of a *goses*. Although the Gemara presumes that a person who swallows a wasp will die within a very short period of time, there is no evidence, and indeed no reason to presume, that such a person loses control of bodily functions immediately. Quite to the contrary, the concern expressed by the Gemara is that he be enabled "to set his house in order," an endeavor that is presumably beyond the capacity of one who is in a debilitated state such that he cannot even bring up secretions from his chest. The position of *Shevut Ya'akov* requiring medical treatment on behalf of a *goses* is espoused by *Mishnah Berurah, Bi'ur Halakhah* 329:4, and by R. Eliezer Waldenberg in a number of his writings, including *Ramat Raḥel*, no. 28; *Ẓiẓ Eli'ezer*, VIII, no. 15, chap. 3, sec. 16; *ibid.*, IX, no. 47; and *Assia*, Nisan 5738, p. 19, reprinted in *Sefer Assia*, III (5743), p. 458.

Although talmudic sources for this interpretation of *Sefer Ḥasidim* and Rema are elusive, the declared principle seems to be that both the obligation of *pikuaḥ nefesh* as well as direct license to intervene in physiological processes derived by the Gemara, *Bava Kamma* 85a, from the verse "and he shall cause him to be thoroughly healed" (Exodus 21:19), does not extend to a patient *in extremis* once the actual process of dying has begun. Conceptually, however, any life-saving act can be denoted either as "prolonging life" or as "interfering with the process of dying." Those disparate descriptions parallel the description of a single glass of water as either half full or half empty. In both instances the chosen depiction may be indicative of a certain attitude on the part of the perceiver but the differing descriptions do not reflect different empirical realities. In the case of the glass of water it has often been said that one description marks the speaker as an optimist, while the other marks him as a pessimist. In a related manner, to describe an act of intervention as life-prolonging is emotively to express approval whereas to describe it as interference with the process of dying is likely to reflect a negative moral and/or theological judgment. Recognizing this to be the case, it is important to emphasize that Rema's ruling (if understood in this manner) is limited to the case of a *goses* and that this term has a precise technical meaning when employed in a halakhic context. Life itself is a terminal condition and the process of dying begins with the moment of birth. Identification of any point along the continuum of life as the beginning of the process of dying is, in the logical sense, entirely arbitrary. Similarly, identification of the state of *gesisah* as denoting the onset of dying is nothing more than a halakhic construct, and hence definition of *gesisah* as the process of dying is tautologous, i.e., a patient in the physiological state termed *gesisah* is treated as being in the process of dying, not because of any incontrovertible empirical considerations, but because Halakhah declares it so.

Needless to say, it is self-evident that if the *goses* can be restored to good health, or even if the state of *gesisah* can be reversed, the obligation of *pikuaḥ nefesh* mandates that the requisite medical intervention be instituted. It is also clear that there exist many patients who, in the past, would have been described as *gosesim* but who today can be treated. In effect, there are conditions in which contemporary medicine is capable of reversing the state of *gesisah*. Or, to state it somewhat differently, since a *goses* is a moribund patient manifesting specific clinical criteria who will die within a specific period of time despite administration of all known medical treatment, identification of patients as members of the class of *gosesim*, and hence the denotation of the term, is relative and will vary with the state of medical knowledge and technology.

This conclusion is not at all surprising if it is remembered that Rambam espouses an identical view with regard to the concept of *treifah* as applied to human beings. Rambam, *Hilkhot Roẓeaḥ* 2:8, rules that, unlike the definition of *treifah* as applied to animals whose meat is prohibited by the dietary code, the definition of a human *treifah* varies from generation to generation. Animal *treifot* are identified and described by the Oral Law given at Sinai. An animal identified as a *treifah* remains a *treifah* regardless of the present-day ability of veterinary medicine to prolong the animal's life indefinitely. Not so, declares Rambam, with regard to identification of *treifot* in human beings. Classification of a person as a *treifah* is of importance primarily with regard to exoneration of the murderer of a *treifah* from the penalty of capital punishment. The murderer either of a person born with one of a specified number of congenital defects or of a person who has suffered a trauma of a nature categorized as a *treifah* does not incur capital punishment. However, rules Rambam, if the victim, as the beneficiary of the medical expertise of his epoch, is presumed to have been capable of survival for more than twelve months, the murderer is guilty of a capital offense. Rambam clearly maintains that the definition of a *treifah*, insofar as humans are concerned, is relative and varies with the state of medical expertise in any given age.[42] Thus, it is not surprising that this is the case with regard to the categorization of a *goses* as well.

As recognized by these authorities, the limitation upon the obligation to preserve life once the process of dying has actually begun can perhaps be captured in metaphorical expression. Man has the right—and indeed the obligation—to rescue his fellow but man, unless he can prevail, ought not to interfere with, or hinder, the Angel of Death in the latter's discharge of his duties. The Angel of Death may take as long as three days to complete his assigned task. During that period man ought not to interfere and thereby prolong the time the Angel of Death must devote to discharging his duty unless he anticipates being able to take the Angel of Death by the scruff of the neck and eject him from the sick room, thereby cancelling his mission.

3. *Nonwithdrawal of Medical Treatment from a Goses*

As has been noted, according to the authorities who rule that prolongation of the life of a *goses* is permissible and indeed mandatory, Rema's ruling permitting cessation of wood chopping and his statement in *Darkei Mosheh* prohibiting an act designed to impede the departure of the soul from the body are highly problematic.[43] It is noteworthy that the examples given by Rema are limited to termination of wood-chopping and removal of salt from the tongue of the patient. Explicitly prohibited by Rema in the same gloss is removal of a cushion or comforter from beneath the patient because the presence of the feathers of some fowl impedes death and because of the fear that such removal would necessarily entail prohibited movement of the *goses*. Rema does not offer the simple and obvious example of withholding life-sustaining medication from the patient.

Elsewhere[44] this writer has drawn attention to the distinction between natural remedies of demonstrated efficacy involving readily recognizable causal relationships and nonscientific *segulot* of undemonstrable causal efficacy, e.g., consuming a portion of meat taken from an area surrounding the liver of an attacking dog as protection against rabies. The obligation of *pikuaḥ nefesh* is limited to utilization of drugs and medications that are in the realm of rationally explainable, causally effective procedures. Use of remedies that are nonnatural or of undemonstrated efficacy is never mandatory. The presence of a persistent clattering noise, salt on the tongue or feathers of certain fowl under a patient's body are clearly in the latter category. Since their use is not mandatory for purposes of *pikuaḥ nefesh* such measures need not, or perhaps should not, be utilized to prevent departure of the soul. However, according to this second understanding of Rema, normal forms of life-prolonging therapy must be administered to a *goses* just as they are administered to any other patient.[45]

This analysis is supported by the phraseology employed by *Shevut Ya'akov* in his comment that one who is not proficient in medicine should not attempt to treat a *goses* but that there is no basis for restraining a person who is proficient in medicine from doing so. The ministrations of a practitioner who is not proficient in medicine are in the category of a *refu'ah she-einah bedukah* and hence forbidden, as are Rema's examples of *segulot*; the ministrations of a competent medical practitioner are entirely different and hence mandatory even if the patient is a *goses*.

Further support for this distinction may be found in the talmudic passage cited by *Shevut Ya'akov*. The Gemara advises a person who has swallowed a wasp to drink strong vinegar so that he may put his affairs in order. *Shevut Ya'akov* fails to comment upon the obvious difficulty posed by advancement of that rationale. If prolongation of the life of a terminally ill patient, or even of a *goses*, is permissible, such prolongation of life should be mandatory as a form of *pikuaḥ nefesh*. The rationale cited by the Gemara, *viz*., "so that he may put his affairs in order" is thus entirely superfluous. If, however, as would seem to be the case, vinegar is not a *refu'ah bedukah*, its use is not at all obligatory. Hence the advice that vinegar be utilized because perchance (*efshar*) the remedy *may* help and the victim may survive long enough to place his affairs in order.[46]

4. *Withdrawal of Treatment in Cases of Intractable Pain*

R. Moshe Feinstein, *Iggerot Mosheh*, *Ḥoshen Mishpat*, II, no. 74, sec. 1, advances an entirely different analysis of Rema's position. *Iggerot Mosheh* expresses amazement at the suggestion that impediments to the departure of the soul from the body may be removed and states that, on the contrary, it would stand to reason that such measures should be introduced in order to prolong life. *Iggerot Mosheh* asserts that the sole consideration governing Rema's ruling is that there is no obligation to prolong the life of a patient who is in a state of pain. *Iggerot Mosheh* further asserts that a *goses* invariably experiences increased suffering by virtue of prolongation of the departure of the soul from the body and, acknowledging that it is not at all obvious that all moribund patients experience pain, comments that "certainly our teachers, Rema and his predecessors, had a tradition with regard to this."[47] Thus, for *Iggerot Mosheh*, the rule formulated by Rema with regard to a *goses* is two-fold in nature: (1) all treatment may be withheld from a patient who suffers "pain;" (2) every *goses* must be regarded as suffering pain of a nature that he is not required to endure. The suffering to which *Iggerot Mosheh* refers is not pain as that phenomenon is conventionally understood. It is readily acknowledged that not all patients experience suffering at the time of death; comatose patients, for example, do not experience pain. Absence of pain can be confirmed by lack of response to pain stimuli such as a pin prick as well as by more sophisticated neurological procedures. Persons who are in pain manifest particular and unique brain waves; brain waves associated with the experience of pain are totally absent in comatose patients. Accordingly, the "pain" described by *Iggerot Mosheh* as an unvarying concomitant of the departure of the soul from the body must be understood as a metaphysical or spiritual pain experienced by the soul rather than by the body.[48] Moreover, there is no explicit reference in rabbinic writings to the fact that prolonging the process of dying prolongs or intensifies such pain.[49] That principle is postulated by *Iggerot Mosheh* as a premise in formulating a hypothesis to explain the ruling cited by Rema.[50] Acceptance of an alternative explanation of that ruling serves to negate any support for such a presumption.

The basic principle that it is not obligatory to prolong the life of every patient is developed by Rabbi Feinstein in an earlier responsum, *Iggerot Mosheh, Ḥoshen Mishpat*, II, no. 73, sec. 1. In that responsum *Iggerot Mosheh* cites the narrative recorded by the Gemara, *Ketubot* 104b, describing the sickness and pain suffered by R. Judah the Prince. As has been noted earlier, when R. Judah's maidservant saw that the prayers of his disciples did not effect either a cure or relief of his suffering, she successfully prayed for his death. *Iggerot Mosheh* concludes that, in circumstances in which the physician has determined that the patient cannot be cured and that his or her life cannot be prolonged without concomitant suffering, further medication should not be administered.[51] By the same token, Rabbi Feinstein declares that medications must be administered to alleviate pain provided that the medication does not foreshorten life even briefly. He also insists that oxygen be administered as needed on the assumption that failure to administer oxygen will increase the suffering of the patient. In *Iggerot Mosheh, Ḥoshen Mishpat*, II, no. 74, sec. 1, Rabbi Feinstein again states that a cancer patient should be informed if medication will merely prolong his life with suffering and that such therapy should not be administered without the consent of the patient. In that responsum he emphasizes that sanctioning the withholding of therapy in cases of extreme pain should not be confused with decisions based upon "quality of life." *Iggerot Mosheh* emphatically declares that the life of a mentally incompetent person, and even of a patient in a permanent vegetative state, must be prolonged to the extent possible so long as the patient does not suffer extreme pain.

A similar pronouncement by the late R. Shlomoh Zalman Auerbach was published in *Halakhah u-Refu'ah*, II (Jerusalem, 5741), 131, and reprinted with a minor linguistic change in his collected responsa, *Minḥat Shlomoh*, no. 91, sec. 24. The following is a literal translation of that statement:

> Many struggle with this question concerning treatment of a *goses*. Some are of the opinion that just as the Sabbath must be desecrated for ephemeral life (*ḥayyei sha'ah*) so is it similarly obligatory to compel the patient with regard to this since he is

> not a proprietor with regard to himself [with the right] to relinquish even a single moment.[52] However, it is reasonable that if the patient experiences great pain and suffering, or even extremely severe psychological pain, [although] I think that it is mandatory to give him food[53] and oxygen for breathing even against his will, it is permissible to withhold medications that cause suffering to the patient[54] if the patient so demands. However, if the patient is God-fearing and is not mentally confused, it is extremely desirable to explain to him that a single hour of repentance in this world is more valuable than all of the world-to-come as we find in tractate *Sotah* 20a that it is a "privilege" to suffer seven years rather that to die immediately.

Noteworthy is the fact that Rabbi Auerbach refers to two distinct situations, *viz.*, the case of a patient who steadfastly refuses treatment and the case of a patient who can be consulted with regard to his wishes, but ignores the situation of the incompetent patient who lacks decision-making capacity. Similarly, the earlier cited statement dated 29 Kislev 5755 speaks only of obligatory forms of treatment but fails to indicate whether, in the absence of an announced desire on the part of the patient, other forms of treatment are prohibited or whether they may be administered at the discretion of the family and/ or physician. *Iggerot Mosheh* speaks of prolongation of pain to the patient as being prohibited other than with the patient's consent. Also noteworthy is Rabbi Auerbach's emphasis upon pain as a spiritual "benefit" or "privilege" and his strong recommendation that the patient be encouraged to accept prolongation of life to the extent medically possible despite accompanying suffering.

The rulings of *Iggerot Mosheh* and Rabbi Auerbach present two distinct but related problems: (1) The threshold level of pain and suffering that serves to permit withholding of treatment. Assuredly, the prospect of inconvenience, albeit lifelong in nature, or of mere discomfort is not sufficient to extinguish the obligation to preserve life. Indeed, *Iggerot Mosheh* carefully refers to "suffering" rather than to mere discomfort or ordinary pain and Rabbi Auerbach is even more precise in speaking of "great pain and suffering." What, then, are the criteria that serve to distinguish "great pain" or "suffering" from ordinary pain? (2) What are the sources and/or the underlying rationale upon which that distinction is based?

The underlying principle is not at all difficult to discover and is indeed expressed by *Iggerot Mosheh* in response to an entirely different query. Rabbi Feinstein was apparently asked whether it is permitted to remove an organ from a cadaver for purposes of a life-saving transplant against the wishes, or without the consent, of surviving relatives. In *Iggerot Mosheh, Yoreh De'ah*, II, no. 174, *anaf* 4, Rabbi Feinstein responds by indicating that it is forbidden to do so. His line of reasoning is most interesting. *Tosafot, Shabbat* 44a, indicate that a person may be presumed to suffer greater distress at the prospect of ignominous treatment of the corpse of a loved one than at the prospect of the loss of his entire fortune. *Tosafot* reach that conclusion on the basis of the fact that, although the Gemara permits removal of a corpse on *Shabbat* from the path of a fire, it does not similarly permit the removal of material possessions that may not generally be transported on *Shabbat*. The Gemara explains that, in cases of fire, the Sages abated the rabbinic prohibition against moving a corpse on the Sabbath because failure to grant such dispensation would result in wilful extinguishing of the fire since a person is likely to become agitated and confused upon confronting the sight of the body of a loved one becoming cremated or disfigured in a conflagration. Since similar dispensation is not granted for the rescue of material objects, no matter how valuable they may be, *Tosafot* conclude that a person does not generally experience the same anguish at the prospect of losing even his entire fortune.

The general rule with regard to expenditure of resources in order to avoid transgression as recorded by Rema, *Oraḥ*

Ḥayyim 656:1, is that a person is not obligated to expend more than twenty percent of his net worth in order to fulfill, or to avoid transgressing, a positive commandment[55] but is obligated to expend even his entire fortune in order to avoid transgressing a negative precept.[56] As cited by *Ḥiddushei R. Akiva Eger, Yoreh De'ah* 157:1, and *Pitḥei Teshuvah, Yoreh De'ah* 157:4, there is some controversy with regard to whether the distinction depends upon the phraseology in which the command is couched, i.e., whether it is expressed in negative rather than in positive terms, or whether the fundamental distinction is with regard to whether the transgression involves an overt act or is merely the result of passive nonperformance.[57] According to the first view, the distinction is based upon the consideration that negative prohibitions are inherently more stringent; according to the latter view, transgressions involving overt acts of commission are more severe in nature because they entail active involvement on the part of the transgressor. Those two views lead to diverse rulings in situations in which a negative command mandates a positive act and hence violation of the commandment occurs through passive nonfulfillment. A case in point is expenditure of funds to preserve life. The obligation is expressed as a negative command, "and you shalt not stand idly by the blood of your fellow," but transgression involves, not an overt act, but passive non-intervention. Thus, according to one opinion, a person is obligated to expend no more than twenty percent of his financial resources in order to rescue a person from death while, according to the other opinion, he is obligated to expend his entire fortune in order to preserve a life.[58]

The financial obligation, however, is limited, at most, to expenditure of one's entire fortune; one is under no obligation to expend more than an entire fortune in order to avoid transgression of even a negative commandment.[59] *Iggerot Mosheh* explains that it is for this reason that *Shakh, Yoreh De'ah* 157:3, concludes that a person need not sacrifice a limb in order to avoid transgressing a negative commandment. Similarly, *Te-*

shuvot Radvaz, III, no. 627, rules that a person need not allow a limb to be amputated in order to preserve the life of another person. The loss of a limb, these authorities rule, is more onerous than loss of an entire fortune. It then follows that, since one need not expend more than one's entire fortune to preserve the life of another person, one need not sacrifice a limb to do so.[60]

Basing himself upon these precedents, *Iggerot Mosheh* reasons that, since desecration of the corpse of a close relative may cause greater anguish than loss of an entire fortune, a person need not permit such desecration in order to avoid violation of a negative commandment and, similarly, a person need not assume such anguish in order to preserve the life of another.[61] However, emotional distress, at least for some people, is subject to control. Therefore, *Iggerot Mosheh* adds that a person should be counseled not to be distressed by the removal of an organ from the body of a loved one for the purpose of transplantation. Indeed, if a person does not actually experience such extreme distress the emotional cost is less than that comparable to expenditure of an entire fortune and, accordingly, for such a person, consent to the procedure would be mandatory. Moreover, *Iggerot Mosheh* notes that Radvaz regards the sacrifice of a limb in order to rescue another person as a fitting act of piety. Accordingly, *Iggerot Mosheh* urges that, in all circumstances, next of kin be encouraged to grant consent for life-saving transplants.

Precisely the same argument can be formulated with regard to physical pain, assuming that there exists intractable pain of such severity that a person would willingly surrender his entire fortune in order to rid himself of such pain.[62] Since a person need not expend more than his entire fortune in order to preserve his life, he need not accept pain of such magnitude in order to do so.[63] Since a person has no obligation to accept intractable pain even for the purpose of preserving life, others have no right to inflict it upon him without consent.[64]

The application of a closely related concept with regard to inordinate pain finds expression in the comments of an early-day authority. As recorded in the Book of Daniel 3:12–21, in allowing themselves to be cast into a fiery furnace, Hananiah, Mishael and Azariah (identified in Daniel as Shadrach, Meshach and Abed-nego), accepted martyrdom rather than agreeing to worship a pagan deity. In a remarkable statement, the Gemara, *Ketubot* 33b, declares that, had those personages been subjected to torture rather than immediate death, they would have succumbed. The classical talmudic commentators understand that statement as expressing a normative rule rather than as a reflection of human weakness. Accordingly, they question, if martyrdom is required in face of idolatry, why is acceptance of torture not required as well? *Tosafot*, for example, resolve the problem by postulating that the act in question was not really an act of idolatry at all and hence Hananiah, Mishael and Azariah chose to accept martyrdom, not as a normative obligation, but as an act of piety.[65]

Shitah Mekubeẓet, Ketubot 33b, cites an anonymous scholar (*u-be-kuntreisin piresh*) who responds to this question by noting that the obligation to sacrifice one's life rather than engage in an act of idolatry is based upon the verse "And you shall love the Lord, your God, with all your heart, and with all your soul, and with all your might" (Deuteronomy 6:5). "With all your soul" is understood as meaning with one's very life. The obligation, then, is to sacrifice even one's life rather than to commit the sin of idolatry—but there is no obligation, argues this anonymous authority, to sacrifice more than one's life. Sustained torture, concludes this authority, represents a sacrifice greater than martyrdom and hence is not required even in order to avoid idolatry. Since, according to this authority, the burden of torture need not be accepted in situations requiring martyrdom, *a fortiori*, it need not be accepted in situations in which the burden imposed for fulfillment of an obligation is limited to expenditure of financial resources.

It may well be assumed that the commentators who resolve the underlying problem in an alternative manner disagree with the halakhic implication inherent in the approach of this anonymous scholar. For them, the obligation to accept martyrdom includes the obligation to accept protracted torture as well. Nevertheless, it is entirely reasonable to assume that their disagreement is limited to situations in which martyrdom is demanded, but that they might well concede that in situations requiring a more modest burden, i.e., expenditure of one's entire fortune, there is no obligation to accept either torture or intractable pain.[66]

As noted earlier, both *Iggerot Mosheh* and Rabbi Auerbach agree that nutrition and hydration[67] as well as oxygen[68] must be provided for all patients. They apparently assume that hastening death by starvation, dehydration or suffocation increases the intensity of the pain and suffering experienced by the moribund patient. However, medical evidence suggests that patients who have permanently lost consciousness do not experience pain or discomfort following the withdrawal of artificial nutrition and hydration.[69] Less information is available concerning the experience of greatly debilitated patients or those suffering from severe illness who are in the end-stage of the dying process. Available information, however, indicates that these patients appear to experience little, if any, discomfort when routine comfort measures are provided.[70] Moreover, in some cases, the provision of artificial nutrition and hydration very close to the time of death may actually increase the patient's discomfort. Some patients are more likely to experience pulmonary edema, nausea and mental confusion when artificial nutrition and hydration are maintained in the last stages of the dying process.[71]

Although the theory espoused by *Iggerot Mosheh* and Rabbi Auerbach is well founded, it seems to this writer that there is little room for its implementation. If the foregoing analysis is correct, those halakhic rulings proceed from the presumption that at least some patients must endure "great pain" or "suffering." While many patients undoubtedly do suffer unspeakable pain, that need not be the case. Recent medical literature is replete with articles and comments deploring the fact that physicians are inadequately trained in palliation of pain or are unwilling to utilize available means to control pain. In rejecting the patient's suffering of unrelieved pain as a valid motive for the practice of euthanasia, Dr. Porter Storey reports on his own treatment of some 2,000 terminally ill patients and asserts that pain "can be effectively palliated by administering narcotic analgesics which can be used safely if the dose is carefully titrated against the symptoms."[72] Moreover, studies conducted over the past decade demonstrate that substantial and sustained doses of narcotics may be administered without risk to the patient.[73] An as yet unpublished report of the Bioethics Committee of the Montefiore Medical Center concludes that "The widespread belief that adequate pain control usually poses high risks of respiratory distress and a consequent hastening of death appears to be based more on longstanding myth than on medical fact." A manual published by the Washington Medical Association reports that "adequate interventions exist to control pain in 90–99% of patients."[74] The American Medical Association has stated that: "The pain of most terminally ill patients can be controlled throughout the dying process without heavy sedation or anesthesia. . . . For a very few patients, however, sedation to a sleep-like state may be necessary in the last days or weeks of life to prevent the patient from experiencing severe pain."[75] From the vantage point of Halakhah, life-prolonging therapy may be withheld only to avoid excruciating pain. However, when pain can be controlled, the obligation to preserve and prolong life remains in full force.

IV. A CONCLUDING COMMENT

A brief comment of the late Rabbi Yosef Eliyahu Henkin, of blessed memory, eloquently captures the Jewish attitude with regard to the emotionally charged issue of treatment of the terminally ill. Many years ago, when I first began to investigate issues of medical Halakhah and when many now commonplace life-prolonging measures were yet novel, I offhandedly asked Rabbi Henkin, "How far is one obligated to go in order to prolong life?" Without the slightest hesitation he responded, "*Azoi lang vi a Yid ken leben, darf er velen leben*" (So long as it is possible for a Jew to live, he ought to want to live). Those words uttered by a blind, frail, saintly individual to whom life had clearly become a burden—but a sacred burden—made a profound impression upon me. That short, succinct statement reflects authentic Jewish values in a way that sometimes becomes submerged in learned responsa. Truly, sometimes one cannot see the forest because of the trees.

NOTES

1. Arthur Hugh Clough, "The Latest Decalogue," *The Oxford Book of Nineteenth-Century English Verse*, ed. by John Hayward (Oxford, 1970), p. 609. These words, when quoted, are almost invariably cited in a literal sense. In actuality, the poet was not endorsing the moral position expressed in this couplet but was engaging in irony. See Maurice Strauss, *Familiar Medical Quotations* (Boston, 1968), p. 159b, note 1.
2. This statement, of course, applies to life as defined by Halakhah. The status of a *nefel*, i.e., a nonviable neonate, requires independent analysis.
3. See *Shulḥan Arukh, Oraḥ Ḥayyim* 329:4.
4. See also *Tosefet Yom Tov, Sotah* 1:9.
5. See, for example, *Schloendorff* v. *Society of N.Y. Hosp.*, 211 N.Y. 125, 129–30, 105 N.E. 92 (1914) (Cardozo J.). ["E]very individual of sound mind and adult years has a right to determine

what should be done with his own body."); *In re Karen Quinlan*, 70 N.J. 10, 355 A.2d 647, *cert. denied sub nom. Garger* v. *New Jersey*, 428 U.S. 922 (1976); *Superintendent of Belchertown State School* v. *Saikewicz*, 373 Mass. 728, 370 N.E.2d 417, 424 (1977); *Satz* v. *Perlmutter*, 379 So.2d 359, 360 (Fla. 1980); *Eichner* v. *Dillon*, 52 N.Y.2d 363, 438 N.Y.S.2d 266, 420 N.E.2d 63, *cert. denied*, 453 U.S. 858 (1981); *Matter of Welfare of Colyer*, 99 Wash. 2d 114, 660 P.2d 738, 741 (1983); *Matter of Conservatorship of Torres*, 357 N.W.2d 332, 339 (Minn. 1984); *In re L.H.R.* 253 Ga. 439, 321 S.E.2d 716, 722 (1984); *Bartling* v. *Superior Court*, 163 Cal. App. 3d 186, 209 Cal. Rptr. 220, 225 (Ct. App. 1984); *Brophy* v. *New England Sinai Hospital, Inc.*, 398 Mass. 417, 497 N.E.2d 626 (1986); *Matter of Conroy*, 98 N.J. 321, 486 A.2d 1209 (1985); *Bouvia* v. *Superior Court of the State of California for the County of Los Angeles*, 179 Cal. App.3d 1127, 225 Cal.Rptr. 297 (Ct. App. 1986); *Rivers* v. *Katz*, 67 N.Y.2d 485, 493, 504 N.Y.S.2d 74, 78, 495 N.E.2d 337 (1986); *Matter of Delio*, N.Y.L.J., June 4, 1987, p. 1, col. 6, p. 35, col. 1 (App. Div., 2nd Dept.); *Randolph* v. *City of New York*, 117 A.D.2d 44, 501 N.Y.2d 827 (1st Dept. 1986); *Hanes* v. *Ambrose*, 80 A.D.2d 963, 437 N.Y.2d 784 (3d Dept. 1981); *Matter of Melideo*, 88 Misc.2d 974 (Sup. Ct. Suffolk Co. 1976); *Matter of Roosevelt Hospital*, N.Y.L.J. Jan. 13, 1977, p. 7 (Sup. Ct., New York Co.); *Matter of Gray*, N.Y.L.J. Apr. 17, 1975, p. 15 (Sup. Ct., New York Co.); *Erickson* v. *Dilgard*, 44 Misc. 2d 27, 252 N.Y.S.2d 705 (Sup. Ct., Nassau Co. 1962); *Cruzan* v. *Director, Missouri Department of Health*, 497 U.S. 261, 110 S. Ct. 2841 (1990); *In re Farrell*, 108 N.J. 335, 529 A.2d 404 (1987); *Workingmen's Circle Home and Infirmary for the Aged* v. *Fink*, 514 N.Y.S. 2d 893 (Sup. Ct., Bronx Co. 1987); *Matter of Chetta*, No. 1086 (Sup. Ct., Nassau Co., May 1, 1987); *Matter of Vogel*, 512 N.Y.S.2d 622 (Sup. Ct., Nassau Co., 1986); *Hazelton* v. *Powhatan Nursing Home*, Chancery No. 98287 (Va. Cir. Ct., Fairfax Co. Sept. 5, 1986); *Rasmussen* v. *Fleming*, 2 CA-CIV 5622, (Ariz. Ct. App., Div. 2, June 25, 1986); *Corbett* v. *D'Alessandro*, 487 S.2d 368 (2d Dist. Fla. 1986).

6. See, for example, *Matter of Application of Winthrop University Hospital*, 128 Misc. 2d 804, 490 N.Y.S.2d 996 (Sup. Ct., Nassau Co. 1985); *John F. Kennedy Memorial Hospital* v. *Heston*, 209 A.2d 670 (N.J. 1971), *overruled in part. In re Conroy*, 486 A.2d 1209 (N.J. 1985); *Norwood Hospital* v. *Munoz*, Mass. Probate Court (Norfolk Div., 5/11/89). Cf., however, *Public Health*

Trust of Dade County v. *Wons*, 541 So.2d 96 (Fla. 1989); *Fosmire* v. *Nicoleau*, 545 N.Y.S. 2d 103 (N.Y. 1990).

7. See, for example, *Matter of Application of Jamaica Hospital*, 128 Misc. 2d 1006, 491 N.Y.S.2d 898 (Sup. Ct., Queens Co. 1985); *Crouse Irving Memorial Hospital* v. *Paddock*, 127 Misc. 2d 101, 485 N.Y.S.2d 443 (Sup. Ct., Onondaga Co. 1985).
8. See also R. Shlomoh Yosef Zevin, *Le-Or ha-Halakhah*, 2nd edition (Tel Aviv, 5717), pp. 318–335; cf., R. Sha'ul Israeli, *Ha-Torah ve-ha-Medinah*, V-VI (5713–5714), 106–111 and VII-VIII (5715–5717), 331–336. See also R. Simchah ha-Kohen Kook, *Torah she-be-'al Peh*, XVIII (5736), 82–58.
9. See R. Shlomoh Zalman Auerbach, *Teshuvot Minḥat Shlomoh*, no. 91, sec. 24; R. Moshe Stern, *Teshuvot Be'er Mosheh*, VIII, no. 239, sec. 4; and R. Aaron Soloveichik, *supra*, p. 71. Cf., however, R. Moshe Feinstein, *Iggerot Mosheh, Ḥoshen Mishpat*, II, no. 74, sec. 1. The Gemara, *Ta'anit* 23a, reports that, upon awakening from his sleep of seventy years, Ḥoni the Circle-Drawer entered the House of Study. Since he was not recognized, he was not accorded proper honor. Becoming distressed, Ḥoni prayed for death and the prayer was granted. Ḥoni was certainly not a *goses* and it is difficult to assume that his psychological pain was so great that, as discussed below, he was relieved of any obligation to preserve his own life. Nevertheless, prayer for death under those circumstances was entirely acceptable.
10. See *Magen Avraham, Oraḥ Ḥayyim* 230:6; *Ḥayyei Adam* 65:1; and *Mishnah Berurah* 230:6.
11. See R. Eliezer Waldenberg, *Ramat Raḥel*, no. 5, and *idem*, *Ẓiẓ Eli'ezer*, IX, no. 47.
12. It is clear that, when halakhically indicated, a patient is not only obligated to seek medical care but may be compelled to do so. See sources cited in *Jewish Bioethics*, p. 43, note 100; cf., *ibid.*, p. 42, note 97. Since the obligation of rescue is phrased as a prohibition against standing idly by "the blood of your fellow" the source of an obligation to save one's own life is somewhat elusive. It is, of course, an uncontested halakhic principle that "A person is his own relative" (*adam karov eẓel aẓmo*). See *Sanhedrin* 9b and 25a; *Ketubot* 18b; and *Yevamot* 25b. By the same token, it may be argued that a person is his own "fellow" and hence owes himself the selfsame duties. See R. Zalman Nechemiah Goldberg, *Moriah*, vol. 8, no. 3–4 (Elul 5738), p. 51, quoted in *Halakhah u-Refu'ah*, ed. R. Moshe Herschler, II (Jerusalem, 5741), pp. 153–54; cf., however, R. Mordecai Jonah

Rabinowitz, *Afikei Yam*, II, no. 40, s.v. *ve-hayah*. Note should also be taken of the fact that the Gemara, *Bava Meẓi'a* 62a, cites the verse "and your brother shall live with you" (Leviticus 25:38) in establishing that preservation of one's own life must be given preference over the rescue of another. An obligation to preserve one's own life may readily be inferred from that definition. Also, Rambam, *Hilkhot Roẓeaḥ* 11:4, cites the verse "take heed of yourself and safeguard yourself" (Deuteronomy 4:9) as establishing an obligation "to be watchful" with regard to any matter that poses a danger as well as the negative commandment "And you shall not bring blood upon your house" (Deuteronomy 22:8) as establishing an obligation to remove a source of danger. See also *Hilkhot Roẓeaḥ* 11:5. The latter verses serve to establish a positive command whereas "nor shall you stand idly by the blood of your fellow" establishes a more stringent negative prohibition for failure to seek life-saving interventions.

Afikei Yam, II, no. 40, s.v. *ve-hayah*, suggests that failure to preserve one's own life may be halakhically equivalent to suicide. Pesikta Rabbati, chap. 24, advances an exegetical rendition of *lo tirẓaḥ* (Exodus 20:13) as *lo titraẓaḥ* in establishing that *felo-de-se* is encompassed in the prohibition against murder. See also *Halakhot Ketanot*, II, no. 231; *Bet Me'ir, Yoreh De'ah* 215:5; *Teshuvot Ḥatam Sofer*, *Yoreh De'ah*, no. 326; Mahari Perla, *Sefer ha-Miẓvot le-Rabbenu Sa'adia Ga'on, miẓvot lo ta'aseh*, no. 59; *Gesher ha-Ḥayyim*, I, chap. 25; and *Torah Shelemah, Parashat Yitro*, chap. 20, sec. 336. Rambam, *Hilkhot Roẓeaḥ* 2:3, declares suicide to be prohibited on the basis of the verse "But your blood of your lives will I require" (Genesis 9:5). The ramifications of citation of that verse are noted by *Minḥat Ḥinnukh*, no. 34. Cf. Mahari Perla's comments on *Minḥat Ḥinnukh, ad locum*. Cf., also, R. Shimon Moshe Diskin, *Mas'et ha-Melekh* (Jerusalem, 5742), *Hilkhot Roẓeaḥ* 2:3, reprinted in *idem*, *Mas'et ha-Melekh* (Jerusalem, 5749), IV, no. 433.

In point of fact, *Afikei Yam*'s position that the obligation to seek a cure for a life-threatening illness and to take other necessary measures to prolong one's own life is based upon the prohibition against suicide may be inferred from comments of Ran, *Shevu'ot* 28a. Rambam, *Hilkhot Shevu'ot* 5:20, rules that one who swears not to eat for seven days has sworn a vain oath and, accordingly, is to be punished immediately for that infraction but may eat whenever he wishes. Ran agrees with Rambam's ruling but not with his reasoning. Rambam regards the oath as vain because it cannot be fulfilled, just as an oath not to sleep for a period of three days is not capable of fulfillment. Ran disagrees and argues that, although a person cannot keep himself awake, he can refrain from eating even though he endangers himself in the process. Nevertheless, Ran regards the oath as vain because "one who has sworn to kill himself has actually sworn to transgress the words of the Torah for Scripture states explicitly 'But your blood of your lives will I require' . . . or also 'take heed of yourself and safeguard yourself.'" Ran explicitly declares that the prohibition against suicide and the obligation to avoid danger mandate active intervention to seek food in order to sustain life. The selfsame obligations require the individual to seek medical treatment as well.

13. *Yated Ne'eman*, 29 Kislev 5755, p. 56. See also *Yated ha-Shavu'a*, 19 Tevet 5755, p. 9.
14. *Shulḥan Arukh, Yoreh De'ah* 339:1.
15. *Loc. cit.*
16. *Shabbat* 151b and *Semaḥot* 1:4.
17. See J. David Bleich, "The Obligation to Heal in the Judaic Tradition: A Comparative Analysis," *Jewish Bioethics*, ed. Fred Rosner and J. David Bleich (New York, 1979), pp. 29–33; and *idem, Judaism and Healing* (New York, 1981), pp. 119–121.
18. See *Jewish Bioethics*, p. 28; *Judaism and Healing*, pp. 116–118; and the more extensive discussion in *Contemporary Halakhic Problems*, IV (New York, 1995), 203–217.
19. See sources cited in *Jewish Bioethics*, p. 43, note 100.
20. See *Ẓiẓ Eli'ezer*, XIII, no. 87. See, also R. Nathan Zevi Friedman, *Ha-Torah ve-ha-Medinah*, V–VI, 229; and R. Iser Y. Unterman, *Torah she-be-'al Peh*, XI (5729), 14.
21. Cf., however, R. Isaac Liebes, *Teshuvot Bet Avi*, II, no. 153, p. 213. Rabbi Liebes cites Rambam's comment in his *Commentary on the Mishnah, Nedarim* 4:4 (see also *idem, Mishneh Torah, Hilkhot Nedarim* 6:8) indicating that the scriptural exhortation with regard to returning lost property also serves to establish an obligation requiring the physician to render professional services in life-threatening situations. See *Sanhedrin* 73a. Rabbi Liebes comments that "on the basis of this derivation, the physician is obligated to restore [the patient's] body, i.e., in a situation in which there is hope to restore the body entirely, but in a situation in which by means of this [treatment] he will not longer restore [the patient's] body but, on the contrary, will

cause him additional pain and suffering, with regard to this he is not at all obligated." Rabbi Liebes' argument is not compelling for two reasons: (1) The Gemara, *Sanhedrin* 73a, applies this obligation to situations involving a person drowning in a river, being mauled by a wild animal and under attack by armed robbers. The "loss" to be restored is life *per se*, not health or well-being. The obligation to restore property is in no way related to the duration of the useful life of the lost item. Hence restoration of the body should be required regardless of the fact that longevity anticipation is limited to even a brief period of time. (2). Although, as indicated by the Gemara, *Bava Kamma* 85a, specific scriptural authorization is required to treat the sick, once such sanction has been granted the obligation with regard to therapeutic intervention is no different from other forms of preservation of life. Failure to intervene constitutes a violation of the commandment "nor shall you stand idly by the blood of your fellow" (Leviticus 19:16). Thus *Shulḥan Arukh, Yoreh De'ah* 336:1, states: "The Torah gave permission to the physician to heal. This is a religious precept and is included in the category of saving life, and if the physician withholds [his services] it is considered as shedding blood." Non-therapeutic rescue as described in *Sanhedrin* 73a, e.g., rescue from drowning or from a wild animal, is mandatory regardless of age, state of health or length of the natural longevity anticipation of the victim. Accordingly, equating medical intervention with other forms of rescue serves to establish an obligation to prolong life even if a complete cure is not possible. See *Perishah, Yoreh De'ah* 336:4; *Ramat Raḥel*, no. 21; and *Ẓiẓ Eli'ezer*, II, no. 25, chap. 7. Cf. *Iggerot Mosheh, Ḥoshen Mishpat*, II, no. 74, sec. 1, s.v. *ve-pashut*. Moreover, the rescuer's monetary obligation is derived from Leviticus 19:6 which establishes an obligation for payment of medical expenses in cases of battery and clearly applies even when a complete cure is impossible.

22. *Ẓiẓ Eli'ezer*, IX, no. 47, sec. 5.
23. There is considerable confusion in some circles regarding the distinction between a *goses* and *treifah*. A *treifah* is a person or animal who, either as the result of congenital anomaly or trauma, suffers the loss or perforation of one or more specified organs and, as a result, is presumed to be incapable of surviving for a period of twelve months. The primary import of classification of a human being as a *treifah* is with regard to punishment for homicide: murder of a *treifah*, although encompassed within

commandment "Thou shalt not kill," is not punishable as a capital offense. For virtually all other determinations of Jewish law the status of a *treifah* is no different from that of normal persons. A *goses*, as defined be Rema, is a moribund person whose demise is imminent. A person suffering from a degenerative, physiological malady may or may not be a *goses* depending upon his clinical state, but in the absence of congenital anomaly or trauma affecting specific organs, such a person is not a *treifah*. Moreover, it must be emphasized that, insofar as the obligation of rescue and the obligation to prolong life is concerned, a *treifah* is treated no differently from any other person. See *Iggerot Mosheh, Ḥoshen Mishpat*, II, no. 73, sec. 4.

24. See, for example, R. Yechiel Michal Epstein, *Arukh ha-Shulḥan, Yoreh De'ah* 339:4, and *Iggerot Mosheh, Ḥoshen Mishpat*, II, no. 74, sec. 1; see also *infra*, note 37 and accompanying text.
25. Cf., R. Ya'akov Yisra'el Kanievski, *Kraina de-Iggarta* (Bnei Brak, 5746), no. 190: "With regard to the basic principle that everything that can prolong the life of a sick person [even for a brief period (*ḥayyei sha'ah*)] must be done, in truth I, too, heard such a dictum in my childhood but I do not know if it [stems from] a reliable person." That statement has been cited by some as reflecting the notion that active intervention on behalf of the terminally ill is not required. However, Rabbi Kanievski's immediately following citation of *Yoreh De'ah* 339:1 and his ensuing discussion make it abundantly clear that treatment may be withheld only because as a result "additional suffering" will be imposed upon the patient or because the patient is a *goses*. In fact, he expresses doubt with regard to the correct interpretation of Rema's position, i.e., whether the active/passive distinction drawn by Rema is predicated upon absence of an obligation to accept inordinate suffering as discussed below or whether it is a distinction relevant solely to the treatment of a *goses*. The clear implication is that he agrees that in all other circumstances it is indeed the case that "everything that can prolong the life of a sick person, even for a brief time, must be done." See also Abraham S. Abraham, *Nishmat Avraham, Yoreh De'ah* 339:1, sec. 2, who declares that all possible therapies must be provided, including cardio-pulmonary resuscitation, "even if there exists only a slight chance that the patient will remain alove and even for *ḥayyei sha'ah* (a brief longevity anticipation)."
26. See also *Tosefet Yom Tov, Arakhin* 1:3. Rambam, in his com-

mentary on *Arakhin* 1:3, describes a *goses* as a moribund person from whose throat a "death rattle" emanates.

27. This is explicitly stated by *Teshuvot Bet Ya'akov*, no. 59, who maintains that it is otherwise forbidden to prolong the life of a *goses*.
28. See *infra*, note 38.
29. See also *Perishah, Tur Yoreh De'ah* 339:5, who writes, "It appears from this that it is the nature of *gesisah* to be three days." Since it is simply not possible to understand this authority as asserting that *gesisah* must always extend for a period of three days, his comment must be understood as stating that the period of *gesisah* extends no longer than three days. See also *Iggerot Mosheh, Ḥoshen Mishpat*, II, no. 75, sec. 5, who states explicitly, ". . . it is also impossible that [a *goses*] live more than three days as is explicit in *Shulḥan Arukh, Yoreh De'ah* 339:2 . . ." See also *Teshuvot Bet Avi*, II, no. 153, s. v. *kol zeh*; *Teshuvot Be'er Mosheh*, VIII, no. 241, sec. 1 and no. 242; and G.B. Halibard, "Euthanasia," *Jewish Law Annual*, I (1978), 198, note 2.
30. See *Bet Shmu'el, Even ha-Ezer* 17:18 and 17:94. Cf., however, R. Ezekiel Landau, *Dagul me-Revavah* on *Bet Shmu'el, Even ha-Ezer* 17:94; *Pitḥei Teshuvah, Even ha-Ezer* 17:13 and *Yoreh De'ah* 339:3; and *Gilyon Maharsha, Yoreh De'ah* 339:2.
31. *Iggerot Mosheh* clearly indicates that the vast majority of those who manifest the criteria of *gesisah*, as determined of those proficient in such matters, cannot survive for more than three days despite medical treatment. This is evident from his statement in the previously cited responsum, *Ḥoshen Mishpat*, II, no. 75, sec. 5, ". . . and it does not come into consideration (*ve-lo shayyakh*) that they might give [the *goses*]) medical treatments" as well as from the further statement ". . . therefore if we see that it seems to the people caring for him that he is a *goses* more than three days and he is alive, we should rather assume that they are not proficient and that they erred in categorizing him as a *goses* even prior to three days; and if those greatly proficient stated that he was a *goses* more than three days earlier, of necessity this person is of the minority. . . ." Thus, consistent with his view that *gesisah* does not occur until additional criteria not mentioned by Rema become manifest, *Iggerot Mosheh* apparently maintains that, even in our day, medical science cannot reverse the state of *gesisah*.
32. Cf., *Hagahot Maimuniyot, Hilkhot Avel* 4:1, and Maharam Rothenberg, *Teshuvot Pesakim u-Minhagim*, ed. R. Yitzchak Zev Kahana (Mosad ha-Rav Kook: Jerusalem, 5723), III, 10.

33. Cf., Maharam Rothenberg, *Teshuvot Pesakim u-Minhagim*, vol. III, no. 1.
34. It has been argued that, in stating that a *goses* cannot survive for more than a period of three days, Maharam of Rothenberg is stating a fact rather than advancing a qualification to the definition of *gesisah*. See R. Gedaliah Rabinowitz, *Halakhah u-Refu'ah*, III (Jerusalem, 5743), 113–114. See also Abraham Steinberg, *Encyclopedia Halakhtit Refu'it*, IV, 371, note 149. It may be presumed that this is the position of some contemporary authorities, who sanction withholding of treatment from a *goses* but who do not explicitly indicate that such treatment is mandatory if life can be prolonged thereby for a minimum period of three days. See, for example, *Mishneh Halakhot*, VII, no. 287. See also *Contemporary Halakhic Problems*, IV, 348, note 56.It might then be argued that, since advances in medical science now make prolongation of the life of a *goses* a distinct possibility, the rule formulated by Maharam of Rothenberg as recorded in *Shulḥan Arukh* regarding commencement of mourning for a person observed to be a *goses* and *Magen Avraham*'s ruling regarding the wife's eligibility to contract a new marriage are no longer valid. Nevertheless, it is quite clear that, even according to those authorities, inability to bring up secretions from the chest as evidenced by their collection in the area of the throat, even when coupled with loss of control over other bodily functions, is not sufficient to render the patient a *goses*. Assuredly, *gesisah* cannot be indefinite in duration. Thus, *Iggerot Mosheh, Ḥoshen Mishpat*, III, no. 73, sec. 3, speaks of *gesisah* as a state readily recognized by experienced members of a *ḥevra kaddisha*. Although *Iggerot Mosheh* felt himself unable to spell out the precise clinical criteria of *gesisah*, it is clear that he regards only moribund patients actually experiencing "death throes" to be in a state of *gesisah*. It is clear that if that state can be reversed there is an obligation to do so. Modern medicine, although at times capable of effecting such reversal, does not presume that a *goses* continues to experience death throes for a significant period of time. Thus it seems that even if Maharam of Rothenberg's comments are regarded as empirical rather than definitional, in practice, a patient who is capable of surviving for any significant period of time is not a *goses*. According to *Iggerot Mosheh* who demands manifestation of clinical criteria beyond those spelled out by Rema, criteria that in his opinion are best recognized by members of a *ḥevra kaddisha*, it must be con-

cluded that even a patient who "brings up secretions in his throat" because of constriction of the chest and who is incapable of surviving for a period of seventy-two hours but who does not manifest the unspecified clinical symptoms to which *Iggerot Mosheh* refers, is not a *goses*. Hence, in the absence of intractable physical pain, such a patient must be provided with any treatment capable of prolonging life provided that such treatment does not threaten to foreshorten the brief period that the patient may be expected to live.

35. Some contemporary writers purport to find talmudic precedent for this position in the talmudic narrative concerning R. Ḥanina ben Tradion and his executioner recorded in *Avodah Zarah* 18a. R. Ḥanina ben Tradion was being burned at the stake and tufts of wool were soaked in water and placed over his heart so that he would not die quickly. His disciples advised him to open his mouth so that the fire might enter and he be spared further agony. R. Ḥanina explained that such an act is forbidden. The executioner then offered to remove the tufts of wool if R. Ḥanina would guarantee him entrance into the world-to-come. R. Ḥanina agreed and the tufts were removed. This, it has then argued, serves to demonstrate that withdrawal of impediments to death is permissible. The argument, however, is based upon a misreading of the text. As recorded by the Gemara, the words of the executioner were: "Rabbi, *if I increase the flame* (emphasis added) and take away the tufts of wool from over your heart, will you bring me to life in the world-to-come?" The executioner did not simply remove the wool tufts that impeded death; he also "increased the flame" by means of an overt act, i.e., he engaged in active euthanasia, an act that is categorically prohibited. Cf., *Yam shel Shlomoh, Bava Kamma* 8:59 and *Teshuvot Be'er Mosheh*, VIII, no. 239, sec. 4. Various hypotheses have been advanced in justification of the conduct of R. Ḥanina ben Tradion; see R. Moshe Feinstein, *Ha-Pardes*, Shevat 5736, p. 12; *idem, Iggerot Mosheh, Yoreh De'ah*, II, no. 174, *anaf* 3, and *Ḥoshen Mishpat*, II, no. 74, sec. 2; R. Eliezer Waldenberg, *Ẓiẓ Eli'ezer*, IV, no. 13, chap. 2, sec. 7; R. Sha'ul Israeli, *Amud ha-Yemini*, no. 32, sec. 2; *Teshuvot Bet Avi*, II, no. 153; *Mishneh Halakhot*, VII, no. 282; R. Moshe Dov Welner, *Ha-Torah ve-ha-Medinah*, VII–VIII, 318; *idem, Torah she-be-'al Peh*, XVIII, 42; R. Simchah ha-Kohen Kook, *Torah she-be-'al Peh*, XVIII, 86–87; and R. Shneur Zalman Reiss, *Ha-Ma'or*, Iyar–Sivan 5734, p. 19. See also *infra*, note 64.

36. The statement of R. Zalman Nehemiah Goldberg, *Moriah*, vol. 8, no. 4–5 (Elul 5738), p. 52, reprinted in *Halakhah u-Refu'ah*, II, 154, to the effect that there is no obligation of rescue with regard to a *goses* "who prefers death to life because of suffering or [because] he has no benefit from life since he has no mental function" is not supported by earlier sources and is not substantiated by halakhic categories governing the obligation of rescue. Unlike *Teshuvot Bet Ya'akov*, no. 89, Rabbi Goldberg permits violation of *Shabbat* prohibitions in order to prolong the life of a *goses*, but only if the patient derives "enjoyment" from, and prefers, such prolongation of his life.
37. See also *Bet Leḥem Yehudah, Yoreh De'ah* 339:1; R. Simchah ha-Kohen Kook, *Torah she-be-'al Peh*, XVIII, 86–87; and *Mishneh Halakhot*, VII, no. 287.
38. *Teshuvot Bet Ya'akov* carefully distinguishes between a *goses* and a person buried beneath the debris of a fallen wall or the like. *Shulḥan Arukh, Oraḥ Ḥayyim* 329:3, rules that Sabbath restrictions are suspended on behalf of such an individual despite the fact that he cannot survive for more than a very brief period of time. The accident victim can be distinguished from a *goses* only by virtue of the fact that he does not as yet manifest the clinical criteria of *gesisah*.
39. See *Or ha-Ḥayyim*, Exodus 31:16, who remarks that the Sabbath may be violated on behalf of a such person only if it is anticipated that he will survive long enough to observe at least one Sabbath. That view is rebutted by *Minḥat Ḥinnukh, Kuntres Mosekh ha-Shabbat*, sec. 39, s.v., *ve-her'ah li lamdan eḥad*.
40. See also *Maḥazit ha-Shekel, Oraḥ Ḥayyim* 329:4; *Teshuvot Ḥatam Sofer, Yoreh De'ah*, no. 338; and *Birkei Yosef, Oraḥ Ḥayyim* 329:4.
41. Indeed the reason advanced by the Gemara for administering a life-prolonging remedy, *viz.*, "perhaps he will live briefly, long enough to set his house in order," far from supporting *Shevut Ya'akov*'s position, would appear to contradict his view since the obligation of *pikuaḥ nefesh*, if it extends even to the terminally ill, is sufficient to require remedies that merely prolong life even in the absence of any possibility of "setting one's house in order." Cf., R. Zevi ha-Kohen Zarkowski, *Bet Shmu'el* (New York, 5740), *ad locum*. Of course, vinegar may have been regarded as a folk remedy of no demonstrated value and hence not a mandatory form of treatment. See also the resolution offered *infra*, note 64. Those analyses do not, however, serve to

explain how the text serves as a proof for *Shevut Ya'akov*'s position.

42. For a critique of Rambam's position, see *Ḥazon Ish, Even ha-Ezer, Hilkhot Ishut* 26:3. For a survey of authorities who adopt positions at variance with that of Rambam, see *Encyclopedia Talmudit*, XXI, 3–7; aee also *Nishmat Avraham, Yoreh De'ah* 29:1.
43. *Ẓiẓ Eli'ezer*, XIII, no. 89, sec. 14, draws a tenuous distinction between the state of *gesisah* and the actual process of dying, i.e., the departure of the soul from the body. The latter state he terms *gemar kelot ha-nefesh*; in *Assia*, Nisan 5738, p. 18, he employes the phrase *sha'at yeẓi'at neshamah* in making the identical distinction.
44. "Experimental Procedures: The Concept of Refu'ah Bedukah," *Contemporary Halakhic Problems*, IV, 203–217.
45. In the course of an oral discussion with this writer, the late R. Jacob Kaminetsky presented this interpretation of Rema as self-evident. This analysis of Rema's positions is also inherent in the position of R. Nathan Zevi Friedman, *Ha-Torah ve-ha-Medinah*, V–VI, 229–32, who rejects the active/passive distinction and insists that medical treatment and medication must be continued even though suffering is prolonged thereby. See Rabbi Friedman's italicized comments, *ibid.*, pp. 229, 230 and 231. Cf., R. Chaim David Halevy, *Teḥumin*, II (5741), 303–305, who recognizes that Rema's examples are in the nature of *segulot* but fails to take cognizance of that aspect of Rema's comments as a possible limiting factor in applying Rema's ruling.
46. For an alternative explanation see *infra*, note 65.
47. It should be noted that *Shulḥan Arukh, Oraḥ Ḥayyim* 339:4, rules that Sabbath restrictions must be set aside on behalf of an accident victim, "even if he is found crushed in a manner such that he cannot live other than for a brief period." It is difficult to understand why the accident victim's pain is less severe than that of a moribund patient. *Teshuvot Bet Ya'akov*'s distinction, *supra*, note 38, is not based upon considerations of pain. Cf., *infra*, note 54.
48. See also R. Chaim David Halevy, *Teḥumin*, II, 305.
49. That there is pain at the moment of death may be inferred from the statement of the Gemara, *Yoma* 20b, declaring that the sound of the soul as it departs from the body is heard from "one end of the universe to the other." See also *Bereishit Rabbah* 6:12. For a discussion of the cause of the anguish see R. Isaac Arama, *Akeidat Yiẓḥak, Parashat ve-Zot ha-Berakhah, sha'ar* 105. See also

Sefer Ḥasidim, cited by *Bet Leḥem Yehudah, Yoreh De'ah* 339:1.

50. R. Shmu'el ha-Levi Woszner, *Shevet ha-Levi*, VI, no. 179, accepting the position of *Shevut Ya'akov*, declares that it is permissible, but not mandatory, to prolong the life of a *goses* and further states that since it is permissible to do so [such treatment] enters into the category of *pikuaḥ nefesh* that takes precedence over *Shabbat*. He further states that even if it is held that treatment of a *goses* is obligatory that is so only if the treatment does not cause greatly enhanced and prolonged suffering. Although *Shevet ha-Levi* asserts that in circumstances of inordinate suffering treatment of a *goses* is not required he does not adopt the position of *Iggerot Mosheh* who asserts that such suffering is always attendant upon a state of *gesisah*.
51. Cf., however, *supra*, p. 68, and *supra*, note 9, as well as the statement of R. Aaron Soloveichik, *supra*, p. 71.
52. See *supra*, p. 65.
53. Cf., *Teshuvot Bet Avi*, II, no. 153, s.v. *u-le-dina* and *sikkum*.
54. There is perhaps some ambiguity with regard to the implication of this statement. The phrase "it is permissible to withhold medications that cause suffering" standing alone, might be understood as limited to suffering caused by the medication, i.e., as a side-effect, rather than by the underlying condition. However, the earlier reference to a patient who "experiences great pain and suffering" seems to indicate that the suffering to which reference is made is not the product of the medication but of the underlying pathology. Moreover, there does not appear to be any halakhic consideration that would support such a distinction between pain that is the result of a malady and pain induced by medication. Indeed, no distinction of that nature appears in the statement of 29 Kislev 5755 to which Rabbi Auerbach was a signator.
55. Cf., *Magen Avraham, Oraḥ Ḥayyim* 656:7, who cites the variant opinion of Rabbenu Yeruḥam who maintains that a person should not expend more than one fifth of his fortune for this purpose but that obligatory expenditure is limited to ten percent; cf. however, *Bi'ur Halakhah, Oraḥ Ḥayyim* 657:1.
56. Cf., however, *Bi'ur ha-Gra, Yoreh De'ah* 257:5.
57. See also *Teshuvot Zera Emet*, II, no. 51; R. Mordecai Schwadron, *Teshuvot Maharsham*, V, no. 54; R. Elijah Feinstein, *Halikhot Eliyahu*, no. 33; *Darkei Teshuvah, Yoreh De'ah* 157:57; R. Israel Meir ha-Kohen, *Ahavat Ḥesed*, chap. 20, sec. 2. Cf., R. Yitzchak Zilberstein, *Assia*, vol. 14, no. 3 (Tevet 5755), pp. 46–50.

58. Cf., however, R. Abraham I. Kook, *Mishpat Kohen*, no. 144, sec. 17, s.v. *amnam be-ikar ha-inyan*, who asserts that all authorities agree that rescue of a person whose life is in danger requires the sacrifice of one's entire fortune. Expenditure of twenty percent of one's fortune, he argues, is mandated by the commandment "and your brother shall live with you" (Leviticus 25:36). Accordingly, he concludes that the additional negative commandment "nor shall you stand idly by the blood of your fellow" must be understood as necessitated in order to mandate expenditure of one's entire fortune in order to preserve a life.

    See also, R. Yitzchak Zilberstein, *Assia*, vol. 14, no. 3, p. 50, who, despite his earlier citation of differing opinions with regard to whether a person is obligated to expend his entire fortune or only twenty percent of his wealth in order to save the life of another, endeavors to demonstrate that he must expend his entire fortune in order to prolong his own life even for a brief period of time. His argument is in the form of deduction from relevant halakhic provisions without an endeavor to present a conceptual basis for that principle.

59. See *Mishpat Kohen*, no. 144, sec. 17, s.v. *amnam be-ikar ha-inyan*.

60. See also R. Moshe Meiselman, *Halakhah u-Refu'ah*, II (Jerusalem, 5741), 116–118.

61. *Iggerot Mosheh*'s conclusion is subject to challenge on the grounds that, although a person may not be obligated to deliver a body for dissection if he thereby subjects himself to inordinate anguish, it does not follow that another party is relieved of his obligation because of the distress caused to relatives of the deceased. Relatives have no proprietary interest in the body of deceased kin. The *mizvah* of *pikuaḥ nefesh* devolves upon those possessing the knowledge and skill required to carry out the procedure. The *sui generis* mental distress of persons not responsible for carrying out the obligation appears to be irrelevant in assessing the obligation of those charged with that duty.

62. See also this writer's discussion of this point in *Contemporary Halakhic Problems*, IV, 282–285.

63. It is undoubtedly this principle that is reflected in the comments of R. Jacob Emden, *Birat Migdal Oz, Even Boḥen* 1:83, who declares that a person is not obligated to accept "severe and bitter pain" in order to preserve the life of another. It is readily understood that excruciating pain constitutes a greater burden than loss of one's fortune. In *Even Boḥen* 1:13, R. Jacob Emden offers a similar analysis of the remarkable statement of the Ge-

mara, *Sanhedrin* 75a, declaring that a woman should not engage in sexually provocative activity in order to save a person from death because of the "dishonor of her family." R. Jacob Emden explains that the degradation and embarrassment engendered by such conduct is more onerous than loss of an entire fortune. See also *Iggerot Mosheh, Yoreh De'ah,* III, no. 179 and *Teshuvot Minḥat Yiẓḥak,* V, no. 8. Cf., however, R. Ovadiah Yosef, *Dinei Yisra'el,* VII, 24, who expresses difficulty in understanding R. Jacob Emden's comments in light of the many sources indicating that a person must suffer discomfort and even pain in order to save the life of another. If R. Jacob Emden's position is understood to be in accord with the foregoing comment the difficulties are resolved: R. Jacob Emden refers only to pain the burden of which is at least equal to the burden of losing one's entire fortune while the sources cited by Rabbi Yosef refer to a much lower level of pain.

64. The difficulty presented by the statement of the Gemara, *Avodah Zarah* 12b, discussed *supra*, p. 81, advising a person who swallows a wasp to drink a quantity of vinegar solely in order to put his affairs in order is readily explained on the basis of this principle if it is assumed that such a person suffers pain of this magnitude.

    The incident involving the executioner of R. Ḥanina ben Tradion cited *supra*, note 35, may also be explained on the basis of this principle. R. Ḥanina ben Tradion neither performed an overt act hastening his own death nor told the executioner that such an act was ever permissible as a matter of Halakhah. He did indeed "place a stumbling block before the blind" in allowing the executioner to do so. Thus, although the executioner's deed was categorically forbidden as an act of homicide, R. Ḥanina himself transgressed a simple negative commandment. Although R. Ḥanina would have been required to expend his entire fortune in order to avoid that transgression he was not obliged to accept the greater burden of prolonged suffering entailed by a slow death at the stake. Cf., *Iggerot Mosheh, Ḥoshen Mishpat,* II, no. 74. The distinction between categorically prohibited homicide and violation of the prohibition against "placing a stumbling block before the blind" in causing a gentile to perform such an act is formulated in a different context by R. Isaac Schorr, *Teshuvot Koaḥ Shor,* no. 20, and R. Moshe ha-Levi Steinberg, *Teshuvot Maḥazeh Avraham,* II, *Yoreh De'ah,* II, no. 19.

65. For an alternative explanation see *Tosafot, Pesaḥim* 53b.

66. Indeed, in developing the thesis that life need not be prolonged

in face of unbearable pain, *Iggerot Mosheh* cites *Ketubot* 33b in establishing that pain is, at times, more onerous than death. It should be noted that *Iggerot Mosheh, Ḥoshen Mishpat,* II, no. 74, sec. 1, declares that a patient's life must be prolonged even against his will, in order that he may be treated by a specialist capable of curing him. That ruling may be understood as reflecting the notion that transitory pain, even when intractable in nature, in anticipation of a cure is far different from intractable pain of the terminally ill. It is to be presumed that a normal person would not expend an entire fortune to avoid transient pain, particularly when a cure is anticipated. That distinction is consistent with *Shitah Mekubeẓet*'s categorization of the pain that one is never required to accept as *yisurin she-ein lahem kiẓvah,* i.e., sustained and interminable pain.

67. See also *Teshuvot Be'er Mosheh,* VIII, no. 239, sec. 4.
68. Cf., however, *Mishneh Halakhot,* VII, no. 287, and R. Chaim David Halevy, *Teḥumin,* II, 304–305. Cf. also, R. Zalman Nehemiah Goldberg, *Moriah,* vol. 8, no. 3–4 (Elul 5738), pp. 55–56.
69. See President's Commission for the Study of Ethical Issues in Medicine and Biomedicine and Behavioral Research, *Deciding to Forgo Life Sustaining Treatment* (Washington, D.C., 1983), p. 181. See also Ronald Crawford, *Seminars in Neurology,* vol. 4, no. 1 (March 1984), p. 151; Brief for Amicus Curiae American Academy of Neurology, pp. 10–29, *Brophy* v. *New England Sinai Hospital, Inc.,* 398 Mass. 417, 497 N.E.2d 626 (1986).
70. See Phyllis Schmitz and Merry O'Brian, "Observations in Nutrition and Hydration in Dying Cancer Patients," *By No Extraordinary Means,* ed. Joanne Lynne (Bloomington, 1986), pp. 29–38; J. Andrew Billings, "Comfort Measures for the Terminally Ill: Is Dehydration Painful?" *Journal of the American Geriatric Society,* vol. 33, no. 11 (November 1985), pp. 808–880. Billings reports that the only troubling and commonly encountered symptoms that can be attributed to dehydration in terminally ill patients are thirst and dry mouth. He suggests that these symptoms can be relieved by small amounts of oral fluid or by keeping the patient's mouth moist with water, ice chips or artificial saliva. See also "Terminal Dehydration," (editorial) *Lancet,* no. 8476 (February 8, 1986), p. 306; and David Oliver, "Terminal Dehydration," (letter) *Lancet,* no. 8403 (September 15, 1984), p. 631.
71. See Joanne Lynne and James Childress, "Must Patients Always Be Given Food and Water?" *Hastings Center Report,* vol. 13, no. 4, (October 1983), p. 19.

72. Porter Storey, "It's Over, Debbie" (letter), *Journal of the American Medical Association*, vol. 259, no. 14 (April 8, 1988), p. 2095.
73. See T.D. Walsh, "Opiates and Respiratory Function in Advanced Cancer," *Recent Results in Cancer Research*, XXXIX (1984), 1115–1117, E. Bruera *et al.*, "Effects of Morphine on the Dyspnea of Terminal Cancer Patients," *Journal of Pain and Symptom Management*, vol. 5, no. 6 (December 1990), pp. 341–344 (December 1990), p. 6; M. Angell, "The Quality of Mercy" (editorial) *New England Journal of Medicine*, vol. 306, no. 2 (January 14, 1982), pp. 98–99. See also R.R. Miller and H. Jick, "Clinical Effects of Meperidine in Hospitalized Medical Patients," *Journal of Clinical Pharmacology*, vol. 18, no. 4 (April 1978), pp. 180–189; R.R. Miller, "Analgesics," *Drug Effects in Hospitalized Patients*, ed. by R. Miller and D.J. Greenblatt (New York, 1976), pp. 133–164.
74. Albert Einstein, "Overview of Cancer Pain Management," *Pain Management and Care of the Terminal Patient*, Judy Kornell, ed. (Washington: Washington State Medical Association, 1992), p. 4. Another study indicates that when treated by skilled practitioners the pain of 98% of patients in hospice care can be relieved. See American Medical Association Council on Scientific Affairs, "Good Care of the Dying Patient," *Journal of the American Medical Association*, vol. 275, no. 6 (February 14, 1996), p. 475. See also C.S. Cleeland *et al.*, "Pain and its Treatment in Outpatients with Metastatic Cancer," *New England Journal of Medicine*, vol. 330, no. 9 (March 3, 1994), p. 592.
75. Brief of the American Medical Association *et al.*, as *amici curiae* in support of petitioners, at 6, *Washington* v. *Glucksberg*, 117 S. Ct. 2258 (1997) (No. 96–110).

4

Life as an Intrinsic Good: Religious Reflections on Euthanasia

"But your blood of your lives will I require; from the hand of every beast will I require it, and from the hand of man, from the hand of a person's brother, will I require the life of man."[1] This earliest and most detailed biblical prohibition against homicide contains one phrase that is an apparent redundancy Since the phrase "from the hand of man" pronounces man culpable for the murder of his fellow man, to what point is it necessary for Scripture to reiterate "from the hand of a person's brother will I require the life of man"? Fratricide is certainly no less heinous a crime than ordinary homicide. A nineteenth century biblical scholar, Rabbi Jacob Zevi Mecklenburg, in his commentary on the Pentateuch, *Ha-Ketav ve-ha-Kabbalah,* astutely comments that, while murder is the antithesis of brotherly love, in some circumstances the taking of the life of one's

---

This paper was originally delivered at a conference on "Life and Death after *Cruzan,*" sponsored by the National Legal Center for the Medically Dependent and Disabled, in New Orleans, April 1992, and is presented, with additions and revisions, as published in *Issues in Life and Medicine*, vol. 9, no. 2 (Fall 1993), pp. 139–149.

ellow man may be perceived as indeed being an act of love par excellence.[2] Euthanasia, designed to put an end to unbearable suffering, is born not of hatred or anger but of concern and compassion. It is precisely the taking of life even under circumstances in which it is manifestly obvious that the perpetrator is motivated by feelings of love and brotherly compassion that the Bible finds necessary to brand as murder, pure and simple. Despite the noble intent that prompts such an action, mercy killing is proscribed as an unwarranted intervention in an area that must be governed only by God himself. The life of man may be reclaimed only by the Author of life. As long as man is yet endowed with a spark life—as defined by God's eternal law—man dare not presume to hasten death, no matter how hopeless or meaningless continued existence may appear to be in the eyes of a mortal perceiver.

Indeed, there is some cogency to the argument that a dogmatic prohibition against homicide is necessary *only* in order to proscribe euthanasia. The Talmud lays down the rule that a person must allow himself to be put to death rather than take the life of his fellow.[3] *Force majeure* cannot, in good conscience, be advanced as justification for an act of homicide. This rule constitutes one of only three exceptions to the general principle in Jewish law that preservation of human life, regardless of the quality or duration of the life saved, takes precedence over all other considerations. The other exceptions are based upon hermeneutic modes of biblical exegesis. No such basis exists upon which the rule might be predicated requiring a person to accept martyrdom rather than allowing himself to be coerced to commit an act of murder. The talmudic justification is that this rule of law is based upon reason alone. It is self-evident that such an act cannot be justified, since, asserts the Talmud, "Why do you think that your blood is sweeter than the blood of your fellow?"[4] That moral judgment is regarded as an *a priori* perception of the human conscience; in effect, it is regarded as a proposition of natural law. It would then follow, *a fortiori*, that man, as a moral creature, is fully capable of recognizing by the light of his own reason that ordinary acts of murder committed for ignoble reasons, or committed wantonly for no reason at all, are heinous in nature. If so, there is no need for a prohibition based upon divine revelation. Revelation is necessary precisely because the act is prohibited even in those situations in which man's moral faculty, if left to its own devices, would not recognize the deed as repugnant, *viz.*, when the taking of human life constitutes an act of euthanasia.

The value of human life is supreme and takes precedence over virtually all other considerations. This attitude is most eloquently summed up in a talmudic passage regarding the creation of Adam: "Therefore only a single human being was created in the world, to teach that if any person has caused a single soul to perish, Scripture regards him as if he had caused an entire world to perish; and if any human being saves a single soul, Scripture regards him as if he had saved an entire world."[5] Human life is not a good to be preserved as a condition of other values but as an absolute, basic, and precious good in its own stead. The obligation to preserve life is commensurately all-encompassing.

Accordingly, life with suffering is regarded as being, in many cases, preferable to termination of life and with it elimination of suffering. The Talmud[6] and Maimonides[7] indicate that the adulterous woman who was made to drink "the bitter waters"[8] did not always die immediately. If she possessed other merit, even though guilty of the offense with which she was charged, the waters, rather than causing her to perish immediately, produced a debilitating and degenerative state that led to a protracted termination of life. The added longevity, although accompanied by pain and suffering, was viewed as a privilege bestowed in recognition of meritorious action. Life accompanied by pain is thus viewed as preferable to death. It is this sentiment that is reflected in the words of the Psalmist: "The Lord had indeed punished me, but He has not left me to die."[9]

This, however, does not necessarily mean that we can understand why life, even when accompanied by suffering, is preferable to elimination of pain through the foreshortening of life. The Talmud[10] presents a remarkable elucidation of the biblical verse "In those days Hezekiah was sick unto death and the prophet, Isaiah the son of Amoz, came to him and said unto him, 'Thus said the Lord: Command your house, for you shall die and not live.'"[11] The Talmud explains that King Hezekiah correctly understood the redundancy inherent in the phrase "you shall die and not live" as meaning "you shall die in this world and not live in the world to come." Going beyond the scriptural text, the Talmud then relates that Hezekiah demanded to know why he deserved so severe a punishment. The prophet responded, "Because you did not engage in procreation." Thereupon King Hezekiah defended himself in saying, "I saw by means of the holy spirit that unvirtuous children would issue from me." To that excuse Isaiah responded, "What have you to do with the secrets of the All-Merciful? You should have done what you were commanded and let the Holy One, blessed be He, do that which is pleasing to Him."

The principle reflected in this talmudic exposition is valid with regard to the declining stages of human life no less so than it is for the generation of human life. The meaning and value of human life is a divine mystery. Man is commanded to procreate, to nurture and sustain life, and to preserve the life that has been entrusted to him until it is reclaimed by the Creator of all life. Whether or not man finds value in the life he is commanded to preserve is, in this fundamental sense, irrelevant; man's obligations vis-à-vis sustaining life are not predicated upon his aptitude for fathoming divine secrets.

Man must hearken to the divine command regardless of whether he understands its purpose or fails to do so, and, assuredly, he may not seek to rescind or modify the divine imperative on the plea that he does fathom the divine intent and is capable of independent decision making in effecting its realization. Nevertheless, man is not constrained from endeavoring to ascertain purposes or values reflected in the divine command provided that he does not become guilty of hubris in allowing his intellect to substitute human norms for the divine imperative. The fourteenth-century philosopher and exegete Gersonides authored a commentary on the Bible in which he incorporated a section entitled *"To'aliyot,"* literally translated as "Benefits" but best rendered as "Lessons." In these vignettes Gersonides offers a list of moral maxims or values that man may derive from a particular section of Scripture. In doing so, there is no claim that man has plumbed the depths of divine meaning and intent or that he has exhaustively discerned the divine purpose. In much the same manner it is possible to discern a reinforcement of values in the preservation and prolongation of life even when that life appears to be bereft of value in conventional human or social terms. Indeed, centuries ago, the Sages of the Talmud, in an entirely different context, compared the human body to Sacred Writ. Lessons and purposes may be derived from divinely ordained experiences just as they are derived from divinely revealed texts. Paradoxically, although the ultimate meaning or purpose of human life remains a divine mystery, strictures against euthanasia serve manifold purposes, some of which are readily perceived.

I. HUMAN LIFE AND DIVINE GRANDEUR

In *Hales* v. *Petit,* a classic sixteenth century case in which the interest of the state in prevention of suicide was first articulated, Justice Dyer wrote that suicide is an offense "against the king in that hereby he has lost a subject, and . . . he being the head has lost one of his mystical members."[12] Suicide may be prevented—and punished—by the king because it constitutes interference with his rights as monarch. Anthropomorphic analogies, by very their nature, can never be completely accurate. Nevertheless, in human terms, honor and glory are often found in sheer magnitude. Royal majesty is perceived as a correlate of the number of subjects over whom the monarch reigns. The more citizens in his domain, the greater the king. Thus, to deprive the king of a subject is to diminish his grandeur; to willfully cause the death of a subject of the king is to be guilty of *lèse majesté.*

Although this, too, is a mystery beyond our ken, God is the supreme king, whose dominion extends over all of mankind. The more numerous the populace, the greater is his grandeur. The loss of even a single life represents a diminution of his kingship. One of the most solemn prayers in the Jewish liturgy is the *Kaddish,* the mourner's prayer. Although recited as memorialization of a loved one, the *Kaddish* contains no reference to the deceased, no hint of reward or punishment, no mention of everlasting life, and no prayer for the repose of the soul of the departed. Its opening phrase, "May His great Name be magnified and sanctified," sets the tenor of the entire prayer as a paean celebrating ultimate universal acceptance of divine sovereignty. Rabbi Meir Shapiro of Lublin explained that the loss of even a single human life represents a diminution of divine sovereignty and hence evokes a prayer expressing the supplicant's yearning for the restoration and enhancement of God's glory.[13]

It is difficult enough for us to comprehend any sense in which mere human existence serves to enhance the glory of the Deity. In anthropomorphic terms, we can readily understand that a monarch's power and glory, both real and perceived, are directly commensurate with the number of able-bodied, healthy, productive subjects over whom he rules. But incremental numbers of aged, nonproductive, ailing subjects hardly enhance royal power or grandeur. Nevertheless, to the extent that the mind can fathom the mystery of human existence, mankind must be perceived as constituting a vast orchestra engaged in a continuous performance in praise of the

Creator. In an orchestra, each musician has an assigned role, and those assigned identical or similar roles are arranged in groups. There are separate sections for musicians playing wind, string, and percussion instruments. Not all the musicians and not all sections play at once. Effective rendition of the musical arrangement requires that, at times, some of the musicians remain silent. Yet even when not actually engaged in playing his instrument, every member remains seated with the orchestra and contributes to the visual magnificence of the performance. Similarly, each and every individual has an assigned role in the divine orchestration of mankind. Not every member is called upon to extol the Deity by fulfilling his assigned role continuously. Some, by virtue of their physical condition, may be quiescent; they are silent members of an orchestra that is nevertheless more majestic by virtue of their presence. Even though an individual in a precarious physical condition may not have the capacity to serve God in an active sense, nevertheless, his very existence constitutes an act of divine service.

II. MAN AS THE CHATTEL OF GOD

Preservation and prolongation of the life of a comatose patient also serve to impress a significant moral lesson upon the human conscience. Much is said in our day regarding patient autonomy and the right of every individual to be master of his or her own destiny. To be sure, no person enjoys rights over the life of another. Nevertheless, the concept of personal autonomy is flawed if it is understood as embodying the notion that man enjoys a proprietary interest in his own life. Our religious heritage teaches us that God is the Creator of man and that he is the Author of both life and death. Thus, even Plato spoke of man as the "chattel of the gods" in denying man's right to foreshorten his own life.[14] Man's interest in his life and in his body are subservient to those of the Creator. It is extremely easy to lose sight of that verity since, in the ordinary course of events, a person's natural desires, self-interest and preservation instinct serve to assure that his natural inclinations coincide with his moral obligation. That is frequently not the case when a person is pain-ridden, debilitated and terminally ill or involved in decision making on behalf of a comatose or nonsentient patient. In such cases, preservation of life does not appear to be at all desirable from a human perspective. But precisely because there is no longer a human will to live does man become cognizant of the fact that he may not make a decision to terminate life because his autonomy is not untrammeled. He is forcibly reminded of the fact that it is the Creator who is the ultimate proprietor of human life—a lesson that man might otherwise be prone to forget.

III. MORAL EFFECT ON HEALTH CARE PROVIDERS

Equally germane in analyzing the purposes reflected in a vitalist policy is an understanding of the negative values it does not allow to take root. In inveighing against suicide, the Court in *Hales* v. *Petit* declared that the deed cannot be countenanced so that "no evil example be given."[155] The taking of human life invites imitation and self-destruction serves as an "evil example" encouraging emulation by other susceptible members of society.[16] Suicide is "a breach of [the King's] peace" because a suicide is not a private act.[17] Quite to the contrary, it constitutes an offense against society because of potential harm to others. Euthanasia, whether active or passive, diminishes commitment to the preservation of life and compromises respect for life which, in turn, constitutes the fundamental underpinning of the social fabric.

Violence and even passive disregard for the preservation of life produce an indelible mark upon human character—as do compassion, concern and prolongation of life. In a remarkably incisive discussion in the *Nicomachean Ethics,* Aristotle asserts that both virtue and vice must be defined as character traits rather than as categorizations of discrete acts.[18] A virtuous person is not simply one who performs virtuous acts but one in whom the act flows from an ingrained character trait. Virtue is a habit, spontaneous and unbelabored, somewhat akin to a spontaneous reflex. The ability to press keys on a piano in the ordered sequence of a concerto does not render the player a pianist. For one to become a musician, the music must become part of the musician's personality and spring effortlessly from his fingers. Habits and skills are acquired. They are the products of practice and reinforcement.

The virtues that we seek to integrate within our personalities are born of virtuous acts repeated in their performance over and over again. Virtue is a disposition developed by repetition of acts that are objectively virtuous. Habits become ingrained as a result of patterned behavior. Failure to respond in a uniform manner, even when the intention is laudable, disrupts the behavior pattern and unsettles character. Examination of pros and cons, advantages and disadvantages, benefits and burdens of care and treatment on a case by case basis means that the therapeutic response is no longer spontaneous. When forthcoming, the decision to preserve life may be virtuous, but it is not the product of a virtuous character. Development of moral character, as Aristotle tells us, depends upon development of ingrained, spontaneous responses.

This should not be confused with the slippery slope argument—not that the slippery slope does not loom as a clear and present danger. The cogency of the Aristotelian position does not lie in the fear that a person lacking a virtuous character will not act in a manner consistent with virtue but in a recognition that an identical act performed by two individuals may be qualitatively different and that development of a virtuous character is integral to man's goal in life.

The development of virtuous character is surely a value society seeks to promote in all of its members. But society has a particular concern with the character development of health care professionals. Persons afflicted by malady or illness have a definite need for assurance that the physician will intuitively do everything possible to preserve life and promote well-being. Such trust cannot be reposed in a physician who is schooled in decision-making calculi that weigh the quality of life to be preserved. In an earlier time in American judicial history courts recognized that such considerations represented a societal interest of a magnitude weighty enough to override patient autonomy. Thus, the physician's paramount objective to preserve life was affirmed in *John F. Kennedy Memorial Hospital* v. *Heston*[19] and in *United States* v. *George.*[20] Confidence in the physician lies at the core of the physician-patient relationship and has a positive effect upon the therapeutic process. Conversely, lack of confidence has an adverse effect upon the therapeutic process. A positive relationship is possible only when the patient knows with certainty that the physician will always do his utmost and not abandon his patient as being beyond hope.

It is quite common for this aspect of the physician-patient relationship to be recognized even by persons who do not wish their lives to be prolonged under any and all circumstances. A simple and insignificant anecdote will serve to illustrate this point. Several years ago I delivered a paper at a medical ethics conference in which I advocated a strong vitalist position. A member of the audience, who happened to be a nurse, commented to my wife: "I don't agree with everything your husband said but, if he were a physician, I would certainly want him to be my doctor."

IV. EMULATION OF DIVINE LOVE

Moreover, providing care on behalf of a debilitated patient incapable of response or of any meaningful activity represents a unique opportunity for the caregiver precisely because it is, in a fundamental sense, devoid of value to the recipient, at least as value is understood in human terms. In the words "and you shall walk in His ways,"[21] Scripture bids us to emulate God's ways to the extent that it is humanly possible to do so. God loves man, and this love, or *agape,* is of a unique kind. Divine *agape* is fundamentally different from the *philia* described by Aristotle. Aristotle describes three forms of love or friendship, each involving a relationship. Those relationships are rooted in (1) pleasure or delight derived from the object of *philia;* (2) utility or pragmatic benefit derived from the relationship; or (3) a relationship based upon recognition of the virtue, i.e., the worth or intrinsic value, of the object of such *philia.*[22] Divine *agape* can hardly be in the nature of either of the first two forms of *philia.* Divine *agape* cannot be the product of the delight God finds in His relationship with men because God is incorporeal and not subject to emotions; God does not experience pleasure or delight. Divine *agape* cannot be rooted in utility, since, as a completely perfect Being, God is lacking in nothing and can derive no benefit to Himself from his relationship with man. Nor can we be so arrogant as to assume that divine love of man is predicated upon man's intrinsic worth, i.e., that God loves man because man is intrinsically precious. Any such exalted view of the human condition is negated by Scripture in the declaration "O Lord what is man that Thou knowest him or the son of man that Thou art mindful of him."[23] God's love of man flows irrepressibly from this essence.

What then is the nature of God's love for man? God's love can only be *sui generis,* unmotivated and not predicated upon any consideration. It is an act of *caritas,* i.e., of charity in the pristine sense of that term, To understand divine *agape* in even a remotely approximate manner, one must draw an analogy by examining one's love for oneself One's love of oneself is not based upon pleasure: even a person whose existence is tormented and who experiences life as an unmitigated state of anguish continues to love himself Similarly, the love one bears toward oneself is not the product of utility, i.e., of benefit that one derives from oneself, since that love endures even when one becomes an unrelieved burden to oneself. And, surely, self-love is not born of a recognition of self-worth. Indeed, the sinner, although fully aware of his deficiencies, is likely to love himself more intensely than the saint. Love of the self is uncaused and, indeed, often undeserved. "Love thy neighbor as thyself"[24] constitutes a mandate to love one's fellow in exactly the same manner, i.e., to love him, not for any particular reason, but for no reason. *Agape* must be freely offered without expectation of reciprocation and must be nonjudgmental. Manifestation of that quality of love for one's fellow is a reflection of divine *agape;* it is man walking in the ways of God and emulating His love of mankind.

Actions commonly described as acts of charity are generally motivated, at least in part, by one or another of Aristotle's modes of *philia.* To be sure, only the cynical or the naive act on grounds of utility, i.e., anticipation of reciprocation. But it is entirely noble to perform acts of charity because of a sense of the human worth of the beneficiary or in anticipation of enjoying the unique sense of self-satisfaction that may be derived from the altruistic nature of a charitable act. Paradoxically—or perhaps not so paradoxically—it is precisely our failure to perceive a rational purpose in prolonging the lives of patients whose continued survival seems to be devoid of meaning that enables our acts on their behalf to rise to the level of *agape.* Such an act cannot be based upon love generated by the precious nature of the life that is being preserved because we fail to recognize any intrinsic value in such life. Nor can the act be motivated by the self-satisfaction born of altruistic behavior. Altruism entails acting on behalf of another. However, if the other person derives no benefit from the act, one can hardly derive a glow of satisfaction from having acted on his behalf One may indeed feel that one has done one's duty, but that feeling is accompanied by a sense of hollowness. And precisely therein lies its purpose. Its purpose lies in the fact that it has no purpose. Of all human acts of charity it most closely approximates the divine because, of all expressions of human love, it most closely represents *agape*. Its value lies in the fact that it has no cause; it is an expression of man's endeavor to become God-like and hence godly.

V. A VEHICLE FOR MIẒVAH

The Sages of the Talmud went beyond recognition of illness as an opportunity accorded to the healthy for expression of *caritas*. They saw in illness an opportunity for the sick to gain merit by virtue of being instruments for expression of loving-kindness. The Gemara, *Nedarim* 39b, states in the name of R. Simeon ben Lakish:

> Where is there a biblical allusion to [the *miẓvah* of] visiting the sick? "If these will die in the manner of the death of all men and the visitation of all men be visited upon them, then God did not send me" (Numbers 16:29). How is this inferred? Said Rava, "'If these will die in the manner of the death of all men.' [i.e.], they become ill and are confined to bed and people visit them, what will people say? 'God did not send me.'"

The term *pekudah* in Scripture and its associated verb forms usually connote "remembering," in the sense of remembering to perform an act or to satisfy a need, e.g., "And God remembered Sarah" (Genesis 21:1). The term acquires the connotation of "visitation" when associated with the act that is prompted by remembrance. Thus, for example, Genesis 21:1 is rendered by *Targum Onkelos* as "And God remembered Sarah" while the verse cited in *Nedarim* 39b is rendered by Onkelos as "the visitation of all men." The conventional understanding of the "visitation" of which the latter verse speaks is the visitation of death to which reference is made earlier in the same verse: "If they will die in the manner of the death of all men." The Gemara, presumably troubled by the obvious redundancy in the verse, interprets the "visitation" to which reference is made as connoting visits paid to the sick patient by family and friends rather than as connoting the visitation of death.

The problem, however, is what is Moses trying to prove? If, as Moses predicts, Korah meets an unnatural death resulting from a supernatural event, that miraculous phenomenon will serve to reinforce Moses' stature as a prophet and as the bearer of divine instruction, contrary to the allegation of Korah. Moses is putting his credentials to the test in the manner of a prophet who proves his prophecy by means of a miracle. Thus, if the announced miracle does not occur, Moses will be exposed as a fraud. Accordingly, the reference to the manner of Korah's impending death is entirely understandable. But how would visits by family and friends prior to his death disprove the claims of Moses? If, for some reason, death can be attributed to a supernatural cause only if it is sudden in nature, Moses could readily have announced that his authority should be regarded as having been confirmed only if Korah dies miraculously and suddenly. The reference to visits by family and friends seems to predicate Moses' claim upon a particular phenomenon that is of no intrinsic relevance.

The Gemara's interpretation of the cited phrase should be understood as reflecting an assertion on the part of Moses to the effect that Korah and his company are totally evil and possess no redeeming merit whatsoever. Their challenge to Moses and to his office is entirely insincere in nature. As the epitome of evil, Korah and his company, declares Moses, lack the merit even passively to provide others with an opportunity for a *mizvah*. If they die, not only miraculously but suddenly as well, that will be a sign that they possess no redeeming merit, as Moses claims. If they do not die instantaneously, with the result that others are afforded the opportunity to perform kindnesses on their behalf, that, declares Moses, will be proof that he has falsely accused them of being bereft of all redeeming qualities.

This remarkable bit of talmudic exegesis does not merely uncover a new level of meaning in a biblical verse but serves as a vehicle for the enunciation of an important value: Even when the life of a person on his deathbed seems to be devoid of benefit, meaning or purpose, the patient retains unique human value by virtue of the role he plays in providing an opportunity for love and compassion. Moreover, to be placed in that role is itself a mark of divine favor.

VI. HUMAN LIFE AS A BONUM PER SE

Finally, difficult as it may be to accept rationally, it must be recognized that, on a different level, human life does represent a purpose in and of itself, i.e., sheer human existence is endowed with moral value. If human life in any of its guises represents a value, that value must logically be either an instrumental good or a *bonum per se.* If human life constitutes only an instrumental good, it follows that life becomes devoid of value when it no longer leads to or promotes that value. When that quality of life has degenerated to the point that it is considered to be devoid of value, there is no compelling reason to distinguish between passive and active euthanasia. If life *per se* does not represent a value, then the taking of life can be wrong only because it extinguishes other goods that are made possible only by the presence of life. When those goods are no longer attainable, the underlying human life can hardly continue to be an instrumental good.

Again, this is not a slippery slope argument. The slippery slope argument seeks to persuade that, although *x* is morally innocuous, if *x* is sanctioned it will rapidly lead, through desensitization, inability to make fine and precise moral distinctions, outright malice, or whatever, to *y*, with *y* representing something that, at least upon reflection, is clearly unacceptable. The problem with the notion of human life as an instrumental good rather than a *bonum per se* is not that it creates a dynamic in which acceptance of passive euthanasia today improperly leads to condoning active euthanasia tomorrow but that the two are morally indistinguishable. Hence acceptance of one logically entails acceptance of the other. The intuitive repugnance of the conclusion of this moral syllogism should serve to demonstrate not that the reasoning is faulty but that its major premise is faulty.

Moreover, if human life is merely an instrumental good, it becomes necessary to define the nature of the good that constitutes the *telos* of human existence. No doubt that may become the subject of disagreement and may variously be defined as the capacity for rational thought, awareness of personhood, the ability to engage in interpersonal relationships, the capacity to experience pleasure etc. It rapidly becomes evident that the absence of such a *telos* is not associated only with the terminal, comatose condition or even with the permanent vegetative state but is also absent in some states of insanity and mental deficiency. If that line of reasoning is pursued to its logical conclusion, it results in the assertion that, *mutatis mutandis,* the life of any person not capable of experiencing that *telos* may be snuffed out with moral impunity. Euthanasia would then become morally acceptable in situations not involving terminally ill persons. Applying such criteria, permanently and severely mentally disabled or retarded persons would be candidates for euthanasia. We intuitively recognize that such an argument constitutes a *reductio ad absurdum*. Yet the only way to escape that conclusion is to accept the alternate formulation of the disjunction with which we began, *viz.*, that all human life constitutes a *bonum per se*.

NOTES

1. Genesis 9:5.
2. *Ha-Ketav ve-ha-Kabbalah* (5th ed., 1946), p. 20.
3. *Sanhedrin* 79a.
4. *Loc. cit.*
5. *Sanhedrin* 37a.
6. *Sotah* 22b.
7. *Hilkhot Sotah* 3:20.
8. Numbers 5:11–31.
9. Psalms 118:18.
10. *Berakhot* 10a.
11. Isaiah 38:1.
12. 1 Plowden 253, 262, 75 Eng. Rep. 387, 400 (Q.B. 1562).
13. *Be-Mishnah be-Omer u-be-Ma'as* (Bnei Brak, 1967), ed. Aaron Soraski, II, 122.
14. Plato, *Phaedo* 62b–c, reprinted in Plato I, 215–17 (Harold North Fowler, trans., 14th ed., 1971) (Loeb Classical Library, vol. 36).
15. 1 Plowden at 262, 75 Eng. Rep. at 400.
16. *Loc. cit.*
17. *Loc. cit.*
18. Aristotle, *Nicomachean Ethics,* Book II, 1130b (reprinted in *The Basic Works of Aristotle,* pp. 952–53) (Richard McKeon, ed., 25th ed., 1941).
19. 279 A.2d 670 (N.J. 1971).
20. 239 F. Supp. 752 (D. Conn. 1965).
21. Deuteronomy 28:9.
22. Aristotle, *Nicomachean Ethics,* Book VIII, 1156–57 (reprinted in *The Basic Works of Aristotle,* pp. 1065–12)(Richard McKeon, ed., 25th ed., 1941).
23. Psalms 144:3.
24. Leviticus 19:18.

5

AIDS: Jewish Concerns

I. IDEOLOGICAL ISSUES

Societal responses to the very serious problems posed by the scourge of AIDS (acquired immune deficiency syndrome) reflect, at least in part, the epidemiological association that exists between the rampant spread of that deadly disease and homosexual activity. The fact that AIDS has disproportionately affected members of the homosexual community has certainly had an impact upon how the problems associated with AIDS are viewed in our society. In some sectors, there is a strong tendency to ignore the fact that not all instances of AIDS infection are the product of homosexual conduct, or even of heterosexual promiscuity or intravenous drug abuse. Unfortunately, many cases of AIDS are directly attributable to blood transfusions, as is reflected in the relatively large number of hemophiliacs who have contracted that disease, and to other entirely innocent forms of contact with the blood or, possibly, body fluids of previously infected persons.

There are individuals who have adopted a moralistic posture in asserting that, since the condition is presumed to be self-inflicted in nature and the product of odious conduct, society is relieved, in whole or in part, from the obligations usually associated with alleviation of suffering. Alternatively, the disease is regarded as the visitation of divine punishment upon those who engage in perverse and unnatural conduct. For some, perception of AIDS as an entirely deserved punishment serves to mitigate feelings of compassion that would ordinarily be evoked in relating to victims of a debilitating illness.

Members of the gay community, on the other hand, regard themselves as victims of prejudice and discrimination. They fear that measures that might be taken by society to prevent the spread of AIDS will serve to brand them as pariahs. Precautions instituted by health-care professionals to protect themselves from contagion are regarded by homosexuals as inherently discriminatory. It is against this backdrop that the attitude of Judaism vis-à-vis treatment of AIDS victims must be assessed.

It should be superfluous to state that Judaism regards homosexual conduct as a serious transgression of divine law. Papers, statements and resolutions emanating from Reform, Conservative and Reconstructionist clergy notwithstanding, Leviticus 18:22 makes it unambiguously clear that homosexual behavior cannot be accepted with equanimity. Even more pertinent to current changing socio-cultural mores regarding homosexuality is a statement recorded in the Gemara, *Ḥullin* 92b. In general, the Sages of the Talmud had very little of a positive nature to say regarding pagan societies of antiquity. One of the very few positive comments that one finds is the statement recorded in the name of Ulla to the effect that, despite the many serious transgressions that were rampant in those societies, and despite the fact that members of those societies engaged in every conceivable form of deviant sexual behavior, including homosexuality, they nevertheless had the grace not to draft a marriage contract as a means of validating a homosexual relationship.

Reflected in that statement is a keen assessment of the mores that were prevalent in antiquity. Homosexual acts certainly took place. Indeed, the cited talmudic statement appears to reflect the fact that relationships that we would describe as stable homosexual unions were relatively commonplace. The Sages of the Talmud certainly did not approve of homosexual conduct. But even though, in antiquity, people did engage in homosexual activity and there appears to have been no attempt to restrict such conduct, society nevertheless refused to bestow an official imprimatur upon homosexual relationships. In days of yore it was clearly recognized that such relationships do not deserve societal commendation. The peoples of antiquity earned the approbation of the Sages because, despite their rampant immorality, they recognized that society cannot bestow its Good Housekeeping seal of approval and pronounce a blessing upon homosexual unions.

One of the classical commentators, R. Isaac Arama, *Akeidat Yiẓḥak*, *Bereishit*, *sha'ar* 20, observes that the homosexual conduct of Sodom was punished much more severely than the homosexuality that was rampant in other cities. He asserts that the inhabitants of Sodom were singled out for censure and punishment because they had institutionalized the form of deviant sexual activity that has become associated with the very name of their city. As recorded in *Bereishit Rabbah* 50:10: "The people of Sodom agreed among themselves that any stranger entering the city would be subjected to homosexual intercourse." Sodomy was not unique to Sodom. But only in Sodom was it accepted as a matter of course; only in Sodom did it become *de rigueur*. In other societies such acts were forbidden by statute, although the law was honored only in the breach. In Sodom, declares *Akeidat Yiẓḥak*, not only was such conduct decriminalized but it was ritualized as well. Removal of the odium associated with a transgression is potentially more serious a matter than the transgression itself and it was for that reason that the people of Sodom were punished so severely.

The current demand for recognition of homosexual relationships as an acceptable alternative lifestyle is based, in large measure, upon a claim that there are some people who, genetically, or as a result of environmental influence, or both, are not heterosexual in orientation but, on the contrary, are homosexual by virtue of natural disposition. Hence it is argued that their behavior is not at all deviant; rather, for those individuals, homosexuality is entirely normal and natural.[1]

The present efforts on the part of the homosexual community to secure recognition of their sexual conduct as a morally acceptable lifestyle lends new poignancy to rabbinic exegesis of Leviticus 18:22. Read literally, the verse declares, "And with a man you shall not lie as one lies with a woman; it is an abomination." The Gemara, *Nedarim* 51a, renders the concluding portion of that passage as "*to'eh atah bah*—you go astray in it." The rabbinic interpretation is not intended to confute the plain meaning of the verse. For the vast majority of humanity, homosexual activity is deviant behavior; it is unnatural and repugnant—an abomination. To speak of such conduct as losing one's way—"going astray"—is almost to minimize the infraction. It may not be reading too much into the rabbinic text if it is understood as directed to homosexuals who feel no repugnance regarding their conduct. A person burdened by a homosexual orientation "goes astray" if he believes such activity to be acceptable because it does not appear to him as an abomination. Countenancing a homosexual lifestyle as morally or socially acceptable constitutes deviation from divinely established norms and hence social institutions legitimizing such arrangements cannot be accepted with approbation.

The validity or non-validity of the claim that homosexuality is natural rather than aberrant, or a normal state rather than an illness, is irrelevant to Jewish teaching regarding this matter. Not everything that is normal and natural is also licit and morally acceptable. Monogamy, for example, is probably not natural to the human species. There is very little evidence, if any, that, were man left to his own inclinations, he would adopt a monogamous lifestyle. Yet Western society has commonly maintained that adultery is to be eschewed and that monogamy represents a moral value despite the fact that a monogamous life-style is not dictated by emotional, physiological or sexual impulses. Divine commandments, by their very nature, are designed to curb and to channel human desires. They are not necessarily reflective of that which comes naturally to man.

Rambam makes this point quite forcefully in his *Shemonah Perakim (Eight Chapters)* which serves as the introduction to his commentary on the *Ethics of the Fathers*. Among modern philosophers it was Kant, in his *Groundwork of the Metaphysics of Morals*, who grappled with the question of whether, ideally, one should act in a virtuous manner out of a desire to do so or whether it is a greater virtue to behave morally in defiance of natural desire. Rambam, in addressing essentially the same question, distinguishes between various categories of commandments and points out that while the Torah does, of course, proscribe certain forms of behavior that are unnatural and instinctively abhorrent there are also many commandments that serve to forbid conduct that is entirely normal and natural. There is no natural repugnance associated with eating the flesh of swine; nor is there any reason to regard carnivorous birds as naturally repulsive. The prohibitions contained within the dietary code are not designed to condition us to react negatively to forbidden foods. Quite to the contrary, the Sages teach that, when confronted by that which is forbidden but desirable, one should not at all endeavor to develop repugnance or distaste. All reports indicate that French cuisine is a gastronomical delight. A Jew is under no obligation to declare that he has no appetite for such food because authentic French cooking requires the mixing of meat and dairy products in preparing sauces and the like. Quite to the contrary, the appropriate response is "*Afshi, aval mah e'eseh? Avi she-ba-shamayim gazar alai!*—I wish to eat it, but, what can I do? My Father in heaven has bound me by His decree!"[2] The appropriate response is a frank and candid recognition that in the absence of a divine command one would naturally be inclined to enjoy such delicacies.

Man is a corporeal being and as such is subject to various and sundry desires. Some objects of desire are forbidden to man; others are consecrated and commanded; virtually all are subject to regulation. Man, by nature, is a sensual and sexual being. Fornication, extramarital liaisons and adultery would not necessarily be foresworn by heterosexuals if not for divine decree. It may well be the case that, for some persons, homosexual conduct is an entirely analogous orientation. If so, such individuals are confronted by yet another potential stumbling block which they must circumvent. Their homosexuality is yet another aspect of human nature in which natural tendencies must be confronted and subdued and represents an additional—and perhaps more difficult—trial. The challenge may be onerous in the extreme, but it may not be ignored. Others, more fortunate in not having been burdened in this manner, are duty-bound to exhibit compassion and solicitude and to provide all possible support to those endeavoring to overcome such inclinations.

For some, the challenge is undoubtedly greater than for others, but the standard is enunciated with utmost clarity for all. Commendation of pagans who did not regularize homosexual liaisons by drafting a marriage contract reflects an awareness that there is a difference between engaging in illicit conduct even while recognizing that such conduct is wrong and between regularizing and formalizing that type of conduct. We may—and indeed must—recognize that the flesh is weak and be understanding of human frailties. But to understand is not to condone, to be solicitous is not to approve.

The sharp distinction that Judaism makes between sinners and their sins is eloquently expressed by the Gemara, *Berakhot* 10a, in an exchange between R. Meir and his wife Beruria. There were a number of wicked men in R. Meir's locale who molested him in some way and caused him severe grief. R. Meir prayed for their death. Beruria assumed that her husband regarded such prayer as justified on the basis of Psalms 104:35

which is conventionally rendered "Let sinners cease out of the earth." But Beruria objected, "Is it written *ḥot'im*? It is written *ḥatta'im*!" The Psalmist carefully calls for the eradication of sin, not of sinners. Beruria adduced further proof for her understanding of this term from the concluding phrase of the verse, "and let wicked men be no more." If sinners have been eradicated then of course there are no longer any wicked men. Hence, according to the conventional interpretation, the concluding words are entirely superfluous. However, explained Beruria, if "*ḥatta'im*" is rendered as "sins" the concluding phrase is entirely cogent: "Let sins cease out of the earth" and when that is accomplished "wicked men" will be no more. Accordingly, Beruria counseled her husband, "Rather pray for them that they should repent and they will no longer be wicked!" The Gemara reports that R. Meir prayed as his wife directed and the wicked individuals who had abused him did indeed repent. Beruria was one of the greatest women in Jewish history and this is clearly an instance in which her insight was accepted by Judaism as expressing a normative teaching.

I remember very vividly an incident that occurred a number of years ago. A young lady in my community called my home the day after *Rosh ha-Shanah* and requested an appointment to speak to me. When I indicated that since this was an extremely busy time of the year I would prefer to see her a week or two hence, she responded by saying that it was absolutely essential that she see me before *Yom Kippur*. Of course, I arranged to see her immediately.

The young lady came to visit me and said, "Rabbi, this is the time of year when Jews become afflicted by pangs of guilt. Their consciences begin to bother them." I answered, "Yes. Is there any way that I may be of help to you?" To this she responded, "No. It's not I who needs help; it is my boyfriend who needs your help."

The young lady proceeded to tell me that she had been having an affair with a young man who, it turned out, was an occasional worshipper in my synagogue. And then she asked for my help. Naive as I was, I assumed that she was about to solicit my assistance in hastening the process of their becoming bride and groom and thereby regularizing and legitimizing their relationship. Not at all! She proceeded to tell me: "Rabbi, I want you to speak to him so that he won't feel guilty about it. A guilt complex isn't healthy. This is the time of year when he becomes overwhelmed by guilt and his guilt is tormenting him."

The plight of a guilt-ridden person properly evokes empathy. Guilt, too, must be recognized and dealt with in terms of the emotional turmoil it may bring in its wake. Yet it is assuredly the case that one dare not bestow an ecclesiastic imprimatur upon an arrangement that is not, and cannot be, condoned by Judaism. No matter how much sympathy one may have for the individuals involved, one cannot lend support to such a lifestyle.

Certainly, in our associations with individuals who are afflicted with AIDS we must react with compassion and love insofar as those individuals are concerned. However, that acceptance need not, and dare not, encompass any form of illicit conduct that may lie at the source of the affliction.

A distinction must be noted between homosexuality and homosexual activity. The former is an inclination, a predisposition that may or may not express itself behaviorally. The latter is an act that may be engaged in by a person who is homosexually oriented or by a heterosexual who has no such predisposition but chooses to perform homosexual acts because he wishes to experiment, because he finds such acts enticing precisely because they represent a form of forbidden fruit or simply because he seeks to flout accepted mores.

To be sure, Judaism provides for punishment to be meted out to transgressors. However, in Judaism, punishment is not designed to serve as retribution but rather as a deterrent. Punishment as a deterrent, as a means of containing the spread of conduct regarded by society as abhorrent, is entirely consistent with the highest degree of sympathy for the perpetrator. Society may even recognize that the perpetrator is himself, in a sense, a "victim" of genetics and/or of his environment and nevertheless proceed to impose sanctions for the express purpose of discouraging imitation on the part of others who cannot plead such mitigating circumstances. Moreover, for the past 2,000 years, punishment for infraction of such transgressions has been a dead letter. Even prior to the destruction of the Temple and the advent of the present exile, we lost the ability to impose penal sanctions as prescribed by Jewish law. By virtue of its own provisions, Jewish law regards reinstitution of the sacrificial order and restoration of the Sanhedrin to its chamber within the sanctified precincts of the Temple Mount as necessary preconditions that must be fulfilled in order to make possible the administration of biblically prescribed punishment for infractions of such nature.

Accordingly, the question of punishment is one that should not arise with regard to our relationship vis-à-vis individuals who engage in deviant sexual behavior or, for that manner, with regard to our relationship vis-à-vis any person who violates any of the commandments of the Torah. Insofar as our attitude is concerned, the act must be deplored, but the person who commits such acts remains a Jew to whom our hearts and arms are open. Such a person remains a brother and our relationship to him must be the fraternal relationship one has with a brother who has strayed from the values and mores of the family, i.e., a brother to whom one's arms are always open and who will be warmly and affectionately welcomed at all times.

Punishment, to be sure, comes not only at the hands of man but at the hands of Heaven as well. It is not surprising, therefore, for a malady to be regarded as a divine visitation in the nature of punishment for misdeeds. This is true not only with regard to AIDS but with regard to other forms of affliction as well. Nevertheless, no one, other than a prophet, can declare with certainty that there is a direct cause and effect relationship between a specific misdeed and any particular misfortune. Who knows when God chooses to punish and what means He utilizes for that punishment? But at the same time the Sages admonish, "If a person perceives afflictions coming upon himself, he should scrutinize his deeds" (*Berakhot* 5a). Judaism, without pointing a finger of accusation, blame or guilt, has always regarded any form of adversity as a divine beneficence, as a form of prodding initiated by God and designed to rouse the afflicted person from complacency so that he will stand back, scrutinize his deeds and examine his lifestyle in order to identify those aspects of his conduct, behavior and lifestyle in which there is room for improvement. And if, as King Solomon informs us, there is no person on earth who consistently does good and never transgresses,[3] there must always be at least some room for improvement. Accordingly, it is impossible to declare with certainty that misfortune or affliction is totally unrelated to one's prior conduct. One ignores what is even merely a possible divine admonition only at one's own peril.

Nevertheless, there certainly are situations in which what may be perceived as a punishment is, in reality, not a punishment at all. The Gemara, *Ketubot* 30a, declares: "Everything is by the hands of Heaven except chills and heat, as it is said: 'Chills and heat are in the way of the stubborn; he who safeguards his soul distances himself from them' (Proverbs 22:5)." A person who goes out in the heat of the day and suffers a sunstroke or a person who does not seek shelter in inclement weather and suffers the results of exposure has only himself to blame. A phenomenon of such nature is not necessarily punishment for misdeeds but is quite likely the necessary result of a cause and effect relationship inherent in nature. Surely, if a person puts his hand into a fire he should not expect God to work a miracle so that the hand will not be burned. One would have to be an extraordinary individual to merit divine intervention in natural processes in order to escape the necessary effect of a physical cause. This consideration applies to AIDS as well. Exposure to contagion, whether through transfusion of contaminated blood or sexual intercourse with an infected person, is no different from exposure to extreme heat or cold in a sense that the resultant disease is the product of man's own folly or negligence. Indeed, the Palestinian Talmud, *Shabbat* 14:3, attributes the vast majority of deaths to human negligence in declaring, "And the Sages say, 'Ninety-nine die as a result of negligence and one at the hands of Heaven.'"

At the same time, one must not forget that even the laws of nature are the product of divine authorship. Although, for the individual victim, AIDS maladies may be natural rather than providential, nevertheless, it is incumbent upon society to examine the present day AIDS epidemic in order to determine what can be learned from it. From a global perspective, perhaps mankind is being taught a lesson. Were our societal standards in conformity with divinely mandated norms the opportunity for individual contagion would simply not arise. In the ultimate sense, every phenomenon is a manifestation of Providence. There can be no doubt that it is divinely intended that we take stock of our social standards and practices and realign them in a manner consonant with divine teaching.

But at the same time we dare not forget that, even insofar as any individual victim is concerned, homosexual conduct and drug abuse are certainly not the only means of AIDS transmission. There are countless individuals who have contracted AIDS in a manner which leaves them totally and completely blameless. Many individuals have contracted AIDS as a result of blood transfusion during the period after the disease first became manifest and before screening of prospective blood donors for the presence of HIV (human immunosuppressive virus) became commonplace, i.e., approximately between 1978 and 1985. Some few victims are members of the health-care professions who have led an exemplary lifestyle, individuals who have never had contact with controlled substances or engaged in deviant sexual behavior, but who have unfortunately contracted this disease as a result of a needle prick, scalpel wound or exposure of skin lesions to infected body fluids.

A response based upon the notion that AIDS victims are simply suffering the just results of their immoral actions is entirely inappropriate and, in many cases, is based on a fundamental error. How, then, should society relate to AIDS victims? Society is duty-bound to treat victims of AIDS as it treats the victims of any other infectious disease. Specifically, society is obligated (1) to do everything in its power to eliminate the suffering of individuals who are afflicted; (2) to prevent the spread of the disease; and (3) to commit its resources to discovering a cure.

II. PRACTICAL ISSUES

1. *Screening Programs and Confidentiality*

The rampant spread of AIDS gives rise to a number of practical issues that must be addressed from a Jewish perspective. In particular, society's obligation to prevent the spread of AIDS gives rise to a moral issue that must be addressed forthrightly. Whether or not society should engage in screening programs in order to identify HIV carriers and, if yes, the scope of such programs are questions that must first be referred to epidemiologists for evaluation. On a primary level, the question is whether such testing is necessary or effective. But clearly, in some areas and for some segments of our population, the answer must be in the affirmative. Presumably, experts in such matters can analyze data and identify sociological and demographic criteria to be used in identifying classes of individuals for whom testing is indicated.

Assuming this to be the case, the moral issue that must be confronted is whether individuals may be compelled to submit to such testing against their will. Compulsory testing is certainly a gross violation of individual liberty. Should a possible HIV carrier be permitted to assert a right to personal autonomy in refusing to participate in such testing programs?

A resolution of this question must be sought within a much broader conceptual framework. Every culture and every society develops a matrix of values and ideals by which it seeks to define itself. The notions of freedom and personal autonomy figure prominently among the great American ideals to which our society subscribes. In a democratic country it is assumed that no one is told how to order his personal life or what risks he may or may not assume. Although individuals are restrained from committing antisocial acts, generally speaking, no one is compelled to perform positive acts against his will, even for his own good.

There is an unfortunate tendency among Jews to engage in a certain form of behavior that is best described as "me-too-ism." This behavior consists of asserting that whatever truths others have taught, we taught much earlier than they; whatever moral or social values they profess, they acquired from us. Of course, democracy and freedom are wonderful; indeed, everyone subscribes to those values. Ergo, they must be values that Judaism taught the world.

This point is illustrated by a German biblical scholar, Benno Jakob, in an intriguing monograph entitled *Auge um Auge*. His discussion focuses upon the concept of *lex talionis*—an eye for an eye, a tooth for a tooth, a hand for a hand, a foot for a foot. Jewish law never understood the biblical passage describing such punishment in a literal manner. There is no evidence whatsoever that such punishment was ever imposed by a Jewish court, no rabbinic text that advocates such punishment and no hint in talmudic sources that the text is to be understood in a literal manner. Halakhic Judaism has consistently interpreted the verse in question as demanding monetary compensation in the form of the value of an eye for an eye, the value of a tooth for a tooth etc. Nevertheless, over a period of millennia, this biblical passage has been cited repeatedly by individuals intent upon excoriating Jews and Judaism. Jews are depicted as a cruel and vengeful people. The law of the Pentateuch is decried as being excessively harsh and punitive in demanding retribution in the form of "an eye for an eye, a tooth for a tooth, a hand for a hand, a foot for a foot" (Exodus 21:24). How could such a widespread calumny arise if the doctrine of *lex talionis* was never part of Jewish teaching?

The misconception with regard to Jewish teaching was imparted to the nations of the world via the highly influential writings of Philo of Alexandria. Philo certainly cannot be described as a great halakhic scholar. But Philo was not a total ignoramus either. He certainly must have known that, in terms of Jewish tradition, his rendition was a gross misinterpretation of the biblical verse in question. How, then, could he portray this doctrine so erroneously and allow the nations of the world, through his writings in the vernacular, to acquire such a distorted view of rabbinic teaching? The answer, asserts Benno Jakob, is very simple. Philo was an Alexandrian Jew. In the Hellenistic society in which he lived, turning the other cheek was not regarded as a character trait worthy of emulation. To be the victim of a bad turn and not to respond in kind was viewed as a mark of weakness, as a sign of a lack of manliness. A real man demands his pound of flesh. In that society, virility demanded standing upon one's rights and insisting upon retribution, measure for measure. Apologists of antiquity assumed that if such is the value to which society at large subscribes, if such is the accepted ideal, than it must be a Jewish value, a Jewish ideal and a Jewish goal as well. Accordingly, in order to demonstrate that Jews were no less Hellenistic than the Greeks, Philo cited a biblical verse and interpreted it in a literal manner.[4] Jews could then engage in "me-tooism"; Jews could claim to have been the ones who taught this value system to the rest of the world.

However, the values of the world, indeed, of any particular

society, change not simply from generation to generation and from decade to decade, but from month to month and even from week to week. Values that were accepted and lauded yesterday are rejected and decried today. In sharp contradistinction, the teachings of Judaism are eternal; those eternal verities are not subject to change. One must be extremely careful to spell out Jewish values with precision and fidelity and not attempt to tailor them to what happens to be in vogue during any particular historical epoch.

This insight is particularly germane with regard to the right to privacy. The right to privacy was first recognized by the U.S. Supreme Court in 1965 in *Griswold* v. *Connecticut.*[5] It took American jurists more than one hundred and seventy-five years to discover a constitutionally guaranteed right to privacy. And even then the members of the nation's highest court could not agree with regard to which of the various provisions of the Bill of Rights serves as the locus of that right. Nevertheless, prominent Jewish thinkers have asserted that the notion of a fundamental right to privacy is something that Judaism taught 2,000 years ago.[6] Such a statement may not be totally erroneous, but, if the statement is intended to connote a right of privacy whose boundaries are as far-reaching as those enunciated by American courts, it is far from totally correct.[7] Certainly, there exist a plethora of rabbinic enactments that were promulgated over the ages that are designed to preserve and to protect particular rights of privacy. For example, if my neighbor and I enjoy adjacent courtyards, I have the right to compel him to contribute fifty percent of the cost of erecting a fence so that each of us may enjoy the use of his respective backyard in privacy (*Bava Batra* 2a). To be sure, *Sema, Ḥoshen Mishpat* 154:10, asserts that, according to some authorities, this is a biblically mandated requirement based upon rabbinic interpretation of the verse "And Balaam lifted up his eyes and he saw Israel dwelling tribe by tribe" (Numbers 24:2). "What did he see?" queries the Gemara, *Bava Batra* 60a. "He saw that the doors of their tents were not aligned one facing the other," answers the Gemara. But even according to these authorities, the requirement reflects, not a right to privacy, but an obligation of *ẓeni'ut* (modesty) as evidenced by the fact that these authorities rule that this requirement cannot be forgiven by agreement of the parties. Rights can be waived; religious obligations are not subject to disposition by acquiescence of the parties. Other scholars maintain that the underlying rationale is that interference with another person's use and enjoyment of his property constitutes a tort[8] and hence reflects a property interest rather than a personal right to privacy. If this provision of Jewish law is to be regarded as reflective of a right to privacy, it could be so only as the result of a specific rabbinic ordinance establishing a particular right of such nature.[9]

Similarly, in approximately the year 1000, Rabbenu Gershom promulgated an ordinance forbidding a person to read his neighbor's mail. Prior to that enactment there was no general right to privacy that served to assure a person that his correspondence would be inviolate. Specific rabbinic legislation was required in order to establish such a right and specific legislation is required in order to expand such rights.[10] Were we privileged to live in an organized Jewish community having duly appointed rabbinic authorities vested with legislative power they would presumably recognize the need to promulgate decrees banning nonconsensual wiretapping. But, in the absence of such legislation, it is far from obvious that matters such as wiretapping or electronic surveillance are proscribed by Jewish law under the general rubric of a right to privacy inherent in Jewish law.[11]

Obviously, an individual's right to privacy may come into conflict with the needs and concerns of society. American constitutional jurisprudence recognizes that there must be a balancing of interests and that, when there exists a sufficiently significant state interest, protection of that interest takes precedence over the rights of the individual.

Personal liberty may be compromised for promotion of the general welfare of society; but fundamental rights may be infringed only in the presence of a compelling state interest.[12] Judaism posited something akin to the notion of a compelling state interest long before that concept arose in American constitutional law. In the case of an individual who poses a threat to society, the individual's rights to autonomy and integrity of his person are subordinated to the needs of society to the extent necessary to eliminate the perceived threat. That is the case even if the individual in question is in no way morally culpable. In its most extreme form, the irrelevance of legal or moral culpability in such instances is manifest in "the law of the pursuer" (*rodef*), a provision of Jewish law that pertains in situations in which an individual endangers the life of another. Such an individual must be restrained in order to eliminate the threat to others. Most significantly, if the only manner in which the aggressor may effectively be restrained is by putting him to death, it is not only permissible but mandatory to take the life of that individual in order to preserve the life of the innocent victim. Unlike American law, which recognizes only a right to self-defense vested in the potential victim, Jewish law posits an obligation to eliminate the aggressor in order to save the victim and regards that obligation as binding not only upon the putative victim but also upon a bystander or a third party who is in no way personally threatened. The obligation to prevent the aggressor from carrying out his planned act of aggression mandates the intervention of every individual—and hence of society as the aggregate of its members—provided that it is possible to rescue the victim. As a duty owed the victim, the discharge of this obligation is in no way contingent upon moral turpitude on the part of the aggressor.

In his classic formulation of the law of the pursuer, Rambam, *Hilkhot Roẓeaḥ* 1:9, posits a situation in which the fetus threatens the life of the mother as the sole exception to the prohibition against feticide. Elimination of the fetus under such circumstances is justified, according to Rambam, because the fetus is a *rodef*, an aggressor bent upon causing the death of its mother. Assuredly, the fetus intends no harm to its mother. Certainly, the developing embryo is entirely without guilt. But the concern is not with assigning moral culpability or punishing a perpetrator. The concern is the defense of the victim. To say that the putative victim must be defended even against blameless aggression is to recognize the legitimacy of society's exercise of its compelling interest in restraining violence. Judaism clearly recognizes that society has the right to interfere with the exercise of individual autonomy and to infringe upon the liberty of its members in order to protect the lives of members of society at large.

To be sure, the legal system of the country in which we live exhibits far greater solicitude for individual autonomy than does Jewish tradition. Nevertheless, the American legal system also recognizes that liberty is a value that must be subordinated when it comes into conflict with a superior value. Given an appropriate state interest, individual liberties may be restricted to the extent necessary to secure that interest.[13] The concerns that augur in favor of mandatory testing programs for identification of AIDS carriers are certainly quite compelling.[14] Although there are indeed a number of constitutional issues that must be addressed,[15] the crucial problem is practical rather than theoretical; the most significant problem is how to design and implement testing programs that will effectively protect the lives and health of members of society at large.

That problem is closely related to the second in the series of issues that confront us with regard to AIDS, *viz.*, the question of confidentiality. Even more problematic than establishment of the screening program itself is utilization of information gained as the result of testing. The right to privacy, a firmly established commitment to a code of professional confidentiality and the well-placed fear of a negative economic and social impact upon individuals identified as AIDS victims or HIV carriers combine to militate against any form of disclosure, no matter how restricted.[16] Nevertheless, it would be of only limited benefit to engage in mass screening if the results are to be withheld from the very people who require the information derived therefrom for their protection. Certainly, the minimal step of making that information available to the victims themselves would undoubtedly contribute in some degree to the mitigation of the spread of AIDS. If they are responsible people, individuals who learn that they are afflicted will comport themselves in an appropriate manner and will minimize the risk to others. But, unfortunately, not all members of society behave responsibly. In some circumstances, it is morally imperative to violate confidentiality by divulging such information to other persons who are found to be at risk so that they may be enabled to take precautions in order to eliminate or to minimize the risk of contagion.

Who should be entitled to know that a particular person is an AIDS victim or an HIV carrier? Under what circumstances should that information be divulged? Some time ago, a young man who is a practicing dentist on the staff of a major medical center on the West Coast informed me that only a short time earlier he had examined a patient in his clinic and discovered mouth lesions that he was fairly certain were associated with AIDS. He sent the patient to a laboratory for a diagnostic test but, when he called for the results, he was told that he was not entitled to become privy to that information. The dentist proceeded to explain the obvious. Putting aside the risks assumed by health-care professionals involved in treatment of such patients, some dental procedures are simply inappropriate in the case of individuals who, to put it mildly, do not enjoy a favorable longevity anticipation. It is not at all prudent to devote the time, effort and expense that must be expended in preparing multiple crowns if the patient is also an AIDS victim for the simple reason that such a person's dental needs can be met in a manner that requires the expenditure of far less time, effort and expense, not to speak of a lesser degree of risk to the health-care provider. These concerns are even more germane when treatment involves expenditure of public funds. This may be a relatively trivial example of the relevance of the health-care provider's need to be apprised of the diagnosis in order to provide proper treatment for the patient, but it is an important example nevertheless. There are health-care decisions for which a total medical evaluation is a necessary prerequisite. It is simply not good medicine to make such determinations on the basis of incomplete information.

Furthermore, the medical practitioner is entitled to information necessary to protect his own health and life. A physician should not be required to expose himself to risk in performing an elective procedure designed to effect a marginal enhancement of the quality of life of the patient. Even if a physician is foolhardy enough to agree to assume the risks to himself that such a procedure may involve, he has no right to create a situation in which nurses and support staff are exposed to risks over which they have no control. Moreover, even in situations in which the physician acknowledges that he would perform the procedure regardless of the risks of contagion because that situation warrants assumption of the risks involved, the physician is entitled to avail himself of precautions designed to minimize the risks to himself and to others. Such information is essential because a physician cannot be expected to assume that every patient is a potential AIDS victim. Constant vigilance is a human impossibility.[17]

The problems become even more complex when the issue is whether or not to divulge the diagnosis to individuals not directly involved in the treatment of the patient. What are the physician's obligations in the case of a patient who is afflicted with a sexually transmissible disease and the physician knows that the patient is engaged to be married but the patient refuses to reveal this information to his prospective spouse?

In general, the teachings of Judaism are most protective

with regard to confidentiality. There is probably no other ethical, moral or religious system that regards innocent gossip concerning another individual's affairs to be a serious transgression of divine law. "You shall not go as a bearer of tales among your people" (Leviticus 19:16) prohibits gossip-mongering even if the information divulged in no way results in substantive harm or prejudice to the interests of the person whose affairs are divulged. Disclosure of another person's private affairs without prior authorization is clearly forbidden.[18] Nevertheless, consistent with the hierarchical ranking of values that is reflected throughout the wide spectrum of Jewish law, those prohibitions are suspended on a "need to know" basis in situations in which disclosure of such information is required in order to avert a threat to life, health or even financial loss.

Consider the case of a patient who has consulted a physician and the physician becomes aware of the fact that the patient is subject to periodic epileptic fits which cannot be controlled by medication. The physician is also aware of the fact that this patient holds a driver's license that he refuses to surrender voluntarily. What are the obligations of the physician under such circumstances?

The answer is quite clear. The physician is obligated to bring the matter to the attention of the appropriate officials in the Department of Motor Vehicles so that they may take action to remove a potential menace from the highways. Indeed, the American legal system recognizes such principles as well. In most states, if not all, physicians are under legal obligation to report instances of child abuse as well as occurrences of sexually transmissible diseases to designated authorities. The privileged nature of the physician-patient relationship is not absolute. Under some circumstances, breach of professional confidentiality is not only warranted, but mandated. Professional confidentiality cannot in itself be used as an excuse to withhold information with regard to the danger of AIDS contagion in circumstances in which there is a pressing need for particular individuals to be aware of the fact that a certain person is afflicted with AIDS. Presently accepted codes of ethics adhered to by members of both the medical and legal professions recognize an exception to the obligation of maintaining professional secrecy when the patient or client plans to endanger others. In a number of cases, courts have ruled that disclosure of such information is required by law.[19] An AIDS victim's determination to continue to engage in unprotected sexual acts is entirely analogous to a marksman's announced intention to engage in Russian roulette with a person other than himself on the receiving end of the bullet. Surely, under such circumstances, protection of human life should take precedence over preservation of professional secrecy.[20]

There is, however, one significant consideration that must be assessed with regard to the issue of whether or not to disclose information of this nature to sexual partners of AIDS victims. There is an ongoing debate within the medical community with regard to whether disclosure on a routine basis will save lives or, in terms of total impact, actually cost lives. It may well be the case, as some contend, that a significant number of possible AIDS victims will refuse to submit to diagnostic testing unless they are assured of complete and absolute confidentiality with regard to the results of such tests. Accordingly, it is argued, in order to assure maximum success for proposed screening programs and to guarantee that all people at risk will indeed be tested for the presence of AIDS, confidentiality must be scrupulously respected. Otherwise, a significant number of people will refuse to be tested; even if the testing program is mandatory in nature, fear of disclosure will inevitably lead to evasion. Revealing a diagnosis of AIDS infection to sexual partners would certainly result in the saving of lives. But, it is contended, such a policy will lead to the loss of a greater number of lives since, once existence of a disclosure policy becomes a matter of public knowledge, undiagnosed victims of AIDS will avoid testing because of their fear of disclosure. Many of those undiagnosed victims, if they were made aware of their condition under conditions of confidentiality, would act in a responsible manner, i.e., they would desist from further conduct that places others at risk and might also be induced to inform spouses or other sexual partners of possible infection that may already be present so that those partners might also be tested. If, because they refuse to submit to testing, such AIDS victims or HIV carriers remain unidentified there is every likelihood that those undiagnosed individuals will infect others unknowingly. Hence, goes the argument, the net effect of a policy of involuntary disclosure would be a greater toll in terms of lives lost to AIDS infection. If this argument is factually correct, a policy of disclosure would itself create a menace to public health. I am not entirely convinced that such a prognosis is correct, but if it were shown to be empirically accurate, it would generate a genuine moral dilemma.[21]

There is a strong temptation to dismiss the argument peremptorily on the grounds that the danger to a present, already identified sexual partner is clear and imminent, while the potential danger resulting from lack of future success in securing the cooperation of possible victims of AIDS in submitting to testing is vague and hypothetical. Moreover, the sexual partner is clearly identifiable as a person who is endangered by another. As such, the sexual partner has a clear moral claim to rescue. In contradistinction, disclosure does not yield any identifiable victim. Moreover, the person who declines to be tested is responsible for his own fate and, since the screening program is available to him, he has no further claim upon others. Sexual partners of unscreened victims exist only as a statistical probability. Hence, no particular individual is in a position to present a moral demand for rescue from contagion.

However, on closer examination, such a conclusion can be rebutted. There can be little doubt that, under ordinary circumstances, in a hypothetical situation in which one is confronted by two groups of individuals whose lives are endangered and it is impossible to rescue both groups, preference should be given to saving the lives of the greatest number of people. Insofar as Jewish law is concerned, the crucial issues with regard to the problems under discussion are whether the group of potentially undiagnosed AIDS victims and the individuals to whom they may transmit the disease are to be classified as individuals whose lives are endangered and, if so, whether specificity versus lack of specificity in identification of victims plays a role in such determinations.

In rabbinic literature, discussion of the definition of danger occurs in the context of suspension of ritual prohibitions in an endeavor to save the life of an endangered person. It is well established that such strictures are suspended on behalf of an individual who can be described as a *ḥoleh le-faneinu*, a term that is literally translated as "a patient before us." Thus, R. Ezekiel Landau, *Noda bi-Yehudah, Yoreh De'ah*, II, no. 210, ruled that, although all Sabbath prohibitions are suspended on behalf of a patient who is already ill, nevertheless, a mother may not boil milk on the Sabbath on the plea that perhaps her young child may suddenly become seriously ill and may immediately require a hot beverage in order to promote recovery.

The concept of a *ḥoleh le-faneinu* was formulated by *Noda bi-Yehudah* in the context of a ruling concerning autopsies. He declared that a post-mortem examination, involving, as it does, violation of the prohibition against defiling a corpse, may be performed in anticipation of deriving medical information of potential value in treating a patient already afflicted with a similar malady but that such a procedure may not legitimately be performed simply in order to advance scientific knowledge.[22]

Nevertheless, it is not necessary that a patient actually occupy a hospital bed in order to satisfy the criterion of *ḥoleh le-faneinu*. Consider the situation in which there is an epidemic that is spreading but has, as yet, not reached a particular locale, although it is anticipated that it will do so. May restrictions pertaining to the observance of the Sabbath or of Holy Days be violated in instituting prophylactic measures necessary to prevent the spread of disease even though the disease is, as yet, not rampant in that locale? *Ḥazon Ish, Oholot* 22:32 and *Yoreh De'ah* 208:7, rules unequivocally that such procedures are permitted and, indeed, that their implementation must be regarded as mandatory.[23] It is not necessary that a particular patient actually be stricken and lie before us; it is sufficient that the danger be identifiable. The distinction lies in the fact that the sick patient is already endangered whereas the possibility of the child becoming ill is merely statistical and hypothetical in nature.[24]

Yet another question was posed by the late Chief Rabbi of Israel, Rabbi Iser Yehudah Unterman, concerning a battlefield situation.[25] Although the issue raised by Rabbi Unterman concerned possible establishment of organ or tissue banks in time of war, the question can readily be reformulated in a more basic form. May an army regiment setting out to do battle on the Sabbath take with it a field hospital to be set up before engaging in battle? In that situation, infraction of Sabbath restrictions is required long before there is a single casualty and even before there is any actual danger of casualties. Rabbi Unterman ruled that even such a situation is tantamount to that of a *ḥoleh le-faneinu*. Warfare, by its very nature, entails casualties; it must be assumed that soldiers will be wounded in the course of battle. Therefore, the decision to engage in military hostilities, in and of itself, generates a danger even though a single shot has as yet not been fired. Although it is quite true in the battlefield situation that there is no "patient before us" in a literal sense and, prior to commencement of hostilities, no actual danger can be said to exist, nevertheless, the cause of danger is already present. The decision to engage in battle is itself the proximate cause of danger and whenever the cause of danger is present the situation is comparable to that of a *ḥoleh le-faneinu*.

Consider also the case of a far-flung settlement in which it has been statistically determined that there will be a multiple number of medical crises within any given twenty-four hour period. May the sole ambulance driver or nurse accompanying a patient to the hospital return to the settlement on *Shabbat* on the strength of the statistical probability that the services of the vehicle or of the nurse will be required during the course of the day? In such cases as well, there have been a number of rabbinic rulings to the effect that, when statistics indicate that there is a reasonable likelihood of a medical emergency, Sabbath restrictions must be ignored.[26] Those rulings establish that statistical probability of danger constitutes the halakhic equivalent of a *ḥoleh le-faneinu*.[27]

It would appear to this writer that the selfsame principles are equally applicable to triage issues. When faced with an immediate emergency any person capable of preserving a life is obligated to do so. When it is impossible to rescue all who are endangered, time and resources should be allocated with a view to maximizing the number of lives preserved. An emergency-room physician may find himself confronted by a dilemma. Half a dozen victims of a single accident arrive simultaneously. One of the victims has sustained multiple fractures, is in shock and has difficulty breathing. He requires the immediate and undivided attention of the emergency-room physician if he is to survive. The others present have arterial bleeding, but no other life-threatening problems. If left unattended, they will bleed to death; if tourniquets are applied quickly, they will all survive. Certainly the physician will save the lives of those five accident victims even though that course of action entails abandonment of the seriously ill patient who requires more complex treatment. It is equally obvious that the physician may not abandon all of the victims in order to catch a plane to attend a medical conference on the plea that he may conceivably learn something at the conference that will perhaps one day save the lives of even a larger number of patients. Nevertheless, assuming that statistically predictable events are treated as present dangers, ignoring a present patient may be justifiable if that is the sole available method of obviating a future calamity that is otherwise certain to occur.

It has been alleged that British intelligence, making use of a device code-named *Ultra*, was able to decipher German codes and as a result became aware of Nazi plans to bomb Coventry some hours before the commencement of aerial bombardment. There was sufficient time for the citizens of the town to have been evacuated. But Winston Churchill refused to allow information regarding the imminent attack to be divulged and permitted the inhabitants of that city to perish as a result of the bombing. His argument was that, were he to divulge information regarding the impending danger, Nazi intelligence would quickly determine how that information came into British hands and the Germans would immediately take countermeasures to assure the security of their communications. British intelligence concerning German military operations would inevitably have been compromised and, argued Churchill, the net result would have been graver danger and the loss of an even greater number of lives.[28] If it is assumed that a known future danger is to be regarded in the same category as a present, imminent danger, provided that it is certain or virtually certain that the future danger will become actual, there may well be grounds to justify ignoring the imminent danger to a smaller number in order to prevent future danger to a larger number of people.

If it were to be established that identification of AIDS victims and divulgence of that information to sexual partners would ultimately result in the loss of a greater number of lives, a case could well be made for passively refraining from disclosing that information. However, I am not at all certain that loss of an even larger number of lives would be the necessary result of such a policy. Moreover, even if this would be the inevitable result of treating confidentiality as inviolate, it is a contingency that we need not necessarily face if society is prepared to adopt other measures. If we are prepared to demand that individuals at risk for AIDS be tested and to institute compulsory diagnostic programs to assure compliance, there may be a method available that would serve to protect sexual partners without divulging privileged information in violation of patient confidentiality.

The dilemma posed by a choice between preservation of confidentiality and preservation of lives might be avoided by adopting a policy of compulsory AIDS testing analogous to IRS policy regarding income tax evasion. Certain classes of people and persons claiming certain deductions are suspect. Those individuals find that their annual income tax returns are scrutinized, and scrutinized repeatedly. In addition, a certain percentage of returns are randomly selected for audit on the basis of no particular criteria. The net result is that when a person receives a form letter inviting him to a session with an IRS auditor he does not know whether he is one of a group of people who have been randomly selected or whether his invitation came as a result of some aspect of his income tax return that triggered an audit. Together with a program for testing members of high-risk groups, it is possible to institute an accompanying program of random testing as well. The effect of such a combined program would make it possible to select individuals for testing without divulging to them that thay have been selected because they have been identified as sexual partners of AIDS victims.

To be sure, a program of this nature would serve to identify only already existing AIDS conditions contracted as a result of sexual intercourse with victims of AIDS but would not prevent continued, unprotected sexual intercourse with presently diagnosed victims that unwittingly places the sexual partner at risk. It would be necessary to secure a commitment from the patient binding him to refrain from endangering others. The patient would be informed that his confidentiality would be respected only so long as he abided by his commitment.

Such a program affords the possibility for development of a policy that should diminish qualms regarding violation of confidentiality. If the sexual partner is free from infection, the

AIDS victim can be told quite forthrightly that, if he refrains from exposing his partner to further risk, his privacy will be fully respected, but should he fail to do so, it will become necessary to reveal his status as an AIDS victim or as an HIV carrier to the endangered party. It should not prove difficult to fabricate reasons to remain in contact with the potentially endangered party in order to ascertain whether or not an ongoing danger exists. To be sure, the possibility of transmission of HIV before discovery of the carrier's breach of commitment remains. The statistical likelihood of contagion under the contemplated circumstances must be carefully assessed and confidentiality preserved only if the hazard is judged to be minimal.

The threat of disclosure would certainly serve as a strong motive in discouraging hazardous sexual activity with a known, already identified sexual partner. Short of quarantine measures,[29] it is impossible to prevent an irresponsible victim from endangering a newly found sexual partner. There are undoubtably some devious people who, with malice aforethought, will avoid testing because they are determined to continue to engage in unsafe sexual practices even if it might prove to be the case that they are infected. It may, however, be assumed that the number of such thoroughly irresponsible people is relatively small. Most people who would seek to avoid testing would probably do so only because of a dread of the certainty of disclosure regardless of preventive or prophylactic measures they might be prepared to take in the future.

It should be recognized that such a policy would not constitute a panacea and would not eliminate sexual transmission of AIDS totally and completely. Whether or not such measures represent a prudent and acceptable means of limiting contagion probably cannot be determined other than by attempting their implementation.

2. *Use of Condoms*

Transmission of HIV during intercourse can be prevented only by assuring that there is no contact with the body fluids of the carrier. The only effective method of preventing such contact is utilization of a condom during intercourse.[30] For Jewish patients, the use of a condom when engaging in marital relations is a matter for the couple to discuss with a competent rabbinic decisor. Use of a condom, as well as utilization of other contraceptive methods, in situations in which pregnancy constitutes a danger to the life of the female partner is a matter that has received considerable discussion and analysis in rabbinic literature. Some authorities are prepared to sanction a wide variety of other contraceptive measures, but not use of a condom, even in situations in which pregnancy poses a distinct threat to the life of the female partner. Others are willing to permit use of a condom in situations in which pregnancy poses a grave threat to the life of the mother.

A thorough review of the permissibility of contraception in the presence of danger is beyond the scope of this endeavor. In oversimplifying a complex issue it may be said that those authorities who permit the use of a diaphragm and/or a condom in circumstances in which pregnancy poses a significant hazard do so either on the theory that protected intercourse is normal and natural in situations in which pregnancy would endanger the life of the female[31] or on the theory that, since the woman is not required—and indeed is forbidden—to endanger her life, the sole telos of intercourse in such circumstances is the sexual gratification of the female and hence prevention of conception is not prohibited.[32]

Although the classic discussions of this issue focus upon situations in which pregnancy, rather than unprotected intercourse per se, constitutes the danger to life of the female, it appears to this writer that those considerations are equally applicable in siutations in which intercourse itself poses the danger. Moreover, the considerations that serve to render contraception permissible in situations involving danger to the female serve, *mutatis mutandis*, to render contraception equally permissible when the danger is to the male, *viz.*, when it is the husband who is at risk for contracting AIDS from his wife. It must, however, be reiterated that some authorities forbid use of a condom under any circumstances on the grounds that coitus involving use of a condom constitutes an "unnatural" form of intercourse.[33]

3. *The Physician's Self-Endangerment*

Another issue that must be addressed is the question of the physician's obligations to his patients and to himself. Does the physician have a right to refuse to expose himself to an infectious disease? In particular, does the physician have a right to decline to treat a patient who is afflicted with AIDS? The prevailing view in our society is that physicians have special and unique responsibilities. Although they are under no legal obligation to do so, physicians are expected to accept risk to themselves in order to save the lives of others.[34] The American Medical Association's official policy statement regarding AIDS states that "a physician may not ethically refuse to treat a patient whose condition is within the physician's current realm of competence solely because the patient is seropositive."[35] It must however be stated that, according to Jewish teaching, a physician has no greater responsibility than any other individual to jeopardize his own life on behalf of others.[36] To be sure, his responsibility is not lesser in nature than that of any other person, but it is not enhanced by his choice of profession. The crucial moral issue is whether, and under what circumstances, an individual is obligated to expose himself to danger in order to preserve the life of another. Our society views altruistic self-endangerment on behalf of others as commendable and exemplary; our society regards the sacrifice of one's own life to save the life of another as a virtue of the highest order. Not so Judaism. There are, to be sure, examples of such sacrificial conduct in Jewish literature and in rabbinic writing, but those references constitute exceptions rather than the rule and each of the exceptions requires halakhic elucidation and justification.

The basic principle is established in a hypothetical situation recounted in the Gemara, *Bava Meẓi'a* 62a. Two people are wandering in the desert and lose their way. One of them possesses a small container of water. The water in the container is sufficient only to enable one person to survive long enough to make his way out of the desert. If they divide the water equally both will die of thirst. There is a sharp difference of opinion among the Sages of the Talmud with regard to the proper course of action. The normative position enunciated by R. Akiva is that the owner of the water should not sacrifice himself on behalf of his companion but should drink all of the water himself in order to save his own life. The principle is derived from the biblical verse "And your brother shall live with you" (Leviticus 25:36). Man is admonished to do everything possible to preserve the life of his fellow so that both may enjoy life together, but not to surrender his life on behalf of his fellow. The obligation is to enable a brother to live *with you*, but not to give him precedence over yourself. Accordingly, one's own life takes precedence over the life of one's neighbor. A person may not commit what is tantamount to suicide in order to save someone else's life. One should love one's neighbor as much as oneself, but not more than oneself. An individual's obligations to himself take precedence over any comparable obligation that he owes to his fellow.

Fortunately, in the real world, most situations in which one is called upon to preserve the life of another do not require self-martyrdom. Such situations usually do not involve certain death for the rescuer. Most situations involve only the possibility of death. A person who jumps into turbulent water in an effort to save someone who cannot swim may be carried out to sea by an undertow, but it is far from certain that this will happen. One eminent authority, R. Joseph Karo, *Kesef Mishneh, Hilkhot Roẓeaḥ* 1:14 and *Bet Yosef, Ḥoshen Mishpat* 426, asserts that elimination of the certain danger to the life of a fellow takes precedence over possible danger to oneself. Nevertheless, the normative rule posited by Judaism is that no individual is obligated to place himself in serious danger even if failure to do so will result in the certain death of another individual.[37] He may do so if he so wishes, provided that the circumstances are such that it is not certain that his own life will be forfeit. Indeed, in some circumstances, it would be commendable to accept a measure of danger in order to save the life of another, but there is no absolute obligation to do so.

The obligations of a physician are no different from those of any other individual. A physician has no obligation to place his own life in serious jeopardy in order to save the life of another. Assuredly, he may do so if he so wishes, but he is not duty-bound to endanger himself.

That statement must, however, be clarified and made more precise. An individual need not place himself in danger in order to save the life of another. However, the term "danger" requires careful elucidation. Physicians may become victims of automobile accidents, as is the case with regard to all who expose themselves to vehicular travel. May, then, a physician refuse to make a house call or refuse to make rounds in the hospital on the basis of a plea that he does not wish to subject himself to the danger inherent in driving his automobile in order to reach the patient? The answer, I believe, is that, under normal conditions, the level of danger involved in the operation of a motor vehicle is below the threshold of what is recognized as "danger" for purposes of Jewish law. The term "danger" is a technical term in Jewish law and is endowed with a fairly precise definition. A comprehensive analysis of danger as a halakhic concept is beyond the scope of the present endeavor. Suffice it to say that in order to avoid an obligation to rescue the life of another on grounds of self-endangerment, the danger to the life of the person called upon to perform an act of rescue must be actual and significant and must be perceived as such by prudent persons. Actions entailing a level of risk perceived as insubstantial in nature are not within the category of "danger" recognized by Jewish law.

Rabbi Iser Yehudah Unterman presents a brief yet intriguing statement in which he establishes a rule of thumb for delineating the level of danger that must be assumed in rescuing another individual.[38] Rabbi Unterman remarks that if someone wishes to know whether he should accept a certain level of danger or whether that level of danger is sufficiently high that he may legitimately refuse to do so because he does not wish to expose himself to risk, the individual should ask himself a simple question. The individual should imagine to himself that the activity in which he is being asked to engage is not an activity designed to save a human life, but an activity designed to save one of his own cherished possessions. Let him imagine, for example, that it is not a human being who has fallen over the side of a ship but that it is a jewelry case that the wind has blown out of his hands and is now bobbing up and down in the water. If he wishes to determine whether he should jump into the stormy waters in order to save the drowning person's life he should ask himself whether he would do so in order to retrieve some cherished heirloom that had been blown overboard. Would he leap into the water in order to recover this irreplaceable and priceless object or would he regard such action as foolhardy and reckless? If the individual in question would assume that or a comparable risk in order to recover some item of value belonging to himself then he ought to treat the life of a fellow man as being of at least equal value and assume a comparable risk. But, if he can say with honesty that he would be willing to suffer serious financial loss because he deems the risk to be too great, then he can in good conscience similarly refuse to endanger his life for the purpose of rescuing the life of another.

Although Rabbi Unterman's statement may not constitute a definitive halakhic pronouncement to be applied rigorously in each and every situation, it certainly serves as an appropriate general approach. This rule of thumb can readily be applied in a medical context: If a physician wishes to know whether he should expose himself to a certain degree of risk, let him assume that the fee offered for the necessary treatment is an exorbitant one. Would he be willing to accept the risk in order to earn a small fortune? If the answer is in the affirmative he should also regard the preservation of a life as sufficient motive. Under such circumstances it should be anticipated that the physician will subject himself to the same degree of risk in order to preserve a human life without regard for the size of the fee or even the absence thereof. For a medical practitioner treating patients in a clinical setting in which there is some danger to the physician, the appropriate rule of thumb is whether the physician regards the risk as being so grave that no possible fee would make the risk worthwhile to him. But if the same physician is prepared to set aside those concerns for a fee commensurate with the danger, it follows that, even if the patient is a charity case, the physician should be advised to accept the risk as inherent in what is expected of all human beings in terms of their obligations vis-à-vis their fellows.

Formulation of this standard does not imply that a physician can be *compelled* to assume such risk. Nor can it be said that there is no situation in which a physician is under absolute obligation to assume some measure of risk. There are some clinical situations in which a risk does exist but it is so minimal that it must be treated as non-existent. In such circumstances an absolute obligation does indeed exist. At the opposite end of the spectrum are circumstances in which the statistically calculable risk is so great that no one should be asked to place himself in jeopardy. But between those extremes there are instances in which the hazard is of a magnitude such that a physician would be well within his moral rights in declining to treat the patient but in which, recognition of the rights of the physician notwithstanding, society has the right to assure that medical treatment is rendered. It seems to me that society not only has the right but also the obligation to establish institutional structures that will assure its members appropriate medical care even when some hazards must be assumed by health-care professionals providing such care.

It must be recognized that there is a significant difference between the ethical obligations of an individual and the obligations of society as a whole. There is no obligation upon any individual to become a fireman, a policeman or a soldier in a volunteer army. Those professions require their members to expose themselves to an unusually high degree of risk. That is certainly evident from the fact that members of those professions are required to pay inordinately high premiums for life insurance. By the same token, society has both a need and an obligation to safeguard its citizens. The history of civilization indicates that an accommodation is possible that will guarantee both respect for rights of the individual and discharge of societal responsibility. Assuredly, society has a need to maintain law and order and a need to put out conflagrations. In order to achieve those ends society must establish a police force and assure that there are firemen on duty to combat fires. Accordingly, society seeks to do everything within its power to induce individuals to become members of a police force or of a fire department. Although, generally speaking, no particular person can be compelled to serve in such a capacity, society discharges its obligation by encouraging and enticing individuals to enter those professions. Society appeals to its members' sense of altruism in seeking to convince individuals to accept the risks associated with police work and fire-fighting out of a sense of moral responsibility. It also appeals to other less noble but nevertheless entirely legitimate motives in providing material inducements for acceptance of such positions.

Society is similarly in a position to assure that health-care professionals will expose themselves to risks of a similar magnitude in providing necessary medical care. The nature of contemporary practice of medicine is such that extremely few health-care professionals practice solo medicine in a literal sense of that term. Virtually no one can prosper in such a practice. Surgeons require operating theaters; physicians require staff privileges in hospitals and medical centers. Those perquisites are recognized as privileges by the medical community and, as privileges, they carry with them concomitant obligations. Most medical institutions require that members of their staffs spend a certain stipulated number of hours per week on a *pro bono* basis providing care in clinics established for the treatment of indigent patients. Such service is regarded as a form of payment for the privilege of utilizing the facilities of the hospital in treating fee-paying patients.

It is common knowledge that in most hospitals and medical centers there are more applicants for staff privileges than can possibly be accommodated by the facility. That is certainly the case with regard to any prestigious medical center. Society has the right to apportion such benefits in a manner that best serves to promote the discharge of society's own responsibilities. Any individual physician may choose to treat patients who pose a certain degree of risk to himself or he may elect not to treat such patients. But society may also say to the physician that it has an obligation to make a reasoned, rational and principled determination that certain risks must be borne by society as a whole. Accordingly, society may appropriately enter into a contract with a health-care professional in which it undertakes to provide him with certain privileges and benefits, but only on the condition that he agrees to accept a concomitant responsibility for the treatment of patients who do pose certain risks. The physician is, in essence, being asked to shoulder that responsibility as a delegate of society. In return, society makes certain resources and perquisites available to him.

Of course, society does not have the moral right to make

irresponsible demands upon any of its members. It may at times be difficult to determine precisely where the point of demarcation between responsible and irresponsible demands should be drawn. The risks associated with any given medical or surgical procedure can be assessed only by clinicians. But, upon assessment of the risk, rational and moral individuals should be able to reach a consensus in making a determination in any given situation with regard to whether assumption of that risk is responsible or foolhardy. When such risks are prudent, society has the right to seek the services of physicians who are willing to assume such risks and to reward them in an appropriate manner.

Society does not have the right to demand suicidal conduct on the part of the doctor, but society can demand that the physician assume reasonable and responsible risks in return for the privilege of drawing upon the resources of society. The physician, in choosing his profession, does not necessarily commit himself to the assumption of those responsibilities and is at liberty to decline to expose himself to danger, but society in its ongoing contract with the physician is not required to make its resources available to him other than upon a return of a *quid pro quo*.

It must be reiterated that society does not have the right to make unjustified and unreasonable demands upon the physician as part of this reciprocal contractual relationship. There are, for example, clinical circumstances in which a physician is entirely justified in refusing to perform procedures on behalf of an AIDS patient that are dangerous to himself. The first obligation of society may well be the determination of whether performance of a particular medical procedure is justified in light of the risk posed to others. As has been stated earlier, those are determinations that must be informed by ethical sensitivity but which, in the first instance, can best be made by clinicians. Thus, in light of the danger such procedures pose to the plastic surgeon, cosmetic surgery undertaken for purely aesthetic reasons probably would not be justified when performed upon an AIDS victim. Presumably, the benefit to the patient is not of a magnitude that warrants placing the physician's life at risk.

Moreover, in making even only reasonable demands upon a physician, society has a reciprocal obligation to minimize the risk to the physician insofar as possible. Others have drawn attention to the fact that not a single research dollar has been devoted to the perfection of a stick-proof latex glove. In my own discussions with an executive of a plastic manufacturing firm, I have been informed that this is a goal that is quite attainable. I have been assured that it is indeed possible to perfect a synthetic material from which a glove could be fashioned that would not be subject to punctures and perforations in the operating room but which at the same time would allow for requisite tactile sensation on the part of the surgeon wearing the glove. All that is required to turn that *desideratum* into a reality is the dedication of sufficient personnel, sufficient time and sufficient money to the necessary research and development.[39]

Certainly, society has an obligation to engage in research designed to perfect the technology necessary to minimize risks to its physician-agents and to devote its resources to that endeavor. Society has an obligation to minimize the dangers to health-care professionals in any and every way that is possible and practical. Society has an obligation to eliminate risks to health-care professionals no less so than it has a duty to provide treatment for patients whose lives are at risk.

4. *Taharah, Mikveh and Meẓiẓah*

Health-care providers are not the only ones who perceive themselves as being at risk as a result of contact with aids patients. Fear of contracting aids has, in recent years, led to numerous inquiries with regard to a number of areas of religious observance. Many of those questions are based upon an exaggerated fear of contagion. A number of years ago, a gentleman reported to me shortly before Passover that he wished to invite an AIDS patient to participate in his *seder* but was informed by members of his own family that if the invitation were to be extended they would absent themselves. There has been at least one report in an Anglo-Jewish newspaper of a chaplain who refused to enter the hospital room of an AIDS patient.[40] These are but examples of the near-hysteria which pervades our community.

Realization that AIDS can be spread only through direct contact with body fluids serves to dispel much of that fear. For example, there is no scientific basis for neglecting AIDS victims insofar as the *mizvah* of visiting the sick is concerned. Casual social contact simply does not pose any significant danger. There is no valid reason for withholding solicitude and comfort from those afflicted by that disease. Indeed, AIDS victims require such ministration more so than most patients.

Some rabbinic figures have advised that a *taharah*, the ritual washing of the body of the deceased, need not be performed on behalf of a person who has succumbed to complications of AIDS.[41] The underlying rationale is unexceptional, i.e., members of the *ḥevra kaddisha* (burial society) need not expose themselves to infectious disease in discharging their duties. Nevertheless, application of that principle in the treatment of AIDS victims is the product of misinformation and hence is erroneous. It is believed that the AIDS virus does not survive for more than a very brief period of time following the death of the victim.[42] Even assuming that the virus remain virulent, wearing shoes without open toes, rubber gloves and a protective garment effectively eliminates any possibility of contracting the disease. There is no halakhic impediment whatsoever to employment of such precautions.[43] When those precautions are taken, the danger of a member of the *ḥevra kaddisha* endangering himself by slipping on a wet floor and fracturing his skull is exponentially greater than the danger of contracting AIDS from a corpse. Quite apart from denying the deceased the honor and respect that is his due, withholding of a *taharah* from a person who has died of AIDS only serves to reinforce a misplaced but widespread fear of association with AIDS patients and unconscionably contributes to the isolation experienced by those who suffer from that dread disease.

A similar fear has arisen in some quarters with regard to the possible spread of AIDS as a result of immersion in the waters of a *mikveh*. That fear, as well, is greatly exaggerated. Neither potable nor recreational waters have been implicated in the transmission of HIV infections.[44] There is no evidence whatsoever that AIDS can be transmitted by body fluids diluted in the waters of a swimming pool or *mikveh*. Addition of chlorine to the *mikveh* because of this fear is both unnecessary and ineffective. Although chlorination of water may effectively prevent the spread of some bacteriological infections, the concentration necessary to be effective against the AIDS virus is too high to be tolerated under normal circumstances.[45] Fortunately, chlorination in order to prevent AIDS contagion is a totally unnecessary precaution.

Meẓiẓah ba-peh, i.e., oral suction in conjunction with circumcision, presents a much more serious problem. The infected blood of a baby harboring the AIDS virus may enter the blood stream of the *mohel* via a lesion or cut in his mouth. Although there is some evidence showing that saliva serves to protect against transmission of AIDS, the possibility of contracting AIDS in this manner cannot be ruled out at present.[46]

There are extensive discussions in rabbinic literature with regard to whether or not other forms of suction may be substituted for oral suction. A review of that material is beyond the scope of this discussion.[47] Nevertheless, a number of points should be made. Many authorities rule that it is entirely proper to perform *meẓiẓah* by means of a glass tube. However, as formulated by Rambam, *Hilkhot Milah* 2:2, the purpose of *meẓiẓah* is to assure the free flow of blood *mi-mekomot ha-reḥokim*, i.e., from beyond the exposed tissue at the site of the wound. The only way this can be effected is by creating a vacuum by means of suction action over the entire area of the circumcision incision. This can be accomplished only by means of a glass tube that encompasses the entire membrum and is placed tightly over the abdominal area. It cannot be accomplished by means of a pipette or capillary tube. Practically speaking, *mohalim* would need glass tubes of varying circumferences in order to perform *meẓiẓah* properly upon infants of different proportions. The *mohel* must also be knowledgeable and vigilant in creating a seal in which suction from *mekomot ha-reḥokim* can be accomplished.

Parenthetically, some *mohalim*, because of their fear of contracting AIDS, have recently adopted the practice of placing a gauze pad over the glans before performing oral suction. They delude themselves in believing that the danger to themselves is significantly mitigated thereby. Moreover, the interposition of a gauze pad makes it difficult, if not impossible, to cause blood to be drawn from *mekomot ha-reḥokim*.

Quite apart from considerations grounded in Halakhah, oral suction is preferred in some circles because of considerations derived from kabbalistic sources. Such considerations should undoubtedly be ignored were it the case that oral suction presents an unavoidable hazard to the well-being of the *mohel*. Fortunately, the danger to the *mohel* can be eliminated. Contrary to the assertions of some,[48] fear of AIDS should not deter *meẓiẓah ba-peh* in low-risk groups when that form of suction is desired on the basis of either considerations of Halakhah or custom provided that proper precautions are taken.[49]

AIDS is present in a neonate only when it is contracted from the mother. If a diagnostic test is performed upon the mother and the results are negative, the likelihood that the mother may be infected and have passed the virus to her child are extremely remote.[50] A *mohel* who is requested to perform oral suction is certainly within his rights in demanding that the mother be tested for the absence of HIV virus. This diagnostic test can be performed by a commercial laboratory either during pregnancy or after parturition and the results can be made available promptly in order to provide for timely performance of circumcision. This obvious solution to the *meẓiẓah* dilemma has been endorsed by R. Joseph Eliashiv in a letter published in *Sha'arei Halakhot*, no. 15 (Tishri 5749). Moreover, a member of the staff of the Center for Infectious Diseases in Atlanta has assured me in writing that a solution of 70% alcohol effectively destroys the AIDS virus.[51] Accordingly, the *mohel* may protect himself by carefully rinsing his mouth with an alcohol solution prior to circumcision. Use of 151 proof rum, readily available in any liquor store, is appropriate for this purpose.[52]

There is also available a pharmacological agent that has been shown effectively to inactivate the virus. Hiberstat, a topical antiseptic containing 0.5% chlorhexidine gluconate in 70% isopropyl alcohol, has been shown to inactivate HIV produced in all cultures within fifteen seconds.[53] That product cannot, however, be recommended for rinsing of the mouth both because of the toxic effects of isopropyl and because of the the toxic effect of chlorhexidine gluconate itself. However, Peridex, an oral rinse used in treatmentt of gingival inflamation also contains chlorhexidine gluconate. Although Peridex, manufactured by Proctor and Gamble, contains only 0.12% chlorhexidine gluconate in a base containing 11.61% alcohol, it has been shown to be effective against HIV.[54]Thus rinsing the mouth with Peridex for a period of 30 seconds provides a demonstrable level of protection.

For even greater effectiveness chlorhexidine gluconate may be combined with a higher concentration of ethanol alcohol. A preparation containing 0.12% chlorhexidine gluconate in 70% ethanol alcohol will serve to inactivate HIV quickly in a relatively short contact time. Chlorhexidine gluconate is available from pharmaceutical companies in a 20% solution. That solution should be combined with 151-proof rum in a ratio of 6 to 1,000, e.g., 0.12 ounce of chlorhexidine gluconate in 20 ounces of 151-proof rum or 0.24 ounce (a little less than

1/4 of an ounce) in 40 ounces of 151-proof rum. Higher concentrations should be avoided because toxicity studies have not been performed at higher levels. Use of this solution will combine the effectiveness of both alcohol and chlorhexidine gluconate and hence should obviate any lingering doubts concerning use of alcohol alone or of a lower concentration of chlorhexidine. Although no clinical studies have been performed, there is no reason to suspect that the combination will inactivate either agent. It should be noted that extreme care must be taken to prevent any solution containing chlorhexidine gluconate from coming into contact with the eyes or ears.

In summary, on the basis of the published reports and my own consultation with experts in the field, in light of the fact that their exposure is to persons in an extremely low risk group, those who require oral *meẓiẓah* need not abandon that practice because of fear of contracting AIDS. They have even less reason to abandon the practice if they take the precaution of having the mother tested for HIV virus. The *mohel* should, however, rinse his mouth for thirty seconds with Peridex, or for several minutes with 151-proof rum, or optimally, with a solution of chlorhexidine gluconate and 151-proof rum as indicated above.

NOTES

1. Norman Podhoretz, "How the Gay Rights Movement Won," *Commentary* (November 1996), p. 36, astutely notes that "the same logic would confer moral legitimization on pedophiles." Podhoretz presents an insightful analysis of attitudinal change toward homosexuality and of the literature addressing that phenomenon.
2. See *Sifra* to Leviticus 20:26.
3. See Ecclesiastes 7:20.
4. See Benno Jakob, *Auge um Auge* (Berlin, 1929), pp. 77–78.
5. *Griswold* v. *Connecticut*, 381 U.S. 479 (1965).
6. See, for example, Rabbi Emanuel Rackman, "Privacy in Juda-

ism," *Midstream*, vol. 28, no. 7 (November 1982), pp. 31–34; Rabbi Norman Lamm, "The Fourth Amendment and its Equivalent in the Halakhah," *Judaism*, vol. 16, no. 3 (Summer 1967), pp. 53–59; and Haim H. Cohn, *Human Rights in Jewish Law* (New York, 1984), pp. 64–67.

7. Rather than speaking of a general right of privacy, a more felicitous manner of describing privacy in Jewish law would be to say that specific prohibitions and prerogatives posited by Jewish law give rise to concomitant particular rights of privacy.

8. See, for example, R. Iser Zalman Meltzer, *Even he-Azel, Hilkhot Shekhenim* 2:16.

9. Thus, in discussing the type of material to be used in erecting a fence between adjacent properties, *Teshuvot R. Eliyahu Mizraḥi*, no. 8, writes that the material need not be of a nature that prevents eavesdropping by one neighbor upon the other "for we have not found in the entire Talmud a harm of such nature. . . . We are not concerned with 'hearing.'"

In a decision of the *Bet Din ha-Gadol le-Irurim* regarding the halakhic status of evidence obtained by wiretapping, R. Shlomoh Dichovsky asserts that Me'iri, *Bava Batra* 2a, espouses an opposing view in asserting that even the thinnest of walls is sufficient "and we are not at all concerned with the harm of 'hearing' for ordinary people are careful with regard to their utterances." Rabbi Dichovsky deduces from Me'iri's explanatory phrase, "for ordinary people are careful with regard to their utterances," that use of an adjacent courtyard is permitted because it poses no harm since a person can restrict his conversation so that private matters will not be overheard, but that activity such as electronic surveillance from which there is no protection is prohibited. See *Piskei Din shel Batei ha-Din ha-Rabbaniyim be-Yisra'el*, XIV, 329.

This writer, however, fails to see any basis for that inference. On the contrary, Me'iri should be understood as heralding the view expressed by R. Eliyahu Mizraḥi. Me'iri's comment is limited to the scope of the edict requiring erection of a fence between adjacent courtyards. Me'iri finds it necessary to explain that the edict was not expanded to encompass prevention of eavesdropping because the Sages found such expansion of their edict to be superfluous. Hence, Me'iri's comment substantiates the view that there exists no rabbinic edict banning the "harm of hearing."

10. There are, however, a number of recent opinions authored by

members of Israeli rabbinic courts in which the writers assert that electronic surveillance is encompassed in the edict of Rabbenu Gershom. Rabbi Abraham Sherman cites R. Chaim Palaggi, *Ḥikekei Lev, Yoreh De'ah*, no. 49, who suggests that Rabbenu Gershom based his edict upon the biblical admonition "And you shall love your neighbor as yourself" (Leviticus 19:18). That consideration, argues Rabbi Sherman, is equally applicable to electronic invasion of privacy. Rabbi Sherman also quotes the views of *Halakhot Ketanot* and *Torat Ḥayyim*, cited *infra*, note 11, and ascribes to the latter authority the view that "a person has proprietorship over all personal information and others have no right to take such information against his will and without his knowledge; such [action] entails [a violation of the] prohibition of 'a borrower without consent is a thief.'" In the opinion of this writer, that statement is conclusory and goes far beyond any statement found in the comments of *Torat Ḥayyim*. See *Piskei Din shel Batei ha-Din ha-Rabbaniyim be-Yisra'el*, XIV, 292–293. R. Chaim Shlomoh Rosenthal also cites one of the considerations advanced by *Ḥikekei Lev* as the rationale underlying the edict of Rabbenu Gershom in arguing that Rabbenu Gershom's edict is equally applicable to electronic surveillance. Rabbi Rosenthal, however, carefully notes that many authorities regard Rabbenu Gershom's edict as not applicable in situations involving potential harm or financial loss, although some authorities require destruction of the letter rather than reading its contents. See *Piskei Din shel Batei ha-Din ha-Rabbaniyim be-Yisra'el,* XIV, 307. Rabbi Dichovsky similarly cites *Ḥikekei Lev* in reaching the same conclusion. See *Piskei Din shel Batei ha-Din ha-Rabbaniyim be-Yisra'el,* XIV, 330.

Ḥikekei Lev advances four possible considerations in explaining why Rabbenu Gershom prohibited reading another person's letter: (1) "And you shall love your neighbor as yourself." (2) Seeking to discover the secrets of another person is a violation of the prohibition against tailbearing. This concept is formulated by *Halakhot Ketanot*, no. 276, but is not related by that authority to the edict of Rabbenu Gershom. (See *infra*, note 11.) (3) The prohibition against "stealing the mind" (*geneivat da'at*) of another. (4) The position of *Torat Ḥayyim*, III, no. 47, to the effect that reading another person's letter is tantamount to borrowing property without consent and, accordingly, is regarded as theft. Rabbi Rosenthal, *Piskei ha-Din shel Batei Din ha-Rabbaniyim be-Yisra'el,* XIV, 307, quite cogently notes that

Torat Ḥayyim's rationale is not applicable to wiretapping.

It is, however, not at all clear that *Ḥikekei Lev* regarded these considerations as establishing a prohibition in the absence of a formal edict. Indeed, each consideration is advanced only as a tentative rationale. *Ḥikekei Lev*, and certainly Rabbenu Gershom himself, may have regarded the opening of mail not as constituting a technical violation of the prohibitions cited, but as a violation of the values reflected in these prohibitions and, accordingly, pronounced a formal ban. If a formal ban was indeed necessary to engender a prohibition, there is no reason to assume that eavesdropping, either natural or electronic, was included in Rabbenu Gershom's edict. It seems certain that, in ruling in a case brought before him, *Teshuvot R. Eliyahu Mizraḥi*, cited *supra*, note 9, did not regard eavesdropping as a prohibited activity.

11. See, however, R. Jacob Hagiz, *Halakhot Ketanot*, no. 276, who prohibits any attempt to discover information concerning another person which that person wishes to remain concealed. *Halakhot Ketanot* regards disclosure of such information to be a prohibited form of talebearing in asserting (rather strangely) that bearing tales to oneself is no different from bearing tales to a third party. Cf., R. Chaim Shabbetai, *Teshuvot Torat Ḥayyim*, III, no 47, who declares that it is forbidden to cause any harm to another person and that "there is no doubt that . . . in the majority of cases disclosure of a person's secret will cause great harm and even if [the harm] will not be financial [it will cause harm] in some other matter."

12. A right is defined as fundamental if its abolition would violate a "principle of justice so rooted in the traditions and conscience of our people as to be ranked as fundamental." See *Snyder* v. *Massachusetts* 291 U.S. 97 at 105 (1933) and *Palko* v. *Connecticut*, 302 U.S. at 325 (1934). Among the rights recognized as fundamental are procreation, marriage, contraception, family relationships, child-rearing and education. See *Paul* v. *Davis*, 425 U.S. at 713. Regulations limiting a fundamental right may be enacted in order to satisfy a compelling state interest provided that the legislation is narrowly drawn to achieve only the legitimate state interest. See *Kramer* v. *Union Free School Dist. No. 15*, 395 U.S. 621.

13. In *Jacobson* v. *Massachusetts*, 197 U.S. 11, 25 (1905) the Supreme Court upheld a Massachusetts statute mandating vaccination against smallpox and ruled that it was enforceable even in face

of religious objections. In that opinion, written by Justice John Harlan, the Court acknowledged the importance of the individual's right to liberty but declared that such interest must yield to the state's right "to secure the general comfort, health, and prosperity," so long as the state does not act arbitrarily or oppressively. For an analysis of epidemic disease and the government's police power to enact reasonable regulations to preserve public health, safety, morals and welfare, as well as a discussion of HIV testing, see Janet L. Dolgin, "AIDS: Social Meanings and Legal Ramifications," *Hofstra Law Review*, vol. 14, no. 1 (Fall 1985), pp. 202–209; and Joanna L. Weissman and Mildred Childers, "Constitutional Questions: Mandatory Testing for AIDS Under Washington's AIDS Legislation," *Gonzaga Law Review*, vol. 24, no. 3 (1988–89), pp. 433–473.

14. Nevertheless, New York law, with certain exceptions, provides that no one may be tested for AIDS without providing informed consent. See New York Public Health Law §§2780–2787 (McKinney Supplement 1990).

15. Quite apart from the issue involving a general right to privacy, in *Schneider* v. *California* 384 U.S. 757 (1966) the Supreme Court found that compulsory administration of a blood test is a search restrained by the fourth amendment. Nevertheless, the Court found that administration of a blood alcohol test in the context of a vehicular homicide was a lawful search. For a discussion of the applicability of the criteria developed in *Schneider* to compulsory HIV testing, see "Constitutional Questions," pp. 454–461; and Paul H. MacDonald, "AIDS, Rape, and the Fourth Amendment: Schemes for Mandatory AIDS Testing of Sex Offenders," *Vanderbilt Law Review*, vol. 43, no. 5 (October 1990), pp. 1617–1627.

Another potential problem is possible violation of the Equal Protection clause of the fourteenth amendment which prohibits government action that discriminates against some individuals. Arguably, testing programs requiring mandatory testing of members of high-risk groups must include all persons who pose a risk to society and exclude all those who do not pose a serious risk. It is however also recognized that all classifications are imperfect. See "Mandating AIDS Testing," pp. 464–471.

For a discussion of these issues in connection with mandatory testing of public employees see Charles D. Curran, "Mandatory Testing of Public Employees for the Human

Immunodeficiency Virus: The Fourth Amendment and Medical Reasonableness," *Columbia Law Review*, vol. 90, no. 3 (April 1990), pp. 720–759.

16. In *Whalen* v. *Roe*, 429 U.S. 589 (1977) the Supreme Court recognized a privacy interest in preventing disclosure of personal medical information but nevertheless upheld legislation requiring pharmacists to report to appropriate state authorities the names and addresses of patients to whom prescription drugs were dispensed.

17. Moreover, mere suspicion of AIDS does not evoke the same vigilance that is aroused by actual knowledge of the presence of disease. That actual knowledge makes possible a higher degree of vigilance than does suspicion is reflected in an entirely different area of Halakhah. An individual who is not proficient in the laws of ritual slaughter may not serve as a *shoḥet* because of the concern that, unwittingly, he may perform the act improperly, e.g., he may stay his hand momentarily, apply pressure upon the knife, etc. If, however, a knowledgeable person stands over him and observes that the act has been performed properly, the animal is kosher, at least *post factum*. R. Akiva Eger, in his gloss on *Yoreh De'ah* 1:3, s.v. *mashma,* declares that this is so only if it is known with certainty before the act that the slaughterer is not proficient. If, however, the individual's incompetence is merely suspected, but not known with certainty, the animal is not regarded as kosher even though a competent observer certifies that the act of slaughter was performed properly. R. Akiva Eger cites comments of early-day authorities in establishing that proper vigilance is possible only when such vigilance is known to be absolutely necessary. When the need for vigilance is not clear, or merely suspected, the observer is simply unlikely to scrutinize the slaughterer's performance with the same attention and meticulousness.

    The identical principle applies, *mutatis mutandis,* with regard to AIDS. The physician who knows that his patient is infected will exercise extreme care. If he knows only that infection is a possibility, or even if he suspects but does not know that the patient is infected, sooner or later he will let his guard down. That is simply how the human psyche operates.

18. See R. Nissim of Gerondi, *Sha'arei Teshuvah*, *sha'ar* 3, no. 225.

19. See, for example, *Brady* v. *Hobber*, F.2d 329 (10th Cir. 1984) in which the Court held that a psychiatrist incurs a duty to warn a third party when a patient makes a specific threat to a partic-

ular person. See also *Taranoff* v. *Regents of the Univ. of Cal.*, 17 Cal. 3d 425, 551 P.2d 334, 131 Cal. Rptr. 14 (1976).

20. A number of states have enacted legislation to accomplish this end. Thus, for example, in 1987 California enacted a partner notification statute which permitted a physician to inform the person believed to be the patient's spouse of the results of a positive HIV test. A 1988 amendment of the statute broadens the category of notifiable persons to include sexual and needle sharing partners but the amendment also permits notification by the physician only after he has attempted to persuade the patient to make the disclosure himself. See *California Health & Safety Code* §199.25 (West Supp. 1990). New York allows disclosure only after the physician counsels the subject regarding the need to notify the contact and has formed reasonable belief that the subject will not inform the contact. The physician must then inform the subject of his or her intent to disclose the information to the contact and give the subject "the opportunity to express a preference as to whether disclosure should be made by the physician directly or to a public health officer for the purpose of said disclosure." See N.Y. Pub. Health Law §2783(4)(a)(3), (4). Rhode Island permits notification of third parties if "the physician has reason to believe that the patient, despite the physician's strong encouragement, has not and will not warn the third party. . . ." See R.I. Gen. Laws §23-6-17(b)(v) (1989). Public health investigators in Washington may reveal the identity of the infected person when the officer believes "that the exposed person was unaware that a risk of disease exposure existed and that the disclosure of the identity of the infected person is necessary." The statute does not state the criteria for determining necessity. See Wash. Rev. Code Ann. §70.24.105(2)(g) (Supp. 1989). For a survey of comparable legislation in a handful of other states, see Harold Edgar and Hazel Sandomire, "Medical Privacy Issues in the Age of AIDS: Legislative Options," *American Journal of Law & Medicine*, vol. XVI, nos. 1 & 2 (1990), pp. 182–196; and Larry Gostin, "The Politics of AIDS: Compulsory State Power, Public Health, and Civil Liberties," *Ohio State Law Journal*, vol. 49, no. 4 (1989), p. 1028, notes 71 and 72.
21. Two separate studies have been conducted comparing anonymous testing and confidential testing in order to determine the relative effect of anonymous testing in encouraging voluntary testing. A study conducted by the Colorado Department of

Health indicates that a policy of anonymous testing has no effect on testing attitudes. See Franklyn N. Judson and Thomas M. Vernon, Jr., "The Impact of AIDS on State and Local Health Departments: Issues and a Few Answers," *American Journal of Public Health*, vol. 78, no. 4 (April, 1988), pp. 387–93. However, an Oregon study indicates that the availability of anonymous testing increased the rate of voluntary testing among male homosexuals by one hundred twenty-five percent, among female prostitutes by fifty-six percent, high-risk heterosexuals by thirty-three percent, IV drug users by seventeen percent and others by thirty-one percent. See Laura J. Fehrm *et al.*, "Trial of Anonymous Versus Confidential Human Immunodeficiency Virus Testing," *Lancet*, August 13, 1988, pp. 379–382. Comparable statistics regarding the effects of a policy of disclosure with regard to persons at risk of contagion are not available.

22. See also *Teshuvot Ḥatam Sofer, Yoreh De'ah*, no. 326.
23. Cf., *Kovez̧ Iggerot Ḥazon Ish*, I, no. 102.
24. See R. Joshua Neuwirth, *Shemirat Shabbat ke-Hilkhatah*, 2nd edition (Jerusalem, 5739), chap. 32, note 2.
25. See R. Iser Yehudah Unterman, *Torah she-be-'al Peh*, XI (5729), 14.
26. See R. Joshua Neuwirth, *Shemirat Shabbat ke-Hilkhatah* 40:67 and *ibid.*, note 159; cf., R. Yisra'el Aryeh Zalmanowitz, *No'am*, IV (5761), 176.
27. For an even more remarkable extension of this principle reported in the name of R. Chaim Soloveitchik see R. Shlomoh Yosef Zevin, *Ishim ve-Shitot*, 2nd edition (Tel Aviv, 5718), p. 65, but cf., *Ḥazon Ish, Oholot* 22:32 and *Yoreh De'ah* 208:7.
28. See Frederick W. Winterbotham, *The Ultra Secret* (New York, 1974), pp. 60–61.
29. In dicta, the Supreme Court in *Jacobson* v. *Massachusetts*, 197 U.S. at 28, affirmed the right of the state to impose a quarantine as a means of protecting public health. Some time later, in *People* v. *Robertson*, 302 Ill. 422, 134 N.E. 815 (1922) the Illinois Supreme Court permitted the quarantine of the proprietor of a boardinghouse who was a typhoid carrier. For a discussion of quarantine statutes see Beth Bergman, "AIDS, Prostitution, and the Use of Historical Stereotypes to Legislate Sexuality," *John Marshall Law Review*, vol. 21, no. 4 (Summer 1988), pp. 787–830. Some commentators have indeed called for the isolation and criminal confinement of recalcitrant AIDS carriers. See James F. Grutsch Jr. and A.D.J. Robertson, "The Coming of

AIDS: It Didn't Start with the Homosexuals and It Won't End with Them," *American Spectator*, vol. 19, no. 3 (March, 1986), pp. 12–15; and Kathleen M. Sullivan and Martha A. Field, "AIDS and the Coercive Power of the State," *Harvard Civil Rights–Civil Liberties Law Review*, vol. 23, no. 1 (Winter 1988), pp. 139–197. For similar demands on the part of political figures as reported in the media see Gostin, "The Politics of AIDS: Compulsory State Powers, Public Health, and Civil Liberties," p. 1017, note 1.

30. The condom heretofore utilized for such purposes is worn by the male and it is that condom that is discussed in rabbinic literature. Recently, however, a panel of experts convened by the Food and Drug Administration has tentatively recommended approval of the newly-developed condom for women for use in disease prevention despite reservations regarding data submitted in support of the claim that the condom is effective in preventing the spread of sexually transmitted diseases. See *New York Times*, February 7, 1992, p. 7. On the basis of available descriptions of this prophylactic device, the halakhic status of the female condom appears to be identical to that of the male condom.
31. See R. Chaim Ozer Grodzinski, *Teshuvot Aḥi'ezer*, I, *Yoreh De'ah*, no. 23.
32. See, for example, R. Moshe Feinstein, *Iggerot Mosheh, Even ha-Ezer*, I, no. 63.
33. See *Iggerot Mosheh, loc. cit.* and *Iggerot Mosheh, Even ha-Ezer*, II, no. 16 and III, no. 21; cf., *Iggerot Mosheh, Even ha-Ezer*, I, no. 70.
34. This was not always the case. Physicians, including Galen in early Rome, often fled cities in time of plague. Many of those who remained either refused to treat seriously ill patients or charged exceedingly high fees for doing so. See Daniel M. Fox, "The Politics of Physicians' Responsibility in Epidemics: A Note on History," *Hastings Center Report*, vol. 18, no. 2 (April-May 1988), p. 5.
35. *AMA Policy Compendium* (1989), p. 9. For an analysis of the duties of members of the nursing profession under the principles enunciated by the American Nurses' Association Committee on Ethics in its "Statement Regarding Risk Versus Responsibility in Providing Nursing Care," *Ethics in Nursing, Position Statement* and *Guidelines* (1988) see D. Anthony Forrester, "AIDS: The Responsibility to Care," *Villanova Law Review*, vol. 34, no. 5 (1989), pp. 819–821.
36. See R. Eliezer Waldenberg, *Ẓiẓ Eli'ezer*, IX, no. 17, chap. 5.

37. See *Teshuvot ha-Radvaz*, III, no. 1,052; *Pri Megadim, Oraḥ Ḥayyim, Mishbeẓot Zahav* 328:7; *Pitḥei Teshuvah, Ḥoshen Mishpat* 426:2; and *Shulḥan Arukh ha-Rav*, V, *Hilkhot Nizkei Guf va-Nefesh* 7. For further discussion and additional sources as well as dissenting views, see my *Contemporary Halakhic Problems*, IV (New York, 1995), 275–279.
38. *Shevet me-Yehudah* (Jerusalem, 5715), *sha'ar rishon*, chap. 9, p. 23.
39. For a report of progress that has been made in this endeavor see *New York Times*, February 24, 1990, p. 34, col. 6.
40. See *Jewish Week*, July 13, 1990, p. 23, col. 1.
41. See Rabbi Barry Freundel, "AIDS: A Traditional Response," *Jewish Action*, Winter, 1986–87, p. 50.
42. In researching the medical literature, I was unable to discover sources that directly discuss survival of the AIDS virus subsequent to death. This information was provided by the former commissioner of health for the state of New York, Dr. David Axelrod. In several conversations over a period of months, Dr. Axelrod was quite emphatic in his statements indicating that, subsequent to the death of the patient, the virus loses its virulence within a matter of several hours at the most. Precisely because of the absence of data in the published literature I carefully note, "Even assuming that the virus remains virulent, wearing shoes without open toes, rubber gloves and a protective garment effectively eliminates any possibility of contracting the diseaase."
43. See the statement of R. Aaron Soloveichik quoted in the *Algemeiner Journal*, February 5, 1988, p. 1. Cf., the aggadic comment recorded in *Pesaḥim* 57a to the effect that the Temple courtyard raised its voice and exclaimed, "Go from here Issachar of Kefar Barka'i" because he honored himself and profaned the sacrifices by wrapping his hands in silk while performing the sacrificial ritual. Rashi, in one explanation, indicates that this priest's action in covering his hands was an act of disdain. However, since Rashi himself, *Sukkah* 42a, maintains that a person may wrap his hand while grasping the *lulav*, it appears that the comment in *Pesaḥim* 57a applies only to performance of the sacrificial service. See *Iggerot Mosheh, Yoreh De'ah* II, no. 16. Moreover, that consideration certainly does not pertain in situations in which gloves are required in order to avoid a hazard to life or health.
44. Syed A. Sattar and V. Susan Springthorpe, "Survival and Disinfectant Inactivation of the Human Immunodeficiency Virus: A Critical Review," *Reviews of Infectious Diseases*, vol. 13, nos. 1–3 (January–June 1991), p. 432.

45. The levels of chlorination used in swimming pools, 0.5–1.0 ppm (parts per million), are adequate for killing certain infectants, such as the polio virus, but that level of concentration is not sufficient for neutralizing HIV. Recent studies would indicate a need for a level of 50 ppm of available chlorine in order to kill the HIV virus. See Sattar and Springthorpe, p. 444, and a letter from an official of the Centers for Disease Control on file with this writer.
46. Philip C. Fox *et al.*, "Saliva Inhibits HIV-1 Infectivity," *Journal of the American Medical Association*, vol. 116 (May 1980), pp. 635–637.
47. A review of that material may be found in R. Moshe Bunim Pirutinsky, *Sefer ha-Brit*, 4th edition (New York, 5751), pp. 213–226 and p. 418. An earlier survey may be found in R. Chaim Chizkiyahu Medini, *Sedei Ḥemed*, (New York, 5722), VII, 236–281. Further material was published by the author of *Sedei Ḥemed* in a monograph entitled *Kuntres ha-Meẓiẓah ve-ha-Milu'im* (Warsaw, 1902). Unfortunately, that work was not incorporated in later editions of *Sedei Ḥemed*. A most valuable and readily understandable synopsis of opposing views as well as the historical background of the controversy by R. Sinai Schiffer, *Kuntres Miẓvat ha-Meẓiẓah*, was translated from the original German by the author's grandson, R. Sinai Adler, and appended to the latter's *Dvar Sinai al ha-Rambam* (Jerusalem, 5726), pp. 97–112. An English publication in pamphlet form compiled by Dr. Bernard Homa, *Metzitzah* (London, 1960), contains translations of early responsa authored by R. Eliezer Hurwitz and R. Moses Sofer as well as a responsum by the late R. Isaac ha-Levi Herzog.
48. See Rabbi Alfred S. Cohen, "Brit Milah and the Specter of AIDS," *Journal of Halacha and Contemporary Society*, no. XVII (Spring 1989) pp. 93–115 and an unpublished and undated statement of a group styling itself the Orthodox Roundtable entitled "The Orthodox Roundtable: Opinion Concerning Mezizah and AIDS."
49. See R. Moshe Sternbuch, *Teshuvot ve-Hanhagot*, II, no. 503.
50. It should be noted that the presently available tests for the presence of the HIV virus will not reveal very recent infection with the result that there may be significant chance of a false negative if exposure occurred within six months of testing. Families requesting *meẓiẓah ba-peh* are, almost by definition, a low-risk group. In those circles the danger of drug use or of sexual promiscuity during the last weeks or months of pregnancy is virtually nil. The *mohel* may, with some measure of cogency, have

reason to fear that, at an earlier stage of life, the parents may have espoused a far different life-style or that, Heaven forefend, even individuals who have been observant all their lives may have engaged in isolated incidents of youthful indiscretion. The AIDS test does serve to allay such fear.

51. Cf., the studies cited by, and the comments of, Sattar and Springthorpe, p. 439.

52. Although there is some dilution of 151-proof rum by saliva a similar dilution takes place with regard to the virus. Moreover, one reported study shows inactivation of HIV by means of a 50% ethanol solution within ten minutes, the shortest time tested. See L. Martin, J. McDougal and S. Loskowski, "Disinfection and Inactivation of Human T Lymphotropic Viruses Type III/Lymphadenopathy-Associated Viruses," *Journal of Infectious Diseases,* vol. 152, no. 2 (August 1985), pp. 400–403. An earlier study found a 99% reduction in enzyme activity after exposure of the virus to 19% alcohol for five minutes. See B. Spiro *et al.*, "Inactivation of Lymphadenopathy-Associated Viruses by Chemical Distinfectants," *Lancet*, no. 8408 (April 21, 1984), pp. 899–901. In comparison a 70% alcohol solution inactivated the virus within one minute. See L. Resnick *et al.*, "Stability and Inactivation of HIV-IIL/LAV under Clinical and Laboratory Environments," *Journal of the American Medical Association*, vol. 255, no. 14 (April 11, 1986), pp. 1887–1891. Thus it is evident that alcohol is effective in concentrations much lower than 70% but that in greater dilution alcohol may require a longer contact time. A later study does question the efficiency of alcohol in distinfecting HIV but, as indicated by the authors themselves, those studies involved dried blood which the solution could not fully permeate. See P. J. V. Hanson *et al.*, "Chemical Inactivation of HIV on Surfaces," *British Medical Journal,* vol. 298, no. 6677 (April 1, 1989), pp. 862–864.

53. See D.C. Montefiore, W. F. Robinson *et al.*, "Effective Inactivation of Human Immunodeficiency Virus with Chlorhexidine Antiseptics Containing Detergents and Alcohol," *Journal of Hospital Infection,* vol 15, no. 3 (April 1990), pp. 279–282.

54. D. Bernstein, G. Schiff, *et al,* "In Vitro Virucidal Effectiveness of a 0.12% Chlorhexidine (CH) Mouthrinse" (abstract), *Journal of Dental Research,* vol. 67 (1988), Special Issue, p. 404, report a 99% reduction in HIV virus after a 30-second exposure to a 0.12% chlorhexidine mouthrinse.

6

HIV Screening of Newborn Infants

Approximately ten percent of HIV-infected infants succumb to the effects of the disease within the first year of life. Many more die in the early years of infancy. The most frequent cause of death among HIV-infected children is pneumocystis carinii pneumonia (PCP). PCP is an opportunistic infection common among HIV-infected children among whom it is more swiftly and more frequently fatal than among adults.

Fatality at the hands of PCP can be dramatically decreased by prophylactic administration of a common antibiotic, Trimethoprim/Sulfamethoxazole (TMP/SMX). Seventy percent of cases of PCP occur in children who have not received this prophylaxis while only seven percent of children stricken by PCP have received the antibiotic. Thus, the available treatment reduces the occurrence of this frequently fatal infection by more than one half. In order to achieve the greatest benefit, the administration of TMP/SMX is begun at one month of age even in the absence of clinical symptoms of HIV-connected disorders.

HIV-infected infants are also at risk for serious bacterial infections, interstitial pneumonia, gastrointestinal disorders and neuro-developmental impairment. Children known to be HIV-infected are carefully monitored for early symptoms of these diseases as well as for reduction in the level of CD4+ cells that indicate susceptibility to infection. In addition to more rapid diagnosis and treatment of these conditions, patients known to be HIV-infected may be treated with intravenous immunoglobulin (IVIG) to boost the immune system and with other treatment regimens such as AZT and DDI that may both prolong and improve the quality of life.

Moreover, HIV-infected children are immunocompromised and therefore their vaccination schedules must be tailored to their immunodeficient state. In general, live virus vaccines are not recommended for use in immunodeficient patients because replication of live attenuated viruses may be enhanced with the resultant danger that, due to their compromised immune systems, the live vaccine may cause the patient to contract the very disease it is designed to protect against.[1] Nevertheless, the risk for contracting measles, with subsequent progression to measles pneumonia and secondary infection with bacterial pathogens, has led to the recommendation for continued administrations of measles-mumps-rubella vaccine.[2] However, in areas in which the risk of tuberculosis is low, it is recommended that the *Bacillus Calmette-Guérin* vaccine (BCG), a live bacterial virus vaccine, be withheld from children known or suspected to be infected with HIV.[3] Most significantly, it is recommended that inactivated polio vaccine (IPV) be substituted for oral polio vaccine (OPV) since the latter contains a live virus.[4] Moreover, family members of asymptomatic HIV-infected children may also be immunocompromised as a result of HIV infection and may therefore be at increased risk for vaccine-associated poliomyelitis from contact with vaccine virus. Accordingly, inactivated polio vaccine, rather than oral polio vaccine, is recommended for all children residing in the household.[5] Thus, failure to inform the mother of the positive results of an HIV test may pose a danger to other siblings as well.

The State of New York currently mandates that all newborn infants be screened for a series of seven congenitally transmitted diseases, including hepatitis B, syphilis and sickle-cell anemia and a number of metabolic disorders, as well as for sickle-cell trait. Parental consent for the performance of those tests is not required. In the event that a baby tests positive for any of those diseases the parents are informed and any available treatment is provided. Since 1987 New York also tests the blood of all newborns for the presence of HIV antibodies. Originally, the HIV test was a blind test conducted anonymously solely for statistical purposes. Since maternal antibodies freely cross the placenta and newly born infants could have contracted the virus only from the mother, the mothers of all neonates who test positive must be infected by HIV. Thus, tests performed on infants accurately reflect the HIV infection rate and epidemiological trends prevalent among identifiable groups of child-bearing women. According to currently accepted estimates, between fifteen and twenty-five percent of infants who test positive are themselves actually infected by HIV. The remainder carry maternal HIV antibodies which disappear over a period of several months.[66] Similar HIV seroprevalence surveys are conducted in forty-four states and territories.

The New York State Public Health Law forbids HIV testing without the consent of the person tested or, in the case of a minor, of his or her parents and also mandates that appropriate counseling be provided. Accordingly, HIV testing would have violated that legal proscription if not for the fact that the testing is conducted anonymously for statistical and public planning purposes only and infected individuals are not identified. Since discovery of HIV antibodies in a neonate is *ipso facto* a determination that the mother is HIV infected, informing the mother that her baby has tested positive is tantamount to informing her that she is infected by HIV.

A bill introduced by Assemblywoman Nettie Mayersohn of Queens in the 1994 session of the New York State Assembly would have required the Department of Health to notify parents if a child tests positive as is the case with currently administered tests for other congenitally transmitted diseases. A compromise proposal would have required mandatory counselling of pregnant women and new mothers concerning the benefits of early diagnosis of HIV but would not have provided for disclosure of this information to women who decline consent. Indeed, recent studies demonstrate that treatment of pregnant HIV-infected women with AZT significantly reduces the incidence of HIV in their newly born babies. Neither proposal was adopted by the State legislature before it adjourned. Assemblywoman Mayersohn's bill was subsequently enacted as an amendment to the Public Health Law in June 1996.[7]

Opposition to the original legislative proposal focuses upon the inherent violation of the rights and liberties of the mother. Since the presence of HIV antibodies in the neonate is conclusive evidence of infection of the mother any inadvertent breach of confidentiality may render the mother vulnerable to discrimination and stigmatization. The more fundamental of the arguments advanced, however, is that the mother has the right to decline testing and has the right not to know her HIV status.[8] Hence, such involuntary disclosure, even if limited to disclosure only to the mother herself, constitutes a violation of her right to privacy.[9]

Jewish law ordained measures to protect the privacy of individuals long before the existence of a right to privacy was recognized as a fundamental right by democratic societies. Thus the Gemara, *Bava Batra* 60a, remarks that Balaam's exclamation "How goodly are your tents, O Jacob" (Numbers 24:5) was uttered in approbation of the configuration of the tents of the Children of Israel in their encampments in the wilderness and explains that the openings of the tents were arranged in a manner such that the occupants of each were assured complete privacy. This comment serves to elucidate the rule recorded in the Mishnah forbidding invasion of privacy in the construction of doors and windows. In another comment, as cited by Rashi in his commentary on Numbers 3:16, the Sages state that Moses, having been charged with taking a census of the tribe of Levi and with including in his count infants aged one month and older, protested that he could not enter a private abode without invitation. Moses' demurral was accepted and, instead of requiring Moses personally to count the members of each family, the Divine Presence announced the number of occupants as Moses passed by the entrance of each tent. As formulated by the Gemara in the opening section of *Bava Batra*, Jewish law provides that, not only does a householder have a right to quiet enjoyment of his property, but also that the owner of an abutting courtyard has an actionable obligation to contribute to the erection of a physical barrier in order to assure that privacy is total and complete. In the post-Talmudic era, the famed Rabbenu Gershom of Mayence promulgated an edict protecting the privacy of written communications.

Although it would be inaccurate to conclude that these and related provisions of Halakhah constitute a "penumbra" establishing an absolute right to privacy with regard to any and all matters, Jewish law does nevertheless recognize certain rights of privacy that are not parallelled in other legal or moral systems. Most striking is Judaism's recognition of a nearly absolute privilege of confidentiality. The Gemara, *Yoma* 4b, declares: "Whence is it derived that [if] one relates something to one's fellow [the latter is commanded] 'Thou shalt not tell'? For it is said, 'and the Lord spoke to him from the tent of meeting *lo emor*' (Leviticus 1:1)." Rashi, in his commentary *ad locum*, explains that the term employed by Scripture in this passage, *lamed, alef, mem, resh,* and vocalized as "*l'emor,*" i.e., "to say" or "saying", is understood, for purposes of talmudic exegesis, as if it were vocalized as "*lo emor*", i.e., "do not say." Thus, the written word vocalized in two alternative and contradictory ways literally constitutes a *double entendre*: "to say" and "do not say." Prior to their communication to Moses, the contents of revelation were reserved to the Deity and, accordingly, the contents of revelation would have been held inviolate by Moses on the basis of the injunction "Do not say" had he not been commanded explicitly "*l'emor,*" to speak and disclose that information to Israel. This talmudic statement is cited as normative by *Magen Avraham, Oraḥ Ḥayyim* 156:2, and serves to establish a formal obligation to regard the communication of any personal or proprietary information as confidential unless permission for disclosure is explicitly granted.

In Jewish law, the privileged nature of communication is not limited to attorney-client, physician-patient or priest-penitent relationships and hence is far broader than in other moral and legal systems. Nevertheless, the privilege is neither all-encompassing in scope nor is the privilege, when it does exist, absolute in nature.

The most explicit and most readily identifiable exception to privacy of communication is in the area of public health. The Gemara, *Avodah Zarah* 28a, reports that Rav Yoḥanan became afflicted with a certain malady and sought treatment at the hands of a gentile woman. For reasons of his own, Rav Yoḥanan wished to ascertain the pharmaceutical agents employed in the medication administered. The woman regarded that information as proprietary and, at first, declined to comply with his request. Rav Yoḥanan thereupon gave the woman assurances that her secret would be held inviolate; moreover, he led her erroneously to believe that he had taken a solemn oath to that effect. Upon receiving the information from her, Rav Yoḥanan seized the earliest opportunity to disseminate his newly acquired medical knowledge in the course of a public discourse. The talmudic narrative clearly establishes that, whatever right to privacy may exist with regard to such information, it is superseded by the obligation to preserve others from illness. That obligation not only abrogates the duty to respect confidentiality but also renders mandatory the breach of a specific and solemn undertaking of secrecy.

Parents do not have the right to endanger the lives of their children by declining medical treatment on their behalf or even by refusing to allow diagnosis of a condition requiring medical attention. The state may, and does, intervene on behalf of a neglected child when parents do not provide necessary medical care. It is for that reason that the law in the state of New York already provides for involuntary testing of newborns for syphilis and sickle-cell anemia and certain other congenital conditions. Any possible adverse effects upon the mother pale into insignificance when measured against the therapeutic needs of the child.

Moreover, there is no basis for an assumption that Jewish law recognizes a right not to receive information about oneself; if such a "right" does exist it is not a right of privacy. "If one has made a bad purchase in the market, should one praise it in his eyes or deprecate it?" is the rhetorical query posed by *Bet Hillel* as reported by the Gemara, *Ketubot* 17a. *Bet Hillel* make the response "Surely, one shall praise it in his eyes" as a self-evident exception to the admonition "Distance yourself from a false matter" (Exodus 23:7). A "white lie" of such nature is justified as a means of advancing the positive value of promoting pleasantness and a sense of well-being. The sole concern voiced by the Gemara in its discussion is with regard to the telling of a fib; there is no hint whatsoever that a person has a "right" not to be informed of matters of which he would rather remain ignorant. A person who has made a "bad purchase" has displayed poor judgment and, moreover, others perceive that he lacks good judgment. Since the situation cannot be remedied and if an opportunity to learn from a mistake does not exist, this information, if imparted, can only cause distress. Yet, the possibility that the individual in question does not want to know such things regarding himself is not a direct consideration. The sole consideration is avoidance of distress and promotion of well-being. Emotional and psychological equanimity is the governing value, not a "right" of privacy.

Indeed, it is unlikely that American law recognizes a right

not to receive unwanted information. Disclosure of personal information to a third party is an invasion of privacy; disclosure to the person himself is not. Does a person have a right not to be informed against his will of the diagnosis of a serious illness? May a physician reveal to a patient who has indicated that he does not wish such information that the patient bears the gene responsible for Huntington's disease? A physician has performed routine blood tests upon all members of a family and discovers that the husband cannot be the biological father of one of the children. Does informing the child of this fact constitute a violation of the child's privacy? Putting aside moral or prudential considerations, there is nothing at present in American case law that would indicate that the doctor commits a legal wrong in imparting such information.

The legal problems associated with disclosure of the results of an HIV screening test are of a somewhat different nature. A person enjoys a common-law right to the integrity of his body. Merely touching a person without permission, actual or implied, constitutes a battery. Draining blood without consent is certainly not legal. Once blood has been drawn and would otherwise be discarded, performance of serological testing upon the blood sample may or may not constitute a violation of a constitutionally protected right of privacy. It is, however, expressly prohibited by the New York State Public Health Law. Once the test has been performed, legally or illegally, disclosure of the results to the patient is not a violation of the patient's constitutionally protected right of privacy. Neonatal testing for HIV antibodies is performed anonymously in the state of New York, not because disclosure would constitute a violation of the right of privacy but because, in the absence of consent, both the test itself and disclosure of the diagnosis was banned by New York statute. Testing of an unidentified blood specimen was never deemed to constitute such a violation. Thus, the legal problem was readily remedied by amending the statute to permit "unblinding" of the procedure.

The law clearly recognizes the state's right to test newborns for various diseases without consent of the parents as a legitimate application of the *parens patriae* doctrine. Disclosure of the result to the mother is indeed disclosure of her own HIV status. However, disclosure of information to affected parties contrary to their desire is not a violation of a constitutionally protected right of privacy.[10] Indeed, in many states, present HIV testing statutes require that the individual tested be informed of the result, particularly if the result is positive. In some instances, e.g., in situations involving applicants for life or medical insurance[11] or prospective blood, semen or organ donors, the statutes in question provide for mandatory disclosure of results of testing that itself was performed with prior consent.[12] In others, e.g., statutes requiring the testing of prisoners or patients in hospitals or medical institutions, no consent is required for either the disclosure or the testing.[13]

In addition to asserting an absolute right of privacy, opponents of the recently enacted legislation advanced four separate arguments in support of their position: (1) Prenatal testing of the mother is a far more effective means of preserving the health of the child since it enables physicians to institute measures designed to minimize contagion in the course of parturition. (2) Optimal treatment of the infant requires cooperation of the mother. Prospects for such cooperation would be compromised if the mother were to be given information that she does not wish to receive, particularly if she realizes that her privacy has been violated. (3) Despite the best intentions of those concerned as well as the establishment of safeguards to prevent any other disclosure, there remains a distinct possibility that information concerning a diagnosis of HIV infection may come into the hands of others with resultant adverse effects upon the mother. (4) A baby actually infected by HIV will, in any event, succumb to complications of that condition. Available treatment can only prolong the life of the child but will not effect a cure.[14]

The first two arguments constitute a *non sequitur*. The underlying premises are entirely correct and public policy should foster prenatal testing programs and also encourage the seeking of prenatal approval for testing the child. Mandatory counselling of pregnant women and new mothers is certainly a salutary initial step. Involuntary testing of the child and disclosure of the results to the mother are steps to be taken only when other measures have failed.

The third argument is based entirely upon conjecture. A similar concern underlies the policy of not informing the sexual partners of a person afflicted by HIV that they are at risk.[15] A person who does not wish to compromise such a relationship does indeed have a rational motive for avoiding testing. A pregnant woman has no such motive. If postpartum testing of the baby becomes mandatory, the mother will not be able to prevent such testing from taking place. Refusal to be tested during pregnancy will not prevent testing of the baby after birth. Testing and treatment during pregnancy can only prevent infection of the fetus. A pregnant woman may still decline testing because she may hope that the baby will not be affected and she will remain ignorant of her own condition, but awareness of mandatory testing of the baby after birth does not in any rational way itself serve as a reason to decline prenatal testing.

In response to the third argument it must be emphasized that violation of the privacy of the mother can be countenanced only to the degree necessary to discharge the duty owed to the child. The chance of inadvertent disclosure despite safeguards to prevent that from occurring is a risk that must be borne.[16] The final argument reflects an attitude antithetical to Jewish values and teachings. There does exist an obligation to prolong life even when a cure is not within the realm of natural possibility. Moreover, there is ample reason for optimism with regard to future developments in medical science that will make a cure possible. Hence, prolongation of life may, indeed, preserve the child long enough for him or her to benefit from an as yet unavailable cure. In addition, currently available treatment not only prolongs life but also eliminates the pain and suffering associated with preventable complications of HIV infection.

Mandatory counselling is of definite value and is independently warranted but, in itself, it is but an incomplete remedy. Early diagnosis and identification of all babies afflicted with HIV is essential in order properly to treat *every* baby. Consequently, a policy of mandatory testing and disclosure is entirely consistent with Jewish teaching and reflects values fundamental to Judaism.

NOTES

1. See Michael E. Pichichero *et al.*, "New Vaccines and Vaccination Policies," *Pediatric Annals*, vol. 19, no. 12 (December 1990), p. 690.
2. *Loc. cit.*
3. See also Ida M. Onorato *et al.*, "Childhood Immunization, Vaccine-Preventable Diseases and Infection with Human Immunodeficiency Virus," *Journal of Pediatric Infectious Diseases*, vol. 7, no. 8 (August 1988), p. 594.
4. *Loc. cit.* See also *Pediatric Annals*, p. 690. This represents the recommendation of the Immunization Practices Advisory Committee (ACIP) of the United States Public Health Service. The World Health Organization has recommended that OPV be used routinely for all children, particularly in developing countries, on the assumption that the benefits of OPV, including ease of administration and lower cost, outweigh the risks to HIV-infected children. See *Journal of Pediatric Infectious Diseases*, p. 594.
5. *Loc. cit.*
6. The standard HIV test consists of an ELISA test and, if positive, a Western blot test in order to eliminate the possibility of a false positive in the ELISA test. Both the ELISA and the Western blot tests test for the presence of antibodies to the HIV virus but do not test for the virus itself. An HIV-infected mother will develop antibodies to the HIV virus and pass on those antibodies to

her fetus but will not necessarily transmit the HIV virus itself to her child. The child will continue to carry the antibodies for a period of months after birth.

It is now possible to determine whether a baby is actually infected by the HIV virus or whether it merely carries HIV antibodies. A polymerase chain reaction (PCR) test discloses the presence of the virus itself, rather than the presence of antibodies to the virus. Thus, a newly born child will test positive on a PCR test only if it is actually afflicted with the HIV virus. The PCR test is reported to be effective in infants at least one month old. PCR is, however, far more expensive than standard HIV antibody tests.

7. There is also federal legislation governing allocation of federal funds that may, in time, serve as an impetus for nationwide testing of newborn children. The relevant provisions of the Ryan White Care Act, 42 U.S.C.A. secs. 300ff-33–300ff-37, were enacted by Congress in May 1996. The Act now requires that the Secretary of Health and Human Services determine by September 1998 whether newborn testing has become "routine." When and if the Secretary determines that newborn testing has indeed become routine, each state is given eighteen months to demonstrate one of the following: (1) the rate of reported cases of pediatric AIDS has been reduced to no more than 50% of the rate of such cases reflected in 1993 data; (2) knowledge of the HIV status of at least 95% of pregnant women who obtained prenatal care on at least two occasions within the first 34 weeks of pregnancy; or (3) that it has implemented mandatory HIV testing of newborns. If newborn testing is determined to be "routine" and the state cannot demonstrate either (1) or (2) it must implement mandatory testing of newborns or forfeit Care Act funding. See Elizabeth B. Cooper, "HIV Disease in Pregnancy—Ethics, Law and Policy," *Obstetrics and Gynecology Clinics of North America,* vol. 24, no. 4 (December 1997), p. 899.
8. It should be noted that syphilis is among the diseases for which there is mandatory screening in New York despite the fact that discovery of syphilis in the child is tantamount to diagnosis of that infection in the mother. However, syphilis is distinguishable from HIV in that New York requires reporting of a variety of sexually transmitted and commercial diseases. In 1989, four clinical societies in New York, including the New York Medical Society, unsuccessfully sued the commissioner of health to

compel him to define AIDS and HIV infection as sexually transmitted and communicable diseases. See *New York State Society of Surgeons et al.* v. *Axelrod*, 157 A.D.2d 54, 555 N.Y.S.2d 911 (1990), *aff'd* 77 N.Y.2d 677, 572 N.E.2d 605, 569 N.Y.S.2d 922 (1991).

9. The leading case in this area is *Whalen* v. *Roe*, 429 U.S. 589 (1977). In *Whalen* the Supreme Court acknowledged a right to privacy in personal information but held that constitutional protection of medical information is not absolute. In general, the right to privacy cannot prevent disclosure of information if such information serves to advance a legitimate state interest and the state's actions in seeking such information are narrowly tailored to meet that interest. See *Schachter* v. *Whalen*, 581 F.2d 35 (2d Cir. 1978); *United States* v. *Westinghouse*, 638 F.2d 570 (3d Cir. 1980); *In re Search Warrant (Sealed)*, 810 F.2d 67 (3d Cir. 1987) *cert. denied sub nom. Rochman* v. *United States*, 403 U.S.1007, 107 S.Ct. 3233 (1987); *General Motor Corp.* v. *Director of the National Institute for Occupational Safety and Health*, 636 F.2d 163 (6th Cir. 1980), *cert. denied*, 455 U.S. 877, 70 L.Ed. 2d 187, 102 S.Ct. 357 (1981); *Schaill* v. *Tippecanoe City School Corp.*, 864 F.2d 1309 (7th Cir. 1988); *Strong* v. *Board of Education of the Uniondale Union Free School District*, 902 F.2d 208 (2d Cir. (1990), *cert. denied*, 498 U.S. 897 (1990).

Courts have generally recognized a right to privacy with regard to AIDS-related information and have been sensitive to the fact that since AIDS is closely related to sexual activity and intravenous drug use such information is highly personal. See, for example, *Woods* v. *White*, 689 F. Supp. 874 (W.D. Wis. 1978), *aff'd*, 899 F.2d 17 (7th Cir. 1990). Disclosure of an individual's HIV status in cases in which the government asserts an interest in disclosure was the subject of litigation in *Nelley* v. *County of Erie*, 776 F. Supp. 715 (W.D. N.Y. 1991) and *Harris* v. *Thigpen*, 941 F.2d 1495 (11th Cir. 1991). Both cases involved HIV-positive prison inmates who had been segregated in order to protect the general inmate population. The New York court found that segregation did little to protect other prisoners and upheld the plaintiff's position while in the latter case the court ruled in favor of the Alabama Department of Corrections. For a review of the issues involved see Roger Doughty, "The Confidentiality of HIV-Related Information: Responding to the Resurgence of Aggressive Public Health Interventions in the

AIDS Epidemic," *California Law Review*, vol. 82, no. 1 (January 1994), pp. 111–184.

10. Some legal scholars have indeed argued that mandatory disclosure of HIV infection should be regarded as unconstitutional. See, for example, Michael L. Closen, "Mandatory Disclosure of HIV Blood Test Results to the Individual Tested: A Matter of Personal Choice Neglected," *Loyola University of Chicago Law Journal*, vol. 22, no. 2 (Winter 1991), pp. 465–466 and 478. Closen does not claim to find support for his position in current case law. His argument is that such disclosure is "haphazard," that it is "both overinclusive and underinclusive in its application to people who 'should' be informed of their HIV infection" and hence the substance of a law mandating disclosure "is not really appropriate to the accomplishment of its health or welfare goal." He further argues that such legislation "also significantly encroaches on an individual's bodily integrity because a measure that intrudes upon one's psychological or emotional state can be just as damaging as a measure that intrudes upon one's physical or physiological integrity." Whether or not those arguments are cogent with regard to disclosure in general, they are not applicable to situations involving disclosure to a parent who is duty-bound to provide for the medical care of a child.
11. See, e.g., *Florida Statutes Annotated* 627.429(4)(c) (West Supp. 1990); *New York Public Health Law* §§ 2781(5), 2782(1)(a),(j) (Consol. 1990); *North Carolina General Statutes* § 130A-148(g) (1989).
12. *Arizona Revised Statutes Annotated* § 32–483 (1989); *California Health & Safety Code* § 16603.3(a) (West 1990); *Louisiana Revised Statutes Annotated* §§ 1062.1(c), 1299.142(B)(1) (West 1990); *Maryland Health–General Code Annotated* § 18–34(b),(c) (1990); *New York Public Health Law* §§ 27812(1)(a) (Consol. 1990); *Wisconsin Statutes Annotated* § 1466.023(1) (West 1990); see also *North Carolina General Statutes* § 130A-148(g) (1989); *North Dakota Century Code* § 23–07.5–05(1)(d),(e) (Supp. 1989).
13. See, for example, *Maryland Health–General Code Annotated* § 18–38(b),(d),(f) (1990) (allows testing without consent of prisoner if there is a possible exposure of a correctional employee to HIV; and requires counseling if test result is positive); *Missouri Annotated Statutes* §§ 191.653(3), .656(2)(1)(e), .659 (Vernon Supp. 1991); *New York Public Health Law* §§ 2781(5), 2782(1)(1)-(o) (Consol. 1990); *North Carolina General Statutes* §

130A-148(g) (1989); see also *South Carolina Code Annotated* §§ 44–29–100, -110 (Lawyers Co-Operative 1989) (allows testing of prisoners for HIV and denies discharge of those who test positive until release is recommended by health department); *Missouri Annotated Statutes* §§ 191.653(3), .656(2)(1)(e), .662 (Vernon Supp. 1991) (testing and disclosure to individuals in drug treatment programs and mental health patients); *New Hampshire Statutes Annotated* § 141-F:7(II) (1988) (testing of and disclosure to medical patients); *Wisconsin Statutes Annotated* § 146.025(3) (West Supp. 1990) (testing of and disclosure to mental patients who pose risk of transmission of HIV to other patients); see also *California Health & Safety Code* § 199.25b (West 1990); *North Carolina General Statutes* § 130A-148(g) (1989); *South Carolina Code Annotated* § 44–29–230 (Lawyers Co-Operative 1989) (if possible accidental HIV transmission from patient to health-care worker, patient can be tested with consent and must be told of result).

14. Another argument has been advanced by the authors of a study that revealed that 48% of health-care professionals would withhold cardiac resuscitation and kidney dialysis on the basis of the fact that the infant tested HIV positive while 23% would advise against cardiac surgery. In light of those findings the authors contend that testing itself carries the risk of the baby being denied beneficial medical treatment and suggest that this risk be "carefully examined." See B.W. Levin, J.M. Driscoll, Jr., and A.R. Fleischman, "Treatment Choice for Infants in the Neonatal Intensive Care Unit at Risk for AIDS," *Journal of the American Medical Association*, vol. 265, no. 22 (June 12, 1991), pp. 2976–2981. However, since, as these authors seem to agree, withholding of such procedures simply on the basis of the statistical possibility that the baby is afflicted with AIDS is not morally defensible, the lesson to be learned is one that is entirely different: The study serves to identify a serious problem with regard to the ethical sensitivity of many neonatal care-givers. However, even given the sad results of the study, the HIV positive baby is probably more likely to be helped than to be harmed by determination of his HIV status. Relatively few babies are candidates for resuscitation, dialysis or cardiac surgery and only a portion of those will not receive such treatment because of discrimination against HIV-infected babies while it is likely that the proportion of HIV-infected neonates who will benefit from early treatment is large.

15. A halakhic analysis of that policy is presented *supra*, pp. 148–159.
16. Jewish law not only permits but commands disclosure of confidential information to the extent necessary to prevent loss of life or property. See R. Israel Iser of Vilna, *Piskei Teshuvah, Oraḥ Ḥayyim*, no. 156; R. Israel Meir ha-Kohen, *Ḥafeẓ Ḥayyim, Hilkhot Issurei Rekhilut, kelal* 1; R. Samuel Kushelewitz, *Netivot Shmu'el*, I, no. 9; R. Benjamin Silber, *Oz Nidberu*, X, no. 46; R. Iser Yehudah Unterman, *Ha-Torah ve-ha-Medinah*, IX-X (5718–5719), 23; R. Eliezer Waldenberg, *Ẓiẓ Eli'ezer*, XVI, no. 4; R. Ovadiah Yosef, *Yeḥaveh Da'at*, IV, no. 60; and *Piskei Din shel Batei ha-Din ha-Rabbaniyim be-Yisra'el*, V, 153. Such disclosure is required despite the obvious possibility that the information may become available to individuals who are not entitled to receive such information.

7

Artificial Procreation

In a manner closely akin to that of the Moslem speakers who have preceded me, permit me to begin my presentation with three words—three Hebrew words—with which, from time immemorial, it has been the wont of rabbinic scholars and students to begin every paper, every document, and every communication: *Be-ezrat ha-Shem yitbarakh*, meaning "With the aid of God, may He be blessed."

It is a distinct honor for me to have been invited to address you. I regard this invitation as an honor for a variety of reasons. First of all, the reputation of this learned body is already well-known and well-established throughout the world and on those grounds alone it is a privilege to present a paper before you. Secondly, I deem it a distinct honor to be the guest of a country and of a government which has manifested, and continues to manifest, hospitality and friendship to members of the Jewish faith. And finally, as a student of Jewish law, it is a distinct honor and privilege to have been invited to deliver a pa-

---

This paper was originally delivered at a conference of the Academy of the Kingdom of Morocco in November 1986 and is presented, with revisions, as published in volume X of the Proceedings of the Academy, *Ethical Problems Raised by the New Techniques in Human Reproduction*, pp. 137–148.

per on Jewish law in Morocco, the land of the eminent codifier of Jewish law, the birthplace of Rabbenu Yitzchak Alfasi, Rabbi Isaac of Fez, who, in the eleventh century, composed the first comprehensive post-talmudic compendium of Jewish law.

With regard to the specific topic under discussion, it must be stated that Jewish scholars have not welcomed artificial forms of procreation with a great deal of enthusiasm. The question is why? How does one explain this negative reaction? Of course, one could point to the primacy of the value of the family and of familial relationships in Jewish tradition and seek to explain this reaction in that manner. Indeed, Judaism has always had the highest regard and the highest respect for the integrity of the family and of familial relationships. Those are certainly desiderata which, given the contemporary milieu, require emphasis and reiteration. Not too long ago I came upon a cartoon in an American magazine. The picture depicted a man and a woman walking through Central Park in New York City. Behind them were several little children. Hiding behind one of the bushes were two would-be muggers. The caption under the cartoon had one of these individuals turning to the other and saying, "That is a family. The family is an endangered species. We ought to leave them alone."

Certainly, the promotion of family values is a matter of great concern to moralists throughout the world and, assuredly, it is a matter of concern to Jewish scholars. Although Jewish law may not be monolithic in nature, and even within Orthodox Judaism there exist different and diverse opinions with regard to many issues, nevertheless, Judaism is first and foremost a religion of law. As a religion of law, the basic principle is that if a specific act or course of action is not proscribed as a contravention of a divine prohibition, or condemned as a violation of the spirit of the law, then, by definition, the action is permitted.[1] What, then, are the grounds for the prevalent negative attitude toward various forms of artificial procreation ?

Some moralists have decided artificial procreation on the basis of considerations of natural law.[2] However, in light of the very particular and very limited role of natural law in Jewish thought, the lack of receptivity on the part of halakhic scholars cannot be explained in light of considerations of natural law. Perhaps it is necessary for me to emphasize that in the history of Western philosophical thought there are reflected two completely disparate forms of natural law theory. Although it has no claim to chronological priority, I would, for lack of a better phrase, describe the first theory as the secular version of the natural law doctrine. That theory posits the notion that there are certain principles, certain maxims, certain rules of conduct, which are discoverable, to use the Lockean phrase, "by the light of nature," i.e., by reason alone.[3] Or, to phrase the same concept somewhat differently, exponents of this version of natural law assert that there are some basic, elementary rules of ethics which man may discover by means of an introspective search of his own intellect and whose binding normative nature need not be predicated upon divine revelation. "Thou shalt not kill" is recognized as a principle of conduct that man could discover for himself even were he not commanded by the Deity to refrain from killing his fellow man.[4] Secondly, there is what may be termed a theological doctrine of natural law, that is, a theory which quite correctly points to reason and design in the universe and to the phenomenon that all of nature is designed for the fulfillment of specific *teloi,* goals or ends. Exponents of this theory of natural law argue that if there is purpose and design in nature and if man can discover the goals of nature by use of his reason then man ought not to thwart the design and plan which is the expression of the will of the Divine Creator.[5]

Judaism, oddly enough, accepts, at least in a limited manner, what I have termed the secular notion of natural law, that is, the notion that there are certain moral maxims which are discoverable by reason alone. But while it certainly does enthusiastically accept the notion that intelligence is manifest in the laws of nature and that creation is designed for a purpose, it rejects the notion that man may not harness nature or that man may not intervene and manipulate the laws of nature for the betterment of the human condition. In rabbinic thought dispensation for such intervention is derived from Genesis 1:28 which bids man to be fruitful and multiply, to fill the earth and to conquer it, to establish his sovereignty and dominion over the animal kingdom and over the natural order into which he was introduced.[6] Thus while Judaism does recognize the role of natural law, in at least certain instances, in the limited sense of establishing binding *nomoi* on the basis of reason alone, it denies the notion of a natural law which legislates against the thwarting of the *teloi* of nature.[7] Since there can be on opposition on grounds of natural law, why, then, this aversion to artificial forms of procreation ?

To understand the attitude of Judaism properly, one must analyze precisely the verse which has been cited. It is the verse addressed to Adam in which he is bidden to procreate: "Be fruitful and multiply, and fill the earth and conquer it." Rabbinic exegesis establishes the obligation to procreate as a commandment that is directed to the male of the species. Rabbinic exegesis focuses upon the phrase "and conquer it." The Sages of the Talmud, in effect, proceeded to ask, "And who is it that conquers the land, exercises dominion over the animal kingdom and over nature itself?" The resultant dictum, "It is the wont of the male to conquer, but it is not the wont of the female to conquer," when viewed from a socio-historical perspective, constitutes an anthropological truism for it was the male who was destined to tame animals, harvest crops, develop natural resources and harness the forces of nature. Hence, the juxtaposition of the injunction to be fruitful and multiply with a particular role that is regarded as wholly within the purview of the male establishes a concomitant male obligation to populate the universe.[8]

But, of course, since, in its imperative mode, "be fruitful and multiply" is addressed to men it cannot be understood as an injunction to bear children for that is a biological impossibility. Even modern science has not yet discovered an artificial means by which a male can experience the pains of childbirth. Accordingly, in terms of its normative ramification, the divine imperative to be fruitful and multiply addressed to the male is codified by Maimonides as a commandment to engage in sexual activity within the marital framework at certain stipulated intervals until such time as children have been sired.[9] Thus, the essence of the divine command is the sexual act itself. To be sure, if children are sired by other means the father may perhaps be relieved of further obligation with regard to the commandment "be fruitful and multiply" and whether or not he is indeed relieved of further obligation is a matter of considerable discussion and some dispute.[10]

Nevertheless, despite the release of the individual from further obligation, he is not to be credited with the performance of a *mizvah*, i.e., with fulfillment of a divine commandment. This, however, merely serves to illuminate the nature and ramifications of a particular commandment but certainly does not serve to establish a prohibition against engaging in activity which, if not divinely mandated, may yet be within the zone of permissible activity.

It should, however be emphasized that although, in many circumstances, Judaism does command what is at times described as extraordinary means or heroic measures in the preservation of human life, it does not require such measures for the sake of generation of life. The only act which is commanded is the act which is natural; the only mandated form of procreation is that which stems directly from the sexual union. Insofar as the various available artificial forms of procreation are concerned, they must, at least in the narrow legal sense, be regarded as permissible unless a violation of some particular divine command is entailed. And indeed some forms of artificial procreation do involve precisely such transgressions. Chief among the contervailing considerations are:

1. *Violation of Marital Bonds*

For Judaism, insemination of a married woman with the sperm of a donor other than the woman's husband presents a serious problem. The problem does not stem primarily from concern for violation of the marital bonds as conceptualized in a theological or philosophical manner, but arises from the specific nature of the biblical commandment against adultery. Various forbidden sexual unions are enumerated in the eighteenth chapter of Leviticus. In every case, save one, the Hebrew of the original biblical text utilizes a term which is patently a euphemism for sexual intercourse. Jurists are aware that, in virtually all systems of law, the sexual act, whether in the context of rape, incest or the consummation of marriage, is defined as penetration rather than ejaculation. That is true in Jewish law as well and remains true even with regard to the prohibition against adultery. But, surprisingly, the language employed in Leviticus 18:20 (which is mistranslated in the standard English translations of the Bible) in the formulation of the prohibition against adultery speaks specifically of the deposit of semen in the genital tract of a married woman. As noted by Naḥmanides, the thirteenth century biblical commentator and exegete, the prohibition against adultery is founded upon a concern that paternal identity be certain and unambiguous, lest progeny unknowingly find themselves engaged in incestuous relationships.

According to some latter-day authorities, the deposit of the semen of a male other than the husband in the genital tract of a married woman, i.e. artificial insemination with the semen of a donor, constitutes adultery pure and simple;[11] others maintain that, absent a sexual act, there can be no culpable infraction.[12] But even those authorities would agree that artificial insemination with the semen of a donor infringes upon the spirit of the law and hence, *de minimis,* is to be regarded as a form of quasi-adultery[13] or prostititution.[14] Accordingly, no form of artificial procreation which involves the introduction of semen of a male other than the husband into the genital tract of a married woman can receive the imprimatur of Jewish law.

2. *Destruction of the Zygote*

The second problem to be considered is one which exists particularly in the area of in vitro fertilization as it is commonly carried out, *viz.*, the problem posed by the destruction of a developing embryo. Of course, were the fertilized ova always to be implanted in the uterus, no problem would arise. However, if, as is indeed the case, a number of ova are fertilized simultaneously, there results a surplus of fertilized ova which are not reimplanted in the uterus of the mother. Disposal of those fertilized ova presents a serious problem to all moralists.[15] The taking of any life, even that of a fetus, is clearly forbidden by Jewish law.[16] Man does not have the right to destroy even the life which he has created and which would not have come into existence save for his intellectual prowess and technical skill. Elucidation of the underlying reason and the specific nature of the offense is not a matter of significance for purposes of this discussion.

A matter of crucial significance is a possible distinction between various stages of gestation. Professor Dunstan, in his paper presented before this Academy, refers to various stages of gestation and particularly to a point of delineation drawn at the fortieth day following conception.

Whether or not there is a prohibition against destroying a fetus within the first forty days following conception is a matter of ongoing debate and disagreement among contemporary rabbinic scholars.[17] That distinction has as its source texts which have been handed down from antiquity. In particular, the Septuagint does draw such a distinction. In an article published a number of years ago, I sought to draw attention to the fact that there is a significant school of thought which maintains that, in its universal teaching, i.e., in the teachings of Judaism to the nations of the world under the general framework of the Seven Commandments of the Sons of Noah, Judaism posits that the destruction of the fetus within the first forty days of development entails no moral infraction while at the same time maintaining that, insofar as Jews themselves are concerned, the destruction of even a nascent or potential life within that period is forbidden. Recognition of disparate standards imposed upon Jews and non-Jews serves to explain why such a distinction occurs in the Greek translation even though it is not present in the original Hebrew text. The Septuagint, intended as it was for a non-Jewish audience, accurately reflects Jewish teaching directed to the nations of the world.[18]

My own small contribution to this ongoing discussion is the drawing of another distinction with regard to the various stages of embryonic development, a distinction that invokes a concept of law which is well-known in the common law tradition: *De minimis non curat lex*. The concept that the law does not concern itself with trifles finds expression in Jewish law as well. Although, in Jewish law, this principle has an extremely limited application in matters of jurisprudence, a closely related concept is of paramount importance within the context of religious law.

For example, Jews are commanded not to eat creeping animals, including marine creatures that creep in bodies of water. If one takes a small drop of water, places it upon a slide and examines it under a microscope, one will observe the presence of literally thousands of creeping organisms. Yet Judaism does not forbid the drinking of a glass of water. But on what basis can the attendant imbibing of creeping things be sanctioned? The answer must lie in the recognition that Jewish law concerns itself only with gross phenomena. A phenomenon that is sub-visual is of no consequence. An organism that can be seen only by means of a magnifying glass or under a microscope is an organism of which Jewish law takes no notice; for purposes of the Jewish legal system, it is as if it did not exist.[19]

If one applies this principle to the developing human organism, it yields the conclusion that legal cognizance can be taken of the organism only when it becomes visible to the naked eye. However, during its very early stages of development, when the organism is still sub-visual,[20] the law takes no cognizance of its existence. If so, it may well be argued that there is no prohibition associated with its destruction. This point remains a matter under discussion and undoubtedly more will be heard in the future with regard to this distinction.

3. *Primum Non Nocere*

A third consideration, the consideration which to my mind probably represents the most significant reservation that emerges from Jewish teaching with regard to in vitro fertilization, and indeed with regard to certain other experimental forms of human procreation, is a consideration paralleling the medical maxim *"Primum non nocere."* The first principle is to do no harm. It is a fundamental principle of Jewish morality that no harm may be intentionally inflicted by one human being upon another.[21] An individual has no right to place another person at risk of harm or injury. A person does not have the right to cause injury to any other human being even if the person performing that act is the author of the life of the affected party. Man is not morally entitled to create life in order to inflict harm or injury upon the bearer or that life.

A number of years ago, Professor Paul Ramsey, who was a Protestant theologian, very eloquently and very cogently formulated a position which I believe to be entirely compatible with the perspective of Jewish law in declaring that all experimentation upon an unborn fetus is *ipso facto* immoral and unethical. Such experimentation is unethical for the simple reason that one cannot possibly predict in advance whether the techniques that are to be employed will result in the birth of a defective child who otherwise would not have been born.[22] This fundamental ethical principle serves to illuminate what may well be the earliest recorded legislation in the area of genetics. The Talmud declares that a man should not marry a woman who comes from a family of epileptics and that a man should not marry a woman who comes from a family of lepers.[23] In ancient times it was presumed that both epilepsy and leprosy were disorders transmitted by heredity. The injunction against marrying into families in which those diseases are present is clearly born of a concern lest the person entering into such a marriage cause the birth of a defective child. Certainly, artificial means of procreation that could lead to such an untoward result would be frowned upon by Jewish law. Life should not be artificially generated when such generation carries with it the risk of unusual suffering or pain.

Unfortunately, data with regard to the incidence of congenital defects in the more than 3,000 births which have resulted from in vitro fertilization is not available since such information has not been published in the medical literature.[24] Thus there is no reliable information with regard to whether such births have or have not occurred or, if they have occurred, whether they have occurred with a higher statistical frequency than would have been anticipated in normal births; or whether the incidence has perhaps been even lower than in natural pregnancies. But certainly in the early period of employment of this procedure the birth of defective neonates was a phenomenon that had to be anticipated The sheer physical manipulation of the ovum and the zygote and the reinsertion of the developing blastocyst in the uterus of the mother could indeed have lead to genetic accidents. Development of the zygote outside of the uterus for even a limited period of time might have precluded operation of mechanisms employed by nature, often in the early stages of gestation, which serve to eliminate defective fetuses. Such mechanisms could well be circumvented by means of artificial techniques and result in the birth of defective neonates who would not have been born had nature been allowed to follow its natural course.

Of course, it is entirely possible that with the passage of time and the perfection of medical technology and techniques it may be shown that such concerns are misplaced or that, if these concerns were not originally misplaced, they may be dispelled by new advances and new developments. Daniel Callahan has observed that the history of medicine is strewn with instances in which unethical acts have led to significant benefits.[25] It may well be the case that a procedure that cannot be ethically condoned at the time of its original employment may turn out to be morally unassailable or it may lead to refinements whose demonstrated efficacy will lead to moral acceptance without qualm or hesitation. With regard to in vitro fertilization, I suspect that the jury is still out and that it is still too early to make any definitive judgment with regard to the ethical implications of the procedure.

Last, but not least, it should be noted that not everything that is permitted should be embraced with open arms. Concerns born of the psychological impact that may result from certain artificial forms of procreation are entirely cogent. Nor should demographic concerns be dismissed peremptorily. It appears that, for some reason, in vitro fertilization results in a preponderance of female births over male births.[26] Certainly, with the advent of genetic engineering, it is possible that prospective parents may chose to utilize such methods not only for preselection of the sex of their child but also for purposes that are entirely frivolous in nature. It should be clearly recognized that these are areas in which society may legitimately promulgate legislation in order to prevent social evils. Society has not only the power but also the moral obligation to regulate artificial forms of procreation in order to prevent untoward results.

I would emphasize one further point with regard to Jewish teaching pertaining to procreation. The biblical phrase "Be fruitful and multiply" occurs twice in virtually the identical context. This biblical exhortation was first addressed to Adam upon his creation and repeated to Noah after the deluge. In rabbinic exegesis it is understood that one occurrence of that phrase is as a command. The other occurrence is by way of a blessing.[27] "Be fruitful and multiply" is at once both a blessing and a command. Procreation is not only the fulfillment of a divine command and a divine mandate, it is also the invocation of a divine blessing. May we, as members of human society, be granted the wisdom always to harness and utilize the fruits of scientific inquiry in a morally legitimate manner and to employ them in human procreation solely in a manner which is a blessing to mankind.

NOTES

1. Cf., Rabbi Yosef E. Henkin, *Ha-Ma'or*. Tishri-Ḥeshvan 5725, pp. 9–11, who posits a legal basis for the values in question. See, however, R. Chaim Dov-Ber Gulevsky, *Lahat ha-Ḥerev ha-Mithapekhet* (New York, 1976), p. 61.
2. See, for example, the address of Pope Pius XII to the Fourth International Convention of Catholic Physicians in October, 1949, *Orizzonte Medico*, 1950. See also Charles J. McFadden, *Medical Ethics* (Philadelphia, 1967), pp. 60–61.
3. John Locke, *Essays on the Law of Nature*, (Oxford, 1954), p. 123; and *idem*, *An Essay Concerning Human Understanding* (Oxford, 1975), p. 75.
4. See *Sanhedrin* 4a. See also Thomas Aguinas. *Summa Theologica*, Pt. I-II, Q. 94, Art. 5.
5. See *Summa Theologica*, Pt. I-II, Q. 91, Art. 1–2 and Q. 94, Art. 2.
6. See, for example, Naḥmanides, *Commentary on the Bible*, Genesis 1:28.
7. See J. David Bleich, "Judaism and Natural Law," *Jewish Law Annual*, vol. VII (1988), pp. 5–42.

8. *Yevamot* 65b.
9. Maimonides, *Mishneh Torah, Hilkhot Ishut* 15:1. For a fuller discussion, see *infra*, pp. 227–231.
10. See sources cited in *Oẓar ha-Poskim, Even ha-Ezer*, I (Jerusalem, 1947), 1:42; R. Chaim Joseph David Azulai, *Birkei Yosef, Even ha-Ezer* 1:14; and Fred Rosner "Artificial Insemination in Jewish Law" in *Jewish Bioethics*, ed. Fred Rosner and J. David Bleich (New York, 1979), p. 111.
11. See, for example, *Teshuvot Bar Leva'i*, II, no 1, and *Teshuvot Minḥat Yeḥi'el*, no. 7, cited in *Oẓar ha-Poskim, Even ha-Ezer*, I, 1:42; R. Judah Leib Zirelson, *Ma'arkhei Lev* (Kishinev, 1932), no. 23; R. Abraham Lurie, *Ha-Posek*, Ḥeshvan-Kislev 5710; R. Ovadiah Hadaya, "Hazra'ah Melakhutit," *No'am*, I (1958), 130–137; and R. Eliyahu Meir Bloch, *Ha-Pardes*, Sivan 5713, pp. 1–3.
12. See, for example, R. Moshe Feinstein, *Iggerot Mosheh, Even ha-Ezer*, I, no. 10; R. Ben Zion Uziel, *Mishpetei Uzi'el, Even ha-Ezer*, no. 19; R. Joseph Saul Nathanson, *Teshuvot Sho'el u-Meshiv, Mahadurah Telita'ah*, no. 132; R. Shalom Mordecai Schwadron, *Teshuvot Maharsham*, III, no. 268; R. Joshua Baumol, *Teshuvot Emek Halakhah*, no. 68; and R. Aaron Walkin, *Teshuvot Zekan Aharon*, II, *Even ha-Ezer*, no. 97.
13. See R. Eliezer Waldenberg. *Ẓiẓ Eli'ezer*, IX, no. 51, sec. 4.
14. R. Yosef E. Henkin, *loc. cit.*
15. For a discussion of the prohibition against destroying a fetus as applied to an embryo fertilized outside a woman's body see this writer's *Contemporary Halakhic Problems*, IV (New York, 1995), p. 241, note 10.
16. See sources cited by J. David Bleich, *Contemporary Halakhic Problems*, I (New York, 1977), 326–339.
17. *Ibid.*, pp. 339–347.
18. *Ibid.*, p. 344, note 40.
19. See R. Israel Lipschutz, *Tiferet Yisra'el, Avodah Zarah* 2:6 and R. Yechiel Michal Epstein, *Arukh ha-Shulḥan, Yoreh De'ah* 83:15 and 84:36. See also R. Abraham Danzig, *Ḥokhmat Adam*, 38:8; *idem, Binat Adam*, sec. 34; R. Shlomoh Kluger, *Teshuvot Tuv Ta'am va-Da'at, Mahadurah Tinyanah, Kuntres Aḥaron*, no. 53; R. Zevi Hirsh Shapiro, *Darkei Teshuvah, Yoreh De'ah* 18:20; R. Eliezer Waldenberg, *Ẓiẓ Eli'ezer*, VIII, no. 15, chap. 14. sec. 10; and R. Moses Feinstein, *Iggerot Mosheh, Yoreh De'ah*, II, no. 146; *idem, Iggerot Mosheh, Even ha-Ezer*, III, no. 33; and R. Pesach Falk, *Teshuvot Maḥazeh Eliyahu*, no. 91. Cf. also, R. Yom Tov Lipman Heller, *Ma'adanei Yom Tov, Halakhot Ketanot*,

Hilkhot Tefillin 9:40; and R. Dov Berish Weidenfeld. *Teshuvot Dovev Meisharim*, I, no. 1. Cf., however, R. Iser Zalman Meltzer, *Hashkafah ve-He'arot*, appended to R. Yechiel Michal Tucatzinsky, *Sefer Bein ha-Shemashot*, p. 153 and R. Moshe Sternbuch, *Mo'adim u-Zemanim*, II, no. 124.

20. I am told that at the eight-cell stage the developing zygote is roughly half the size of a period that appears at the end of a sentence in the *New York Times*. I am not quite certain whether something of that size is to be characterized as an object that can be perceived by the naked eye. If it is not to be classified as something perceivable by the naked eye, it may well be the case that, at that stage of development, Halakhah takes no cognizance of the zygote and regards it as non-existent for purposes of the prohibition against destroying an embryo and of the prohibition against destroying the male seed.
21. *Shulḥan Arukh, Ḥoshen Mishpat* 378:1 and 420:1.
22. See Paul Ramsey, "Shall We Reproduce?" *Journal of the American Medical Association*, vol. 220, no. 10 (June 5, 1972), pp. 1346–1350, and vol. 220, no. 11 (June 12, 1972), pp. 1480–1485; and *idem, The Ethics of Fetal Research* (Yale University Press, 1975).
23. *Yevamot* 64b.
24. Reports in the medical literature regarding the presence or absence of congenital defects in such children are few and scanty. A recent study of one hundred twenty-five pregnancies conceived in vitro report the birth of 115 babies (including fifteen sets of twins) of whom three had some congenital abnormality. See M.C. Andrews, S.J. Musher *et al.*, "An Analysis of the Obstetric Outcome of 125 Consecutive Pregnancies Conceived in vitro and Resulting in 100 Deliveries," *American Journal of Obstetrics and Gynecology*, vol. 154, no. 4 (April 1986), pp. 848–854. Another study of twenty infants born of in vitro fertilization assessing their developmental status upon reaching their first birthday found an increased rate of preterm delivery, intrauterine growth retardation and cesarean sections. One significant and two minor abnormalities were reported and one infant was slightly under the expected developmental assessment as measured by the Griffiths Developmental Scales. See J.L. Yovich. T.S. Parry *et al.*, "Developmental Assessment of Twenty In Vitro Fertilization Infants at Their First Birthday," *Journal of In Vitro Fertilization and Embryo Transfer*, vol. 3, no. 4 (August 1986), pp. 253–57.

25. *New York Times*, July 27, 1978, p. A16, col. 13.
26. See, For example, René Frydman, Joëlle Belaish-Allart *et al.*, "An Obstetric Assessment of the First 100 Births from the In Vitro Fertilization Program at Clamart, France," *American Journal of Obstetrics and Gynecology*, vol. 154, no. 4 (March 1986). p. 551; P.A.L. Lancaster, "High Incidence of Preterm Births and Early Losses in Pregnancy After In Vitro Fertilization." *British Medical Journal*, vol. 291, no. 6503 (October 26, 1985), p. 1161; D. Mushin, J. Spensley *et al.*, "Children of IVF," *Clinics on Obstetrics and Gynaecology*, vol. 12, no. 4 (December 1985), p. 860; A. Speirs, A. Trounson *et al.*, "Summary or Results," *Clinical In Vitro Fertilization*, ed. C. Wood and A. Trounson (Berlin, 1983), pp. 157–163; and C. Wood, A. Trounson *et al.*, "Clinical Features of Eight Pregnancies Resulting from In Vitro Fertilization and Embryon Transfer" *Fertility and Sterility*, vol. 38, no. 1 (July 1982), pp. 22–9.
27. See *Tosafot, Yevamot* 65b, s.v. *ve-lo ka'amar*; and Naḥmanides, *Commentary on the Bible,* Genesis 1:28. Which of the two occurrences is regarded as the command is a matter of dispute between Maimonides, *Mishneh Torah, Hilkhot Ishut* 15:1, and *Sefer ha-Ḥinnukh*, no. 1. See also the supercommentary of R. Eliyahu Mizraḥi on Rashi, Genesis 9:1; Maharsha, *Sanhedrin* 59a; and R. Moses Schik, *Maharam Shik al Taryag Miẓvot*, (Munkacs, 1895), no. 1.

8

Sperm Banking in Anticipation of Infertility

I. THE HALAKHIC PROBLEM

In some circumstances, radiation or chemotherapy in dosages sufficient to arrest certain forms of malignancy may affect the gonads in a manner that is likely to result in sterility. Hence male patients receiving radiation to the testes or, as is more frequently the case, chemotherapy for conditions such as Hodgkin's disease or non-Hodgkin's lymphoma are unlikely to be able to sire children. As a result some men, particularly those who have not yet become fathers, avail themselves of the option of having their semen frozen and stored in sperm banks. Utilizing a procedure that has been available since the late 1960s, the semen is collected before the patient undergoes treatment and his wife is later impregnated by means of artificial insemination using the husband's previously ejaculated sperm. Sperm can be cryobanked indefinitely. There have been documented pregnancies resulting from semen stored as long as fifteen years. However, some physicians report disappointing results in patients suffering from Hodgkin's disease, presumably because the quality of the sperm has been compromised by that illness. The halakhic propriety of such procedures for unmarried men is the subject of a symposium published in *Sefer Assia*, VII (Jerusalem, 5754), 279–303.

In the case of married men, the halakhic issues involved are precisely those present in all instances of homologous artificial insemination utilizing the husband's semen (AIH). Historically, the first reported employment of this technique in humans was for the purpose of overcoming the physical problem of depositing sperm in the genital tract of a woman whose husband suffered from hypospadias. That procedure was carried out at the close of the eighteenth century in approximately 1790 by the illustrious English surgeon, John Hunter, who succeeded in artificially impregnating the wife of a London linen draper.[1] Typically, AIH is recommended in situations in which the husband suffers from oligospermia, i.e., his sperm count is too low to enable him to father a child in the normal manner. AIH may also be advised when the husband is unable to maintain an erection, the husband experiences retrograde ejaculation due to neurological lesions or other causes, in instances of cervical abnormalities, anatomical abnormalities of the uterus, vaginismus, faulty spermatozoa reception of the vagina or hostility of the mucous secretions of the cervix, as well as when intravaginal coitus is impossible due to a tumor, excessive obesity, or anatomical disparity of the male and female sexual organs.[2] In such procedures, combination of ejaculates and delivery of the collected sperm directly to the uterus compensates for a low sperm count. The primary halakhic question is whether noncoital ejaculation by the husband is forbidden as a form of onanism or whether it is sanctioned in circumstances in which ejaculation is undertaken for purposes of procreation. This matter has been the subject of extensive discussion in rabbinic literature.[3]

Although a number of prominent authorities refuse to sanction the practice,[4] a majority of those who have addressed the issue permit AIH,[5] albeit with varying degrees of enthusiasm, but disagree among themselves with regard to the means of semen procurement that may legitimately be employed.[6] Among contemporary decisors, Rabbi Joseph Shalom Eliashiv as well as the late Rabbi Shlomoh Zalman Auerbach are reported as not being supportive of such procedures, particularly in instances involving unmarried men.[7] *Ḥazon Ish* also expressed a negative view, although it is not clear whether he decried the practice *in toto* or only when the procedure is carried out prior to the wife's immersion in a *mikveh* as a means of circumventing the fertility problem faced by some women who observe the regulations of family purity and experience a short ovulation cycle.[8]

Tosafot, Yevamot 12b and *Ketubot* 39a, demonstrate that normal intercourse is clearly permitted even when procreation is impossible as evidenced by the permissibility of marital relations with a minor and with an infertile woman. Intercourse with a post-menstrual woman is similarly permitted. The question is whether all non-vaginal ejaculation constitutes onanism or whether such forms of ejaculation are permitted when designed to promote procreation. The numerous authorities who permit AIH point to the talmudic discussion recorded in *Yevamot* 76a:

> Rabbi Judah stated in the name of Samuel: If [the membrum] was perforated and sealed in a manner such that it will tear when semen is emitted the man is unfit, but if [it does] not [tear] the man is regarded as fit. . . . Rava the son of Rabbah sent to Rabbi Joseph: Let our Master instruct us how to proceed [to test whether the semen will reopen the closed perforation]. Rabbi Joseph said to Rava: Warm barley bread is brought and placed upon his anus;[9] he emits semen and we observe [whether the wound has reopened]. . . . Abaye said: Colored [women's] garments are passed before him.

The talmudic discussion centers around the prohibition recorded in Deuteronomy 23:2 forbidding intercourse with a man who has sustained certain injuries to his genital organs. Included in that prohibition is a person who has sustained an unhealed perforation of the membrum. In this context healing is defined as closure of the perforation by adhesion of tissues with sufficient strength so that the perforation will not reopen upon erection and ejaculation. Whether or not such healing has indeed occurred would, of course, immediately become evident upon performance of a normal coital act. Intercourse, however, cannot be permitted unless it is known that the perforation has indeed become adequately sealed. As expressed by Rava, the result appears to be a Catch-22 situation: Marital relations cannot be permitted unless it has been demonstrated that the perforation is properly sealed. But since, ostensibly, ejaculation is permissible only in the context of intercourse such healing cannot be demonstrated. R. Joseph and Abaye both respond with advice regarding methods of achieving ejaculation without intercourse. The cogency of their replies, it is argued, is contingent upon antecedent acceptance of the thesis that only ejaculation that "wastes" the seed is prohibited as onanism but that other forms of ejaculation are permissible when undertaken in order to enable procreation to occur. Hence, since no marital relations may take place until the emission of semen occurs, such ejaculation is entirely permissible. Some scholars cite this opinion not only in support of AIH but also as the basis for sanctioning semen testing designed to facilitate treatment of male infertility, at least when there is reason to suspect that failure of the wife to conceive is due to infertility of the husband.[10]

It is clear that at least some form of non-coital seminal emission for purposes of procreation is permissible. The crucial question is whether such dispensation is limited only to the forms of emission specified in *Yevamot* 76a or whether other forms of ejaculation are permitted as well. R. Shlomoh Luria, *Yam shel Shlomoh*, *Yevamot* 8:15, observes that the procedures suggested by the Gemara represent indirect methods of ejaculation, i.e., they are designed to stimulate arousal that will culminate in ejaculation of semen, but do not involve a direct causal act. In general, transgression of a biblical prohibition occurs only if the act performed is the proximate cause of the prohibited effect; an act only indirectly causing such an effect (*gerama*) is generally prohibited by virtue of rabbinic decree. Rabbinic injunctions are often not universal in nature. They are enacted either as a "fence around the law" or to thwart conduct designed to frustrate the *telos* a prohibition is designed to achieve. Such rabbinic edicts frequently exclude situations in which countervailing policy considerations were regarded as paramount. Thus, it is not at all surprising to find that, in the situation addressed by *Yevamot* 76a, the Gemara sanctions sexual arousal as an indirect means of effecting seminal emission. In effect, a rabbinic prohibition is rendered nugatory in limited situations in order to facilitate marriage and thereby promote procreation. According to *Yam shel Shlomoh*, there is no evidence to contradict the presumption that the prohibition against onanism applies to all forms of biblically proscribed non-coital emission; for purposes of the biblical prohibition all acts that do not have direct procreative potential are forms of "wasting the seed."

Thus, according to *Yam shel Shlomoh*, a semen sample for diagnostic purposes may be obtained only by utilization of the methods indicated by the Gemara and by other analogous indirect methods, e.g., reading or viewing pornographic material, a method that is analogous to gazing upon colored female garments. However, at least in contemporary times, it is quite unlikely that such methods will result in a suitable seminal emission.

It may well be argued that, even according to *Yam shel Shlomoh*, direct means may be employed to obtain semen for purposes of AIH. In contradistinction to situations involving ejaculation for purposes of determining eligibility for marriage or for diagnostic purposes in which emission of semen is only indirectly related to the siring of a child, when semen is emitted for purposes of AIH the ejaculate itself is used directly for impregnation of the wife as is the case when ejaculation occurs in the context of sexual intercourse. Hence, it may be argued, the semen is not in any sense "wasted" and, accordingly, the biblical prohibition does not apply.[11]

Other authorities do not make the distinction drawn by *Yam shel Shlomoh* and permit even direct forms of semen procurement for all procreative purposes,[12] including semen testing.[13] However, R. Moshe Feinstein, *Iggerot Mosheh, Even ha-Ezer*, I, no. 70, distinguishes between semen procurement through use of a condom or in the form of coitus interruptus[14] and masturbation. *Iggerot Mosheh* also points to the fact that the Gemara, *Yevamot* 76a, does not advise masturbation as a means of causing ejaculation to occur.[15] But instead of drawing a distinction between direct and indirect acts designed to achieve ejaculation, as did *Yam shel Shlomoh*, Rabbi Feinstein points to a statement of the Gemara, *Niddah* 13b, from which he infers that masturbation constitutes a violation distinct from, and in addition to, "wasting of the seed." In that discussion, the Gemara speaks of a prohibition regarding "licentiousness by hand" and "licentiousness by foot" and by means of talmudic exegesis, relates those acts to biblical verses describing prohibited acts. *Iggerot Mosheh* reasons that the prohibition against onanism reflects a ban against "wasting of the seed" and hence does not apply to ejaculation designed to facilitate procreation even if there exists no direct causal nexus between ejaculation and conception while the prohibition to which reference is made in *Niddah* 13b, he opines, is directed not against ejaculation *per se*, but against physical manipulation involving "licentiousness by hand" or "licentiousness by foot."[16] Since that prohibition is unrelated to the concept of "wasting" the seed *Iggerot Mosheh* concludes that it is forbidden even when undertaken for purposes of procreation.

II. ARTIFICIAL INSEMINATION AND PATERNITY

From the foregoing it would appear that, in principle, AIH is entirely permissible and that the only area of dispute is with regard to appropriate means of semen procurement. That conclusion, however, is not entirely accurate. As has been stated, the authorities who permit this practice predicate their position upon the discussion found in *Yevamot* 76a that serves to establish that ejaculation for purposes of procreation is permitted. More precisely, that source serves to support the conclusion that emission of semen is warranted in order to establish capacity to contract a legitimate marriage in order to fulfill the biblical injunction "be fruitful and multiply" (Genesis 1:28 and 8:17). The selfsame principle would seem to render permissible semen testing necessary to determine treatment for male infertility since the goal is to enable the patient to fulfill the command "be fruitful and multiply." However, somewhat curiously, siring a child by means of AIH may not constitute fulfillment of that obligation. In order for a person to fulfill the commandment he must not only be the biological father of the child but must be recognized as the halakhic father as well. A Jewish male who consorts with a gentile woman is assuredly the biological father of the issue of that union but, since Jewish law does not recognize relationships of that nature, he is not the halakhic father. Similarly, a Hebrew servant is permitted to cohabit with a Canaanite slave but Halakhah does not recognize a paternal-filial relationship between the Hebrew servant and his offspring and, accordingly, in siring such children the Hebrew servant does not fulfill his obligation to "be fruitful and multiply."[17] The issue that must be addressed is whether Halakhah recognizes paternity only with regard to children born of sexual intercourse or whether such recognition extends also to issue born *sine concubito*. In light of the fact that AIH does not involve a coital act there are strong grounds to argue that, if intercourse is a necessary condition for establishing a halakhically recognized paternal relationship, AIH cannot be sanctioned since the birth of a child as a result of the procedure does not constitute fulfillment of the biblical commandment.

Most authorities find a resolution of this question in a statement of R. Peretz ben Elijah of Corbeil in his *Hagahot Semak*, cited by *Baḥ, Yoreh De'ah* 195; *Taz, Yoreh De'ah* 198:7; *Ḥelkat Meḥokek, Even ha-Ezer* 1:8; and *Bet Shmu'el, Even ha-Ezer* 1:10, who states:

> A menstruating woman may lie upon her husband's sheets but should be careful not to lie on sheets upon which another man has slept lest she become impregnated from the semen of another.[18] Why is she not concerned lest she become impregnated from her husband's semen during her menstruation and the child be conceived of a *niddah*? He answered that since there is no forbidden intercourse the child is entirely legitimate even if she becomes impregnated from another, for indeed Ben Sira was legitimate. However, from the semen of another we are particular with regard to determination [of paternity] lest [the child eventually marry] his paternal sister.

There cannot be sibling incest in the absence of a halakhically recognized fraternal relationship. A fraternal relationship exists only when, and because, the siblings share a common parent. Indeed, it is tautological to say that siblings enjoy a common paternal-filial or maternal-filial relationship. In the hypothetical situation discussed by *Hagahot Semak* the brother and sister shared a common, halakhically recognized, filial relationship even though one was born *sine concubito*. That conclusion is accepted by *Bet Shmu'el, loc. cit.*, R. Shimon ben Ẓemaḥ Duran, *Tashbaẓ*, III, no. 263, and most later authorities.[19] Nevertheless, some later authorities, including R.

Chaim Joseph David Azulai, *Birkei Yosef, Even ha-Ezer* 1:14, dispute this view and maintain that a coital act is the *sine qua non* of a halakhically recognized paternal relationship.[20] The view of *Bet Shmu'el* and *Tashbaẓ* is similarly questioned by *Taz, Even ha-Ezer* 1:8. *Ḥelkat Meḥokek, Even ha-Ezer* 1:8, expresses doubt with regard to whether a paternal-filial relationship arises *sine concubito*.[21]

Some scholars, including R. Joshua Baumol, *Teshuvot Emek Halakhah*, I, no. 60, R. Shlomoh Zalman Auerbach, *No'am*, I (5718), 157, and R. Judah Gershuni, *Kol Ẓofayikh* (Jerusalem, 5740), p. 367,[22] assert that although the progenitor of a child born *sine concubito* may not fulfill the commandment to "be fruitful and multiply" he certainly fulfills the mandate expressed in the prophetic verse "He created the universe not a waste, He formed it to be inhabited" (Isaiah 45:18). Ejaculation for that purpose, they contend, cannot be regarded as "wasting" the seed.

III. THE NATURE OF THE OBLIGATION TO PROPOGATE

Assuming that semen procurement by one means or another for purposes of insemination is permissible, is a childless man who faces imminent sterility as a result of radiation treatment or chemotherapy obligated to deposit his sperm in a sperm bank in order to impregnate his wife at a future time? For that matter, is a man who has a low sperm count obligated to avail himself of AIH in order to become a father? Rabbi Eliyahu Bakshi-Doron, the present Sephardic Chief Rabbi of Israel, *Binyan Av*, II, no. 60, correctly notes that, despite the fact that a large number of responsa have been published permitting AIH, in none of these responsa is there a hint that the procedure is obligatory. Dr. Abraham S. Abraham, *Nishmat Avraham*, IV, *Even ha-Ezer* 23:1, quotes a letter written by the late R. Shlomoh Zalman Auerbach in which the latter writes, ". . . the holy Torah did not obligate a person to freeze semen." However, that cryptic statement does not explain why such measures are not obligatory in order to satisfy the obligation of procreation mandated by the commandment "be fruitful and multiply."

The Gemara, *Ḥagigah* 2b, describes the plight of a person whose status is "half Canaanite slave and half free," e.g., the individual was part of an estate inherited by two brothers, one of whom proceeded to execute a bill of manumission while the other did not. Such a person may neither marry a Jewess of legitimate birth nor consort with a female Canaanite slave. The part of that individual's *persona* that is a free man is prohibited from having intercourse with a slave while the part that is a slave may not cohabit with a Jewess. Accordingly, the rule is set down that the master who has a partial interest in the slave must relinquish his title and set the slave free; moreover, if he fails to do so willingly, physical duress may be brought to bear upon him in order to secure compliance.

Tosafot, *ad locum* and *Bava Batra* 13a, question the premises expressed in the dilemma posed by the Gemara. The obligation to "be fruitful and multiply" is a positive commandment; the restriction against cohabitation between freemen and slaves is the product of a negative commandment. The general rule is that when a positive commandment and a negative commandment are in conflict and one or the other must be transgressed, fulfillment of the positive commandment takes precedence (*aseh doḥeh lo ta'aseh*). If so, queries *Tosafot*, why is this individual not permitted to cohabit with a Jewess in fulfillment of a positive commandment even though that fulfillment entails concomitant infraction of a negative commandment? *Tosafot* responds by noting that the rule of *aseh doḥeh lo ta'aseh* applies only if fulfillment of the positive commandment is simultaneous with violation of the negative commandment whereas, in performance of the sexual act, transgression of the negative commandment occurs in the initial stage of penetration (*ha'ara'ah*) while fulfillment of the positive commandment does not occur until a later stage of the sexual act (*gemar bi'ah*).[23] *Tosafot*'s reasoning in applying the relevant principle is unexceptionable and hence the talmudic dilemma is entirely understandable since it is perfectly clear that fulfillment of the precept and transgression of the prohibition do not occur simultaneously. The problem is that the time lapse between transgression of the negative commandment and fulfillment of the positive commandment seems to be far greater than indicated by *Tosafot*. "Be fruitful and multiply" seems to imply propagation of the species, i.e., birth of a child. That event does not take place at the time of intercourse but only subsequent to a period of gestation. The gap is not between the earliest stage of penetration and completion of penetration—a matter of mere seconds—but between intercourse and birth of a child—a period of nine months.

It is abundantly clear that *Tosafot* regard the admonition "be fruitful and multiply" as connoting not the siring of a child, but as a commandment making the procreative act, *viz.*, intercourse, mandatory. Such intercourse is required on a regular basis until the requisite number of children has been born. A gentile who converts to Judaism together with his children is exempt from this requirement because he, in fact, has sired children. The *mizvah* is the sexual act, but the *mizvah* is incumbent only upon those who are yet childless.

This analysis of the nature of the *mizvah* is logically compelling. Halakhah defines the *mizvah* as binding only upon the male, but not upon the female. Speculative science and Hollywood fantasies aside, no male has ever experienced the pain of childbirth. It is axiomatic that God does not command the impossible. Although endocrinologists claim that, with proper hormone treatment, the phenomenon of a male carrying a fetus to term (as portrayed in the 1995 film *Junior*) is theoretically possible, any attempt by a male to bear a child would pose a grave risk to the life of the putative father (or perhaps more accurately, the male mother).[24] No one need assume such risk in fulfilling any *mizvah*. Certainly, when commanded by God, the males to whom the *mizvah* was addressed did not understand it to require them to seek hormone treatment at the hands of endocrinologists. The *mizvah*, then, must be defined as mandating that which is in the province of the male, *viz*., the sexual act that has procreation as its goal.[25]

This thesis is reflected in the precise language employed by Rambam in spelling out the *mizvah* to "be fruitful and multiply." Rambam, *Hilkhot Ishut* 15:1, states that a husband "is obligated to engage in intercourse at each designated interval until he has children for such is the positive commandment of the Torah as it is said 'be fruitful and multiply.'" The commandment requires the male to marry a woman capable of bearing children and to engage in intercourse with stipulated frequency. The essence of the commandment is the marital act; the birth of children represents the *terminus ad quem* beyond which the marital act is no longer mandated by reason of "be fruitful and multiply."[26]

Noteworthy also is the fact that in enumerating the questions put to a person on the Day of Judgment, the Gemara, *Shabbat* 31a, indicates that the first question is phrased in the words "Did you engage in procreation?" rather than "Did you sire the required number of children?" The latter question is not posed because, contrary to a literal reading of the verse, man is not commanded to sire, much less to bear, children; he is commanded to "engage in procreation," i.e., to perform the procreative act that is within his province, *viz*., intercourse. It is thus possible, although highly improbable, for a man who suffers no reproductive abnormality to select a fertile woman as a wife, to marry at the proper age, to engage in intercourse at the stipulated intervals throughout his entire lifetime but yet not to become a father. According to this analysis, such a childless person has nevertheless discharged his obligation to "be fruitful and multiply." Accordingly, a question with regard to the birth of children would not be at all appropriate at the time of judgment; the appropriate question is that formulated by the Gemara, "Did you engage in procreation." Similarly, the Mishnah, *Yevamot* 61b, declares, "A person should not desist from procreation unless he has children." Here, too, the obligation is couched in terms of the procreative act rather than in terms of siring children.

Yet another significant halakhic conclusion flows from this thesis. Were the words of the precept to be construed as a commandment focused upon producing children, the reproductive process employed to achieve that end would be merely instrumental and would not form part of the *mizvah*. Although sexual intercourse is the obvious means of achieving the requisite goal, the same result might conceivably be accomplished by other means. It would then follow that, since the means are not intrinsic to the commandment, a person incapable of siring a child in the usual and natural manner would be obligated to employ artificial means, when and if available, to achieve that end. Procedures such as AIH or other forms of assisted procreation would be mandatory for otherwise infertile males.

However, since intercourse is the essence of the commandment, it is that act alone that is incumbent upon the male. A person incapable of impregnating his wife by means of natural intercourse has no obligation whatsoever to engage in any other practice designed to cause conception to occur. The result is that, although artificial means and "heroic measures" may in at least some circumstances be required in order to prolong life, they are never required in order to generate life. Of course, means such as AIH may be entirely permissible but their use is discretionary rather than mandatory.

IV. SPERM BANKING FOR THE UNMARRIED

Rabbi Bakshi-Doron[27] permits AIH and semen banking only for an already married man. He accepts the notion that ejaculation for purposes of procreation is permissible but argues that it is permissible only for a married man who is "actually obligated" (*ḥayyav be-po'el*) in the performance of the *miẓvah* of procreation but not for an unmarried man whose obligation cannot yet actually be discharged. Dr. Abraham cites R. Shlomoh Zalman Auerbach as declaring, "There is no distinction at all between a married man and a bachelor for even a bachelor is obligated to marry a wife and fulfill the commandment concerning procreation. But, in my opinion, even a married man is not obligated [to freeze semen] for the holy Torah did not obligate a person to freeze semen. The sole matter of doubt with regard to this matter is only whether it is prohibited or permitted."

Rabbi Auerbach's view is entirely cogent. Bachelors are bound by the obligation to "be fruitful and multiply" no less so than married men. Dr. Daniel Melech, writing in *Sefer Assia*, VII, 300, compares the bachelor's obligation to that of a person who has not purchased an *etrog* for use on *Sukkot*. The latter is clearly "actually" obligated in the performance of the *miẓvah*; his obligation "actually" includes taking the necessary measures to acquire an *etrog*. A bachelor is similarly required to fulfill the *miẓvah* of procreation but only in a legitimate manner, i.e., by means of marital relations with a lawfully wedded wife, and must perform the antecedent acts necessary for that purpose.

Accordingly, the consensus of halakhic opinion is that there is no difference between married and unmarried men with regard to semen banking. At the same time, such procedures are discretionary at best; they are certainly not mandatory. The position of authorities such as Rabbi Auerbach and Rabbi Eliashiv who discourage but do not prohibit the procedure is presumably based upon well-grounded hesitation to sanction halakhically controversial methods of semen procurement for a purpose that is entirely discretionary in nature.

NOTES

1. Magnus Hirschfeld, *Geschlechtskunde auf Grund dreissigjähriger Forschung und Erfahrung bearbeitet* (Stuttgart, 1928), II, 404; Hermann Rohleder, *Test Tube Babies: A History of the Artificial Impregnation of Human Beings* (New York, 1934), p. 40; Alan Guttmacher, "The Role of Artificial Insemination in the Treatment of Sterility," *Obstetrical and Gynecological Survey*, vol. 15, ed. by Nicholson J. Eastman (Baltimore, 1960), p. 767; and *idem*, "Artificial Insemination," *Annals of the New York Academy of Sciences*, vol. 97, art. 3 (Sept. 29, 1962), p. 623. The report is attributed to Hunter's nephew, Everett Home, "An Account of the Dissection of a Hermaphrodite Dog etc." *Philosophical Transactions of London*, vol. 89 (1799), p. 157.
2. Wilfred J. Finegold, *Artificial Insemination* (Springfield, 1964), p. 17; Guttmacher, *Obstetrical and Gynecological Survey,* p. 769; Barry S. Verkauf, "Artificial Insemination: Progress, Polemics, and Confusion—An Appraisal of Current Medico-Legal Status," *Houston Law Review*, vol. 3, no. 3 (Winter 1966), pp. 280–281; and Amey Chappell, "Artificial Insemination," *Journal of the American Women's Medical Association*, vol. 14, no. 10 (October 1959), p. 902.
3. A useful survey of that literature is presented in *Ha-Refu'ah le-Or ha-Halakhah,* ed. R. Michal Stern, I (Jerusalem, 5740), part 2, pp. 1–102.
4. *Rav Pe'alim*, III, *Even ha-Ezer*, no. 2; R. Malki'el Zevi Tennenbaum, *Teshuvot Divrei Malki'el*, IV, nos. 107–108; R. Ovadiah Hadaya, *No'am*, I (5718), 130–137, reprinted in *idem*, *Teshuvot Yaskil Avdi,* V, *Even ha-Ezer*, no. 10; R. Ya'akov Breisch, *Teshuvot Ḥelkat Ya'akov*, I, no. 24; R. Shlomoh Epstein, *Teshuvah Shlemah*, II, *Even ha-Ezer*, no. 4; R. Ben Zion Uziel, *Mishpetei Uzi'el, Even ha-Ezer*, no. 19; and others.
5. R. Shalom Mordecai Schwadron, *Teshuvot Maharsham*, III, no. 268; R. Simchah Bunim Sofer, *Teshuvot Shevet Sofer, Even ha-Ezer*, no. 1; R. Chaim Ozer Grodzinski, *Teshuvot Aḥi'ezer*, III, no. 24; R. Abraham Bornstein of Sochachev, *Avnei Nezer, Even ha-Ezer*, no. 63; R. Aaron Walkin, *Teshuvot Zekan Aharon*, I, nos. 66–67 and II, no. 97; R. Zevi Pesach Frank, *Teshuvot Har Ẓevi, Even ha-Ezer*, no. 1; R. Moshe Feinstein, *Iggerot Mosheh, Even ha-Ezer*, I, nos. 70–71, II, nos. 16 and 18 and III, no. 14; R. Ovadiah Yosef, *Teshuvot Yabi'a Omer*, II, *Even ha-Ezer*, no. 1; R. Joshua Baumol, *Teshuvot Emek Halakhah*, I, no. 68; R.

Ya'akov Yitzchak Weisz, *Teshuvot Minḥat Yiẓḥak*, I, no. 10, III, no. 47 and IV, no. 5; R. Shlomoh Zalman Auerbach, *No'am*, I (5718), 145–166; R. Eliezer Waldenberg, *Ẓiẓ Eli'ezer*, III, no. 27 and IX, no. 51, *sha'ar* 4, chap. 6; R. Yisra'el Zev Mintzberg, *No'am*, I, 129; and others.

6. Retrieval of semen from the vagina of the wife after coitus presents no halakhic problem; see *Teshuvot R. Akiva Eger,* no. 72; *Iggerot Mosheh, Even ha-Ezer,* I, no. 70 and II, no. 16; and R. Joel Teitelbaum, *Teshuvot Divrei Yo'el*, II, *Even ha-Ezer*, no. 107, sec. 6. Testicular puncture and aspiration of spermatozoa, sometimes recommended for men whose epididymes or vasa deferentia are occluded, is also acceptable; see *Teshuvot Zekan Aharon*, I, nos. 66–67; *Teshuvot Minḥat Yiẓḥak*, III, no. 108; *Ẓiẓ Eli'ezer*, IX, no. 51, *sha'ar* 1, chap. 2; and *Iggerot Mosheh, Even ha-Ezer*, II, no. 3.
7. See Abraham S. Abraham, *Nishmat Avraham*, IV, *Even ha-Ezer* 23:1. Rabbi Eliashiv's view is reported by R. Eliyahu Bakshi-Doron, *Binyan Av*, II, no. 60.
8. See letter of *Ḥazon Ish* published in R. Kalman Kahana, *Taharat Bat Yisra'el*, 3rd ed. (Jerusalem, 5723), p. 11 and in the Hebrew-English edition, *Taharat Bat Yisra'el: Daughter of Israel* (Jerusalem, 5730), pp. 135–136.
9. This method of stimulation is probably an approximation of rectal massage of the prostate gland and seminal vesicles with pressure on the ampulla of the vas deferens described in medical literature as a means of obtaining semen for artificial insemination. See G.P.R. Tallin, "Artificial Insemination," *Canadian Bar Review*, vol. 34, no. 1 (January, 1956), p. 7.
10. An even more permissive view is expressed by R. Jacob Emden, *She'ilat Ya'aveẓ*, I, no. 43. *She'ilat Ya'aveẓ* understands the talmudic phraseology prohibiting "purposeless emission of seed" (*le-vatalah*) quite literally and hence sanctions destruction of the male seed for any legitimate purpose, e.g., in order to overcome "grave pain." R. Jacob Emden's view is rejected by most authorities as an isolated opinion. Cf., however, *Ẓiẓ Eli'ezer*, XIII, no. 102 and the sharp rejoinder of *Iggerot Mosheh, Ḥoshen Mishpat*, II, no. 69, sec. 4.
11. It seems to this writer that this is the thrust of the point made by *Teshuvot Zekan Aharon*, I, no. 97, s.v. *ve-'al dvar ha-safek ha-sheni.*
12. *Zekan Aharon*, I, no. 67, and *Teshuvot Divrei Yo'el*, II, *Even ha-Ezer*, no. 107, sec. 6, suggest that seminal emission is permitted by the Gemara, *Yevamot* 76a, solely in the case of a person who

would otherwise never be able to marry and hence is likely to experience non-procreative emission of semen on an ongoing basis.

13. See, for example, *Bet Shmu'el, Even ha-Ezer* 25:2, who cites *Yevamot* 76a in connection with coital bleeding which, if from the wife, renders ongoing marital relations forbidden but, if from the husband, is halakhically innocuous. *Bet Shmu'el* tentatively permits non-coital ejaculation in order to examine the ejaculate for the presence of blood but fails to specify that only indirect stimulation is permissible.
14. *Iggerot Mosheh, Even ha-Ezer*, I, nos. 70 and 71, II, no. 16 and III, no. 14, regards use of condoms and coitus interruptus as equally acceptable. R. Chaim Ozer Grodzinski, *Teshuvot Aḥi'ezer*, III, no. 24, sec. 5, permits use of a condom but not coitus interruptus. *Iggerot Mosheh*, in his first responsum, also appears to prefer that method in deference to the views of *Aḥi'ezer*. However, *Teshuvot Zekan Aharon*, I, no. 66, and II, no. 97, and *Ẓiẓ Eli'ezer*, IX, no. 51, *sha'ar* 1, chap. 2, regard coitus interruptus as the preferred method. That conclusion would also flow from the position of *Teshuvot Yismaḥ Levav, Even ha-Ezer*, no. 7; *Teshuvot Ereẓ Ẓevi*, no. 45; and *Teshuvot She'erit Yiẓḥak*, no. 21; see also R. Moshe Sternbuch, *Teshuvot ve-Hanhagot*, I, no. 361. Cf., *Teshuvot Yabi'a Omer*, III, *Even ha-Ezer*, no. 7; R. Moshe Turetsky, *Teshuvot Yashiv Mosheh*, p. 169; R. Joseph Rosen, *Teshuvot Ẓofnat Pa'aneaḥ*, I, no. 115 and III, no. 161; R. Schmaryah Menasheh Adler, *Mareh Kohen, Mahadura Telita'ah*, nos. 48 and 49; and *Oẓar ha-Poskim*, IX, 20:1, sec. 7.
15. Coitus interruptus is, of course, not an option in situations in which intercourse cannot be sanctioned since in all instances in which intercourse is prohibited even minimal penetration is prohibited as well.
16. The prohibition, however, is directed only against "licentiousness" of this nature that leads to emission of semen. For that reason, it appears to this writer that there would be no objection to masturbation for purposes of AIH by a person who suffers from retrograde ejaculation. In such cases spermatozoa are recovered from urine collected subsequent to orgasm. From a halakhic perspective, such recovery of sperm would appear to be no different from testicular aspiration.
17. R. Shlomoh Zalman Auerbach, *No'am*, I, 157, argues that since such liaisons are permissible, halakhically recognized paternity cannot be a necessary condition for permissible emission of seed. In point of fact, this argument is readily rebutted. Natural

intercourse does not constitute "waste of the seed" and is always permitted as evidenced by the absence of a restriction against consorting with a minor, an infertile or post-menopausal woman. Only non-coital ejaculation requires the warrant of procreative potential.

18. In 1905, a German court was asked to consider the case of a woman who claimed that, without her husband's knowledge, she had scooped up fresh semen ejaculated by him on the bedclothes and introduced it into her genital tract causing a pregnancy that resulted in the birth of a baby girl. A trial court in Coblenz ruled that this artificial fecundation was a legal act. See Rohleder, *Test Tube Babies*, pp. 184–185. That decision was upheld in 1907 by an appeals court in Cologne. Shortly afterwards, in a second and remarkably similar case, a woman claimed to have discovered freshly ejaculated semen, probably the result of a nocturnal emission, which she inserted in her vagina. Despite (questionable) medical testimony denying that pregnancy could have resulted from that act, the appeals court in Cologne affirmed the legitimacy of the child. Later, the German Supreme Court took a similar position. See Rohleder, pp. 186 and 197–199. See also Alfred Koerner, "Medicolegal Considerations in Artificial Insemination," *Louisiana Law Review*, vol. 8, no. 3 (March 1948), p. 492; Finegold, *Artificial Insemination*, pp. 67–70; and Anthony F. LoGatte, "Artificial Insemination: Legal Aspects," *Catholic Lawyer*, vol. 1, no. 1 (January 1968), p. 174.
19. See, for example, *Mishneh la-Melekh, Hilkhot Ishut* 15:4; R. Yonatan Eibeschutz, *Bnei Ahuvah, Hilkhot Ishut* 15; *Teshuvot Bet Ya'akov*, no. 124; *Teshuvot Mishpatim Yesharim*, no. 396; *Turei Even, Ḥagigah* 26a; *Arukh la-Ner, Yevamot* 10a; *Teshuvot Divrei Malki'el*, IV, no. 107; *Teshuvot Yaskil Avdi*, V, no. 10; *Ẓiẓ Eli'ezer*, XX, no. 51, *sha'ar* 4, chap. 3; and *Teshuvot Minḥat Yiẓḥak*, I, no. 50.
20. This is also the position of *Teshuvot Bar Leva'i, Even ha-Ezer*, no. 1 and *Mishpetei Uzi'el, Even ha-Ezer*, no. 19; cf., R. Menachem Kasher, *No'am*, I, 125–128; and *idem, Torah Shelemah*, XVII, 242.
21. A number of authorities maintain that, although a paternal-filial relationship may arise *sine concubito*, birth of a child under such circumstances does not constitute fulfillment of the commandment. See, for example, *She'ilat Ya'aveẓ*, II, no. 97; R. Chaim Joseph David Azulai, *Birkei Yosef, Even ha-Ezer* 1:14; *Maharam*

Shik al Taryag Mizvot, no. 1; *Teshuvot Yaskil Avdi, Even ha-Ezer*, no. 15, sec. 8; *Bigdei Yesha*, no. 123; and *Bigdei Shesh, Even ha-Ezer*, no. 1, sec. 11.

22. Rabbi Gershuni's article first appeared in *Or ha-Mizraḥ*, Tishri 5739, pp. 15–22.
23. For an elucidation of the conflicting opinions regarding the precise meaning of these terms see *Encyclopedia Talmudit*, vol. III, 2nd ed. (Jerusalem, 5715), pp. 98–99.
24. For a non-technical discussion of the feasibility of such pregnancy see Dick Teresi and Kathleen McAuliffe, "Male Pregnancy," *Omni*, vol. 8, no. 3 (December 1985), pp. 51–56 and 118, and Dick Teresi, *New York Times Magazine*, November 27, 1994, pp. 54–55. As reported in *Omni*, in experiments conducted upon animals, male mice and at least one male baboon have carried fetuses. There are some two dozen reported cases of women who became pregnant subsequent to undergoing hysterectomies. In 1979, an Auckland, New Zealand woman underwent a hysterectomy in the course of which an errant fertilized ovum lodged in her abdomen and that pregnancy resulted in the birth of a healthy baby girl.
25. It should, however, be noted that this thesis is rejected by *Minḥat Ḥinnukh*, no. 1 and presumably by the authorities cited *supra*, note 21. See, however, *Teshuvot Har Ẓevi, Even ha-Ezer*, no. 1; *Teshuvot Zekan Aharon*, II, no. 97; *Iggerot Mosheh, Even ha-Ezer*, II, no. 18; R. Elchanan Wasserman, *Kovez He'arot*, no. 69, secs. 26–27; and R. Moshe Sternbuch, *Olam ha-Torah*, no. 2 (Tevet-Shevat 5736), pp. 16–23; cf., *Teshuvot Divrei Yo'el*, II, *Even ha-Ezer*, no. 107, sec. 6.
26. Thus, even a non-Jew who has fathered children is not bound by this commandment subsequent to conversion. See R. Joseph Rosen, *Teshuvot Ẓofnat Pa'aneaḥ*, no. 185.
27. Rabbi Bakshi-Doron's responsum first appeared in *Assia*, vol. II, no. 4 (Nisan 5748), pp. 34–39 and is published in his *Binyan Av*, II, no. 60.

9

Surrogate Motherhood

I. INFERTILITY AND THE OBLIGATION TO PROCREATE

Despite the passage of time since the New Jersey case of Baby M[1] captured the attention of millions of Americans, both the human and legal questions posed by surrogate motherhood remain largely unresolved. Medically, the procedure is not at all complex and represents a simple method of coping with female infertility. A woman who is willing to serve as a surrogate, usually in return for a fee, is found and an agreement is reached. She is artificially inseminated with the semen of the infertile woman's husband, carries the baby to term and subsequently surrenders the baby to the couple. In such cases, the husband is the biological father but the wife has no natural relationship with the child. With the development of *in vitro* fertilization, it is now possible, in some limited circumstances, for the wife to be the biological mother as well.[2] If the wife's fertility problem is not related to production of ova, her own ovum can be fertilized in a petri dish with her husband's sperm and then transferred to the womb of the surrogate who serves as host for purposes of gestation. When all parties are content with the terms of the agreement, there is no occasion for public attention to be focused on the arrangement. But, at times, as was the case with regard to Baby M, the surrogate undergoes a change of heart and refuses to deliver the baby to the father and his wife or attempts to recover custody of the child after the child has been surrendered. In either event, the emotional turmoil is readily understandable and the legal dilemma is obvious.

The problems of surrogate motherhood, as issues of Halakhah, must be placed in proper perspective. Perhaps, this can best be done by means of an anecdote. Many years ago, I was approached by the rabbi of a hasidic congregation. The problem concerned a couple in his community. Unfortunately, the man and his wife were unable to have children. The rabbi arranged for the gentleman to meet with me. In the course of our conversation, the gentleman requested my assistance in obtaining a child for adoption. Time went by and several months later this person sought me out again. This time he thanked me for my efforts and proceeded to inform me that he and his wife were no longer seeking a child for adoption. Taken by surprise, I asked him why he had undergone a change of heart. The gentleman, who frequently consulted a hasidic leader or *rebbe* with regard to personal matters, told me that he had informed the *rebbe* of his desire to adopt a child. The *rebbe*'s response in its entirety consisted of a single sentence: "*Vemen vilst du a tova ton, der Ribbono shel olom, oder zikh alein*?—For whom do you wish to do the favor, the Master of the universe or yourself?"

The question prodded the man to whom it was addressed to serious introspection and reconsideration of his motives. Recognition of the fact that he was not really seeking to perform a *mizvah*, and indeed that adoption and conversion of a non-Jewish child does not constitute fulfillment of a *mizvah* incumbent upon a Jew, led him to the awareness that his motives were neither spiritual nor altruistic. To be sure, his desire was entirely natural, quite human and readily understandable; but seen in that perspective he no longer perceived his need to be imperative.

Hasidic mentors often prove to be psychologically insightful. There can be no question that lack of children leaves a painful void. Paternal and maternal inclinations are deeply ingrained in the human psyche and cry out for expression. Such needs should neither be decried nor minimized. Rachel of old cried out in deep anguish, "Give me children, or else I die" (Genesis 30:1). Nevertheless, it is necessary to evaluate the means adopted in satisfying that need. The means must be measured against the results in assessing the propriety of the procedures that must be employed in achieving the desired goal.

Elsewhere[3] this writer has endeavored to demonstrate that the essence of the biblical commandment to "be fruitful and multiply" that is binding upon males is simply to engage in coital activity with the prescribed frequency and that the birth of children is merely the *terminus ad quem* beyond which sexual activity is no longer mandated by virtue of the biblical commandment. Recognition that the commandment to "be fruitful and multiply" (Genesis 1:28 and 9:7) requires only conventional sexual activity within the context of a marital relationship yields the conclusion that no form of assisted procreation is mandatory. Although Halakhah may demand employment of extraordinary and heroic measures in prolonging life, with regard to the generation of life it requires only that which is ordinary, normal and natural. However, so long as the methods employed in assisted procreation do not entail transgression of halakhic strictures such methods are discretionary and permissible.

It is readily demonstrable that even if the husband desires to avail himself of some form of assisted procreation, the wife is under no obligation to cooperate by submitting to procedures that place any unusual and undue burden upon her or expose her to risks other than those associated with natural pregnancy. Assuredly, no person is required to assume the risks associated with a surgical procedure for the purpose of fulfilling any *mizvah*. That principle is clearly reflected in the comments of *Tosafot, Pesaḥim* 28b, s.v. *arel,* who declare that it is reasonable to assume (*mistavra*) that a *tumtum* need not undergo abdominal surgery in order to fulfill the commandment of circumcision. A *tumtum* is described in talmudic sources as a person whose gender cannot be determined due to the absence of external genitalia. It was presumed that incision of the abdomen would reveal the presence of either male or female anatomical structures. It was further presumed that, if the individual was found to be a male, the organs might be released and caused to descend with the result that circumcision would become feasible. Yet, despite the presumed feasibility of the procedure, the authors of *Tosafot* take it for granted that there is no obligation for a person to submit to such measures despite his ongoing failure to fulfill the *mizvah* of circumcision. The obvious consideration upon which this position is predicated is that, although performance of *mizvot* necessarily entails certain burdens both in terms of expenditure of financial resources and in terms of personal inconvenience, the onus of undergoing a surgical procedure is beyond the pale of duty.

Teshuvot Ḥelkat Yo'av, I, *Dinei Ones,* sec. 7, extends this principle to performance of a *mizvah* in face of any significant threat to health in declaring that a person need not assume the risk of falling victim to a serious illness in discharging a religious obligation. That conclusion is readily understood in light of the limit placed upon the financial burden that must be assumed in fulfillment of a *mizvah.* A person need not expend more than twenty percent of his or her net worth in order to fulfill a positive commandment.[4] Indeed, according to some authorities, a person is required to expend no more than one tenth of his fortune for such a purpose.[5] A rational individual would cheerfully spend at least a fifth of his financial resources in order to avoid serious illness or to avoid the burden of a major surgical procedure. Hence it may be stated that, conversely, incurrence of serious illness is tantamount to expenditure of more than a fifth of one's fortune. Accordingly, a person need not assume the risk of succumbing to a serious malady in order to perform a *miẓvah.*

Fulfillment of the commandment to be fruitful and multiply does not require assumption of a burden greater than that required for fulfillment of any other positive commandment. Women, who are not bound by the *miẓvah* of procreation,[6] are held to a different, and indeed lesser, standard in fulfilling reproductive obligations. Although the *miẓvah* to populate the universe (*shevet*) may apply to females as well as to males, that *miẓvah* is not in the character of a mandatory obligation. The Gemara, *Ḥagigah* 2b, declares, "For indeed the universe was created solely for procreation as it is said, 'He created it not a waste. He formed it to be inhabited' (Isaiah 45:18)." Populating the universe is a divine *desideratum* and human activity undertaken to achieve that *telos* constitutes fulfillment of the divine will. Nevertheless, absent an obligation to "be fruitful and multiply," activity designed to achieve that goal is in the nature of a discretionary *miẓvah* (*miẓvah kiyyumit)* rather that in the nature of a mandatory obligation (*miẓvah ḥiyyuvit*). A wife's reproductive obligations are a product of the covenant generated by the marital relationship. As such, they are limited to pregnancy, child-bearing and child-rearing involving risk, stress and emotional anguish no greater than the norm. Thus *Iggerot Mosheh, Even ha-Ezer*, III, no. 12, rules that a woman confronted with an inordinate statistical risk of bearing a child afflicted with a severe congenital abnormality may insist upon utilizing permissible contraceptive measures on the grounds that she is not contractually bound to assume a burden of that nature even though her husband is desirous of doing so. Accordingly, a woman is certainly not required to undergo a laparoscopy in order to remove ova as part of an attempt to overcome infertility. Similarly, she is under no obligation to accept the medical risks inherent in hormone treatment designed to produce multiple ova.[7] For similar reasons, it would seem that a wife is under no obligation to assume the duty to raise the child of a woman with whom her husband has entered into a surrogate motherhood relationship. Thus a wife may effectively veto her husband's desire for a surrogate relationship.

II. ARTIFICIAL INSEMINATION AND ADULTERY

Assuming the consent and desire of all parties, the permissibility of surrogate motherhood hinges upon resolution of a number of halakhic questions. Since surrogate motherhood involves insemination of a woman with the semen of a man who is not her husband, the first halakhic issue encountered is identical to that involved in a far more common means of overcoming male, rather than female, infertility, *viz.*, AID, or artificial insemination using the semen of a donor.

The empirical possibility of conception *sine concubito* was recognized by the sages of the Talmud. In questioning the permissibility of marriage between a high priest and a pregnant virgin, the Gemara, *Ḥagigah* 14b, accepts the possibility that pregnancy might have occurred in a "bathhouse" other than by means of sexual intercourse, i.e., the woman may have been impregnated in the course of bathing in water in which the male had previously ejaculated.[8] One midrashic source, the *Alfa Beta de-Ben Sira,* reports that Ben Sira was conceived in such a manner.[9] His father is reported to have been the prophet Jeremiah. Jeremiah experienced an ejaculation in the course of bathing and his own daughter, who later used the same bathwater, was impregnated.[10]

Although some authorities differ,[11] the consensus of rabbinic opinion is that there is no technical infringement of the prohibition against adultery other than by means of vaginal penetration by a male.[12] That position is confirmed by a statement of a thirteenth-century rabbinic scholer, R. Peretz of Corbeil, in his work *Hagahot Semak*, cited by *Baḥ, Yoreh De'ah* 195; *Taz, Yoreh De'ah* 195:7; *Bet Shmu'el, Even ha-Ezer* 1:10; and *Ḥelkat Meḥokek, Even ha- Ezer* 1:8, cautioning a woman not to recline upon bedsheets used earlier by a male other than her husband lest those sheets be soiled by the man's still moist semen. The concern is expressed in terms of fear that the woman may become pregnant and that in the course of time "a brother may marry his [half-]sister." The fact that *Hagahot Semak* expresses concern for a possible incestuous relationship but is silent with regard to a concern for bastardy and its associated marital disqualification or that the woman be forbidden to her husband on account of an adulterous act is taken by later authorities as evidence reflecting the notion that, since bastardy results only from adultery (or incest), the prohibition against adultery is limited to sexual intercourse.

Nevertheless, Ramban, in his commentary on the verse "And unto the wife of your fellow you shall not give your semen for seed to defile her through it" (Leviticus 18:20), notes that the biblical admonition concerning adultery is couched in language quite different from that found in multiple verses occurring in the same biblical section dealing with consanguineous relationships. In those instances the biblical phrase employed is "you shall not lie with" or "you shall not uncover the nakedness of," each of which is a euphemism for the sexual act, and indeed that biblical section opens with the verse "No man shall draw near to the relative of his flesh to uncover nakedness" (Leviticus 18:6). Only with regard to the concluding prohibition in that section, viz., adultery, does Scripture speak of "semen" and "seed." If that phraseology is taken literally, the essence of adultery would be understood as consisting of the deposit of the ejaculate in the genital tract of a married woman. Ramban explains that, unlike the considerations underlying other sexual prohibitions, adultery is forbidden because of the consequences resulting from the deposit of semen, i.e., conception. A woman who has had multiple sexual partners, explains Ramban, will perforce not be able to ascertain the father of her child with certainty. Thus, for Ramban, the rationale underlying the prohibition against adultery is the blurring of paternal identity and it is that concept that is reflected in the description of adultery as the deposit of semen by a stranger to the marital relationship.[13] Thus it follows that artificial insemination, even if it does not constitute a technical halakhic violation,[14] is contrary to the spirit of the law. Following Ramban's own explication of the biblical command "You shall be holy" (Leviticus 19:2) as an admonition not to be "a degenerate within the bounds of biblical license,"[15] AID, even if it does not constitute actual adultery, must be regarded as quasi-adulterous in nature and hence a prohibited form of procreation.[16]

Rabbi Yosef Eliyahu Henkin asserts that the act of insemination is prohibited on other grounds.[17] The admonition "be fruitful and multiply" occurs twice. In its first occurrence (Genesis 1:28) it is addressed to Adam; the second time (Genesis 9:7) it is addressed to Noah and his sons upon their emergence from the ark. The repetition to Noah, opines Rabbi Henkin, is for the purpose of establishing a limitation upon the parameters of procreation. Addressing Noah, God tells him, "Go forth from the ark, you and your wife and your sons and your sons' wives with you" (Genesis 8:16). That passage underscores the fact that Noah and his sons each emerged from the ark with his wife, i.e., that the inhabitants of the ark emerged as members of family units. It was in that context, i.e., as members of distinct and identifiable families, that Noah and his sons were commanded to "be fruitful and multiply."

Accordingly, procreation, declares Rabbi Henkin, is designed to take place only within the family unit in a manner such that the genealogy of offspring is known in a determinate manner. Promiscuous relationships are to be eschewed because of the resultant ambiguity regarding parental identity. Consorting with multiple males blurs parental identity. Artificial insemination with the semen of an anonymous donor similarly renders identification of the father virtually impossible. That consideration, declares Rabbi Henkin, serves to render AID impermissible for married and unmarried women alike.

Rabbi Henkin similarly points to the terminology employed in the prohibitions "*lo tiheyeh kedeshah*" and "*lo yiheyeh kadesh*" (Deuteronomy 23:18). Those passages are read literally as prohibiting both female and male prostitution. Some rabbinic scholars, including *Targum Onkelos, ad locum*, interpret the verse as prohibiting sexual liaisons between a slave and a freeman or a freewoman.[18] Rabbi Henkin notes that, unlike the terminology employed in the various prohibitions against incestuous unions, there is no direct reference in these passages to the sexual act *per se*. Accordingly, asserts Rabbi Henkin, it must be concluded that the primary concern is not the sexual act itself but rather the concern is with regard to promiscuity and the resultant absence of a halakhicly identifiable paternal-filial relationships. Any act, including artificial insemination, argues Rabbi Henkin, that leads to the birth of a child whose father cannot be identified must be abjured as the moral equivalent of prostitution.

III. ARTIFICIAL INSEMINATION AND BASTARDY

Putting aside the sexual propriety of the surrogate relationship, once parties have entered into such a relationship and a child is born, what is the status of the issue of a surrogate relationship?

The earliest source addressing the underlying issue is the previously cited admonition of *Hagahot Semak* to the effect that a woman should not recline upon the bedsheets of a male other than her husband. The concern expressed is that the woman may become pregnant and, with the passage of time, a brother may unknowingly enter into a marital relationship with his half-sister. That, to be sure, is a significant concern. Equally significant is a consideration that *Hagahot Semak* passes over in silence, *viz.*, that any child conceived in that manner is himself a *mamzer* by virtue of the fact that he or she is the progeny of a married woman and a male who is not her lawful husband

and hence is forbidden to contract a marriage with any woman of legitimate birth. Since that concern is universal and far more immediate than the concern that is expressed by *Hagahot Semak,* the failure of *Semak* to state that concern should presumably be accepted as a clear indication that he did not consider it to be relevant. Accordingly, *Hagahot Semak* must have regarded a child born to a married woman but sired *sine concubito* by a male other than her husband as free of the taint of bastardy. Hence, it must be inferred that *Hagahot Semak* regarded *mamzerut* as attendant solely upon an adulterous or incestuous act. Since physical penetration of the female by the male is a necessary element of adultery, any child born *sine concubito* is not a *mamzer* because the child is technically not the product of an act of adultery.

Conversely, it follows that those few authorities who adopt the position that there can be adultery without an actual act of sexual penetration would regard the child conceived in that manner as a *mamzer.*[19] One authority, R. Ya'akov Breisch, *Teshuvot Ḥelkat Ya'akov*, I, no. 24, cites a statement of *Tosafot, Yevamot* 77b, asserting that bastardy is not necessarily contingent upon transgression of the prohibition against an adulterous or incestuous relationship. *Tosafot* cite the non-normative talmudic opinion that a child of a Jewish woman and a non-Jewish father is a *mamzer.* That relationship entails neither capital punishment nor the biblical penalty of excision (*karet).* Indeed, according to the talmudic opinion that maintains that the commandment "And you shall not intermarry with them" (Deuteronomy 7:3) applies only to members of the seven indigenous nations of the land of Canaan, such acts are not interdicted by an express biblical command. If so, query *Tosafot,* on what grounds can the issue of such a union be declared bastards? In one resolution of that problem, *Tosafot* posit that *mamzerut* flows, not from particular illicit acts, but from any union between individuals disqualified from contracting a valid marriage with one another. *Ḥelkat Ya'akov* argues, in effect, that, since transgression is not a necessary condition of bastardy, there is no independent reason to assume that an antecedent sexual act is such a condition. He argues that, quite to the contrary, bastardy is simply the result of the halakhic status of the parents vis-à-vis one another. It should be noted that this argument is based upon one theory advanced by *Tosafot* in resolution of a particular problem and may well represent a concept not accepted by other authorities who present alternative answers to the query posed by *Tosafot.*

IV. SEMEN PROCUREMENT

There is yet another aspect of the process of artificial insemination that may serve to preclude surrogate motherhood in many, if not most, situations.

The prohibition against onanism serves to proscribe ejaculation other than in conjunction with the act of intercourse. However, many authorities recognize at least some exceptions to the prohibition based primarily upon a discussion of the Gemara, *Yevamot* 76a. Elsewhere[20] this writer has analyzed the reasoning employed by the numerous authorities who permit ejaculation for purposes of AIH (artificial insemination utilizing the semen of the husband) and indeed even for semen testing in conjunction with diagnosis and treatment of infertility. That analysis also discusses the methods of semen procurement sanctioned by Halakhah for such purposes.

The consideration underlying those permissive views is that at least some forms of non-coital ejaculation may be sanctioned when undertaken for the purpose of fulfilling the commandment to "be fruitful and multiply." Left unclear is the question of whether ejaculation for a lesser purpose is deemed to be wanton and hence "for naught." R. Jacob Emden, *She'ilat Ya'aveẓ,* I, no. 43, maintains that ejaculation for any "grave need," including avoidance of severe pain, is not wanton destruction and hence permissible. Most authorities, however, maintain that the *telos* of emission must be procreative in nature.[21] The question is whether any ejaculation that is not designed to fulfill the biblical command to "be fruitful and multiply" constitutes ejaculation "for naught" or whether other forms of procreation that do not serve to fulfill the commandment but do serve to populate the universe in the sense of "He created it not a waste. He formed it to be inhabited" (Isaiah 45:18) also serve to legitimize emission of semen. Ordinarily, those *teloi* go hand in hand; populating the universe *(shevet)* also serves to fulfill the mandate to "be fruitful and multiply." But that need not always be the case. A person who engages in procreation that does not result in a halakhicly recognized paternal-filial relationship has not "multiplied" himself since he has no halakhicly recognized relationship with his biological progeny. Nevertheless, he has certainly contributed to augmentation of the population of the universe.

For those authorities who maintain that only birth of children as a result of natural intercourse serves to fulfill the command to "be fruitful and multiply," permissibility of AIH hinges upon whether non-coital ejaculation is permissible solely for purposes of fulfilling the commandment to "be fruitful and multiply" or whether fulfillment of *shevet* is sufficient to legitimize emission of semen.[22] Assuming that the sexual act is not a necessary condition of fulfillment of the commandment to "be fruitful and multiply" because a paternal-filial relationship exists even in the absence of a sexual act,[23] some forms of non-coital ejaculation may be employed in order to fulfill the biblical command. However, ejaculation for the purpose of inseminating a non-Jewish woman does not serve to achieve that end. The issue of a Jewish father and a gentile mother, even if conceived in a normal, natural manner, is not regarded as the issue of the Jewish father for purposes of Halakhah and hence birth of such a child does not constitute fulfillment of the biblical commandment concerning procreation. Birth of such a child does, however, serve to populate the universe.

If, as is frequently the case, the surrogate is a non-Jewish woman, the child is obviously not Jewish and, presumably, if surrendered to the childless couple, would be converted to Judaism. Nevertheless, the father does not fulfill the commandment to "be fruitful and multiply" even upon conversion of the child. Hence, if non-coital emission of semen can be countenanced only for purposes of fulfilling the biblical commandment regarding procreation, impermissibility of semen procurement for insemination of a gentile woman would itself serve to bar a surrogate relationship with a surrogate who is not Jewish.

V. ARTIFICIAL INSEMINATION AND PATERNITY

A closely related issue is the question of the existence of a halakhicly recognized paternal-filial relationship between the semen donor and the child born of artificial insemination. A host of halakhic matters hinge upon recognition or non-recognition of a paternal-filial relationship, including, but not limited to, inheritance; mourning; exemption of the donor's wife, in the absence of other issue, from levirate marriage; priestly and levitical status; and, most ominous of all, consanguinity. Nor should the question of obligations a father owes a child, including the obligation of financial support, be overlooked.

Once again, the earlier cited comment of *Hagahot Semak* serves as the primary source for resolution of this question. To be sure, *Hagahot Semak* does not directly address the issue of paternal relationship, but his stance with regard to that question is abundantly clear. The concern to which he gives expression is that of a possible consanguineous marriage between a brother and a sister or, to be more precise, between a half-brother and a half-sister. The fear is that a child born *sine concubito* will not know the identity of his or her biological father and hence will be ignorant of a biological relationship with any half-siblings who may exist, i.e., any other children sired by the same man. But, it must be remembered, a fraternal relationship is really epiphenomenal; a fraternal relationship, by definition, is the relationship that exists between two persons who enjoy a common filial relationship with a single father or mother. Thus, if no halakhicly recognized relationship exists between a male who procures semen and the child born as a result of insemination of the ejaculate, a child conceived in that manner could not have halakhicly recognized paternal siblings and hence there could be no fear that the child might marry a paternal sister. From the fact that *Hagahot Semak* regards such a concern as cogent it must necessarily be deduced that he espouses the view that a paternal-filial relationship arises *sine concubito*. Thus, according to *Hagahot Semak*, although the male who ejaculates in bath water or on bedclothes, or who becomes a sperm donor and thereby causes a married woman to conceive, has not committed adultery and, despite the fact that the child is not regarded as the bastard issue of an adulterous union, the male is nevertheless regarded as the father of the child.[24]

Nevertheless, one of the classical commentators on *Even ha-Ezer, Ḥelkat Meḥokek* 1:8, expresses doubt with regard to whether or not a paternal-filial relationship exists in such instances. Moreover, there is some dispute regarding the actual position of *Hagahot Semak*. The primary expositor of the view denying the existence of a paternal relationship is R. Chaim Joseph David Azulai, *Birkei Yosef, Even ha-Ezer* 1:14.[25] *Birkei Yosef* cites a variant manuscript reading of the text of *Hagahot Semak*. According to that reading, *Hagahot Semak* cites the concern regarding prevention of a future consanguineous marriage in the context of the ban against the remarriage of a widow or divorcée within three months of termination of her earlier marriage. That prohibition is expressly predicated upon a concern for certainty in establishing paternal identity and, according to *Birkei Yosef*, is cited solely by way of example or analogy.

According to *Birkei Yosef*, if a child is conceived *sine concubito*, the biological father is not recognized as the halakhic father and *Hagahot Semak* merely expresses the view that the sages of the Talmud would have decried any act that leaves a child bereft of a halakhicly recognized father just as they legislated against relationships that might give rise to ambiguous paternity.

VI. SUPPRESSION OF MATERNAL IDENTITY

Once a child is born as a result of surrogate motherhood, may the identity of the mother be suppressed?

That question, too, has its counterpart with regard to children born as a result of artificial insemination. If, as the vast majority of rabbinic authorities agree, a paternal-filial relationship does exist when a child has been born as a result of artificial insemination, is it necessary to disclose the identity of the father? As AID is customarily practiced in the United States, the donor is assured of anonymity and, in general, there is no way that the child can discover the identity of his or her father. In surrogate mother arrangements, sealing the records, if permitted, would have the same result.

Suppression of paternal identity is one of the considerations that led rabbinic decisors to ban AID. R. Moshe Feinstein, *Iggerot Mosheh, Yoreh De'ah*, I, no. 162 and Even ha-Ezer, I, no. 7, voices a similar concern in decrying sealed adoptions.[26] At least until recent years, adoption agencies and the American legal system joined forces in an attempt to prevent an adopted child from ever learning the identity of his or her natural parents. It would appear that *Iggerot Mosheh* regards any attempt to suppress the parental identity as a violation of a biblical commandment. Although polygamy is biblically permissible, the Gemara, *Yevamot* 37b, declares that a man may not maintain a wife in every port, i.e., he may not maintain multiple families and households whose members do not know of one another's existence. The concern is that, with the passage of time, children of the various households may grow to maturity and contract a marriage without realizing that they share a common father. In prohibiting such arrangements, the Gemara adduces the verse "lest the earth be filled with licentiousness" (Leviticus 19:29) as the consideration upon which the ban is predicated. *Iggerot Mosheh* apparently asserts that the prohibition is not merely rabbinic in nature and simply reflective of the concern expressed in the cited scriptural passage; rather, the ban represents the instantiation of an actual biblical prohibition.[27] According to *Iggerot Mosheh*, any act carrying with it the potential for suppression of a familial relationship of a nature such that it may possibly lead to a consanguineous relationship is biblically proscribed. As such, suppression of the identity of natural parents in adoption proceedings, anonymous sperm donations and surrogate relationships in which the identity of the mother is not disclosed are equally forbidden as a violation of "lest the earth will be filled with licentiousness."

VII. SURROGACY AND BABY-SELLING

Conception by means of artificial insemination presents halakhic problems with regard to the permissibility of the means utilized in causing pregnancy to occur in the context of surrogate relationships. Enforcement of the surrogacy contract providing for custody of the child presents an additional cluster of issues. Although the contract may provide for impregnation in a manner that Halakhah regards as illicit, Jewish law does not regard illegal contracts as *ipso facto* unenforceable.

The enforceability of surrogate motherhood contracts in the American legal system is generally regarded as hinging in the first instance upon the question of whether the agreement is to be construed as a contract for the sale of a baby or as a contract for performance of personal services. Has the surrogate, who receives a fee for her services, simply agreed to make her uterus available for gestation of the fetus or has she contracted for the sale of a baby upon birth? If the latter, not only is the contract unenforceable, but fulfillment of its terms constitutes a penal offense.[28]

However, since baby-selling, while undoubtedly repugnant, is not a criminal act in Jewish law, the question of enforceability of the provisions of an illegal contract need not be addressed. That baby-selling is not a criminal act in Jewish law is poignantly illustrated by a recommendation made by *Sefer Ḥasidim* (Jerusalem, 5720), no. 245.

Jewish tradition recognizes a number of nonmedical and nonscientific *segulot* or remedies in the nature of metaphysical forms of intervention designed to avert the natural result of life-threatening maladies. One of those is *shinuy ha-shem,* changing the patient's name. That *segulah* is based upon the concept that no person dies other than pursuant to a decree of the Heavenly court. The procedures of the Heavenly court, we are told, mirror those of terrestrial courts in their procedural aspects. Change of name is designed to render such a decree nugatory on the grounds that a change of name entails a change of identity. The original decree cannot be carried out because it can be applied only against the named individual. The patient who has undergone a change of name is a different person against whom no decree has been issued. As a different person, he is entitled to a new hearing. In effect, the name change provides the basis for a writ of *habeas corpus* before the Heavenly tribunal. On rehearing, the Heavenly court may find some new merit, presumably not of sufficient strength to abrogate an already entered judgment but sufficient to prevent the entry of an unfavorable decree *de nouveau*.

In Jewish tradition, an individual's name is composed of a combination of his own name and his patronym or matronym. Accordingly, a change of name can be effected either by changing a person's given name or by changing the patronym or matronym. A patronym can be effectively changed by substitution of fathers, i.e., by acquisition of a new father in place of the original, biological father. A matronym can be effectively changed by substitution of mothers, i.e., by acquisition of a new mother in place of the original, biological mother.

Living in an age in which infant mortality was rampant, *Sefer Ḥasidim* provides instructions for changing a person's name by substituting new parents for the original ones. *Sefer Hasidim* advises that parents, concerned because they have had children who have died in infancy, arrange for a close friend to present them with a *shekel*, a loaf of bread, a piece of meat and a jug of wine and to acquire the child from them in return. From that point on, declares *Sefer Ḥasidim*, the infant will be deemed, at least for purposes of the Heavenly court, to be the child of the adoptive parents. The procedure involves what is at least *pro forma* the sale of a child. Were a person to undertake such a procedure today, and were he to do nothing more, the district attorney would certainly have no interest in the matter. However, Jewish law, unlike other systems of law, concerns itself with form no less than with substance. Hence, were baby-selling recognized as a crime by Jewish law, even a purely formal and indeed sham sale of a child could not be countenanced.

VIII. ENFORCEABILITY OF SURROGATE CONTRACTS

There are nevertheless other considerations that serve to render surrogate motherhood contracts unenforceable in Jewish law.

Typically, for reasons that are obvious, the contract is executed before the woman is inseminated. At that point, the fetus is not yet in existence. Halakhah does not recognize the validity of the conveyance of an entity that is not yet in existence. Hence, were the contract to be construed as a sale, the sale would be void with the result that the woman has the prerogative of reneging on her undertaking. If, on the other hand, the agreement is to be construed as an employment contract that provides for compensation for services rendered, apart from the right of a worker to abrogate such a contract, provision of such services at the behest of the father does not serve to convey a proprietary interest in the child.

More significantly, children are not property and do not represent a property interest that can be transferred. Child custody, although often a matter of dispute between a couple no longer living together as man and wife, is regarded by Judaism primarily as an obligation rather than a right.[29] To the extent that child custody involves an issue of the rights of an individual, the rights involved are those of the child. The duty of a parent to care for and to support a child may be said to give rise to a concomitant right vested in the child to receive such care and support. Thus, although both conceptually and for certain aspects of Jewish law, there may well be a distinction between a duty and a resultant right, in general, duties and rights may be regarded as two sides of the same coin.

Since determination of which spouse shall be the custodial parent is, in effect, adjudication of how a child's right can best be exercised, any contract between the parents must be regarded as a nullity if it in any way prejudices the rights of the child. It is self-evident that two contracting parties do not have the power to dispose of, or in any way prejudice, the rights of a third party who is not a party to the contract. It is for that reason that *Teshuvot Mabit,* II, no. 62, cited by *Be'er Heitev, Even ha-Ezer* 82:6, rules that a woman who, as part of a divorce settlement, enters into an agreement in which she renounces custodial prerogatives may subsequently renege and is not bound by her initial undertaking.[30]

Similarly, a surrogate contract providing for surrender of the baby by the natural mother represents an agreement by the natural mother not to seek custody. As such, it is unenforceable with the result that, if the mother declines to surrender the child voluntarily, the *Bet Din* must perforce treat the controversy as a dispute between two parents each of whom asserts a prerogative to custody of the child. Thus, the case before the *Bet Din* is not a contract dispute but a custody dispute to be resolved on the basis of halakhic canons governing matters of custody.

Halakhah posits a number of general rules governing award of custody. Mothers are presumptively entitled to custody of girls on the theory that the mother is better qualified to serve as a role model and to provide the type of practical and moral guidance necessary in the rearing of a daughter, while the father is presumptively entitled to custody of male children because it is the father's obligation to teach his son Torah.[31] The latter principle is, however, tempered with a tender years doctrine reflecting the consideration that children below the age of six, both male and female, require nurturing care that can best be provided by a mother. As stated by *Teshuvot Maharashdam, Even ha-Ezer,* I, no. 123, and Rema, *Even ha-Ezer* 82:7, those principles are merely the reflections of a simple, more general principle, namely, that custody is to be determined on the basis of the best interests of the child. Those particular provisions simply reflect the presumption that, in the generality of cases, both parents are equally fit and competent in all other respects. Hence, *ceteris paribus*, the factors that are enumerated must be regarded as determinative of the child's best interests. However, in the real world, seldom, if ever, are all other matters equal. Consequently, there is a long list of responsa, beginning with the earlier cited *Teshuvot Maharashdam* and *Teshuvot Radvaz*, I, nos. 64, 226, 263 and 360 as well as *Teshuvot Ri mi-Gash*, no. 71; *Teshuvot ha-Meyuḥasot le-Ramban*, no. 38; *Teshuvot Maharam Padua*, no. 53 and including, *inter alia*, numerous decisions of the Israeli rabbinic courts[32] indicating that custody must be determined on the basis of the best interests of the child and that such determination must be made on a case by case basis and only upon the weighing and balancing of all relevant factors.[33]

IX. A SOLUTION TO THE SOCIETAL DILEMMA

For reasons that do not necessarily parallel the mores of Judaism, there is a strong inclination in many sectors of contemporary society to prohibit, or at least to discourage, surrogate motherhood arrangements.[34] Criminalization of the arrangement accompanied by appropriate penal sanctions might be one way of dealing with the problem. Yet criminalization is regarded as too harsh and, in any event, is not likely to be effective.

The halakhic considerations entering into an analysis of surrogate motherhood contracts suggest a solution to the societal problems posed by the specter of such arrangements, a solution that recommends itself equally well to a society whose institutions are not necessarily predicated upon the provisions of Halakhah.[35]

As has been shown earlier, most rabbinic authorities are of the opinion that there exists a paternal-filial relationship between a semen donor and a child born of artificial insemination. It then follows that the donor is obligated with regard to financial support of his biological child. Halakhah also provides that the father is liable for child support whether or not he is awarded custody of the child. Moreover, if the mother is awarded custody, she is entitled not only to reimbursement for expenses incurred on behalf of the child but also to compensation for her services as a wet nurse. Although Halakhah does not provide for payment of alimony *per se*, it does provide for financial assistance to the mother of young children.

The financial responsibility for raising a child devolves upon the father. When the mother is awarded custody it is because such is in the best interests of the child. However, as recorded in *Shulḥan Arukh, Even ha-Ezer* 82:7, a custody award in favor of the mother does not extinguish the father's financial responsibility. Since the mother is no longer married to the child's father, she is not required to provide child-rearing services without remuneration. Payment to the mother as guardian of the child, since that too is necessary for the child's welfare, is an expense that may be assigned to the father.

Adoption of the policy inherent in these provisions of Jewish law with regard to child support and custody would have a chilling effect upon surrogate agreements. As recorded in *Shulḥan Arukh, Even ha-Ezer* 82:5 and 82:8, a mother has the prerogative of refusing to accept custody. Hence, in a surrogate arrangement, if the neonate suffers from a congenital defect or abnormality, the mother may well decline to accept custody and thereby leave responsibility for the child entirely in the hands of the father. In every case, if the woman who has agreed to surrender the child as part of the surrogate agreement undergoes a change of heart and seeks custody, she may very well prevail. If awarded custody, she is entitled both to child support and to a fee for her services in rearing the child. As a result, a male contemplating such an arrangement has no guarantee that he will actually have a child to raise. However, he will be absolutely certain of incurring financial obligations to the child born to the surrogate as well as, should custody be awarded to the surrogate, of incurring an obligation for what constitutes, in effect, alimony payments to a woman who was never his wife. Thus, the man is assured of financial responsibilities but has no guarantee of custody of the child. The prospect should be sufficiently onerous to discourage most people from pursuing such an agreement.

In point of fact, in the early days of recourse to artificial insemination as a remedy for infertility, legislation was enacted in most American jurisdictions for the direct purpose of rendering sperm donors immune to financial claims for support of progeny born as a result of artificial insemination. Such legislation reflected a societal decision to encourage AID as a means of coping with infertility. If society is determined to discourage surrogate relationships, that goal can be achieved by amending existing sperm donor legislation to make it clear that the immunity from financial claims conveyed by such statutes does not extend to persons entering into written or oral surrogate agreements.

X. A FINAL COMMENT

One further observation is in order. Surrogate relationships are often described as a modern-day counterpart of concubinage that was prevalent in days of yore. There is no question that, in antiquity, and in the biblical period in particular, when a woman proved to be barren, her husband frequently took a concubine for purposes of procreation. The biblical narrative concerning Abraham and Hagar seems to be a case in point. Ramban, in his commentary on Genesis 16:2, offers the following observation:

> "And Abraham hearkened to the voice of Sarah." Even now [Abraham] did not intend that he be fulfilled through Hagar by having progeny through her. Rather, his sole intention was to do the desire of Sarah so that she be fulfilled through [Hagar], that she derive happiness of spirit from the children of her handmaiden.

Hagar is here described as the surrogate who will bear the children while Sarah will experience the gratification and pleasure of raising those children.

Ramban, however, offers a second observation as well. Commenting on the verse "And Sarah oppressed her" (Genesis 6:6), Ramban remarks: "Our mother [Sarah] sinned in this matter." Sarah is described as having desired to displace Hagar and to raise Hagar's child as her own. But, in practice, the arrangement does not succeed. The child is not Sarah's; it is Hagar's. People may believe that they are capable of transcending biological realia but, in practice, they find that they cannot.[36] Despite the best intentions of all concerned, biological facts give rise to psychological consequences and human beings frequently find it impossible to rise above, or to suppress, natural instincts and emotions.

The phenomenon of a mother who reneges on a surrogate

agreement should not be at all surprising. The woman may be a surrogate wife or a surrogate reproductive partner, but the term "surrogate mother" is a misnomer. There is nothing in the nature of surrogacy in her maternity; she is a natural mother, both biologically and psychologically. At the time when she enters into the contractual relationship the surrogate may believe herself capable of renouncing her motherhood and of surrendering the child. However, when confronted with the reality of her motherhood, she may understandably find herself incapable of doing so. Men and women are human, not superhuman, and should not be called upon sacrificially to deny natural human instincts and emotions.

NOTES

1. Matter of Baby, 217 N.J. Super. 313; 525 A.2d 1128 (1987), *aff'd in part and rev'd in part,* 109 N.J. 396, 537 A.2d 1227 (1988).
2. The primary focus of this discussion will be upon surrogacy arrangements in which the gestational mother is the biological mother. The question of maternal identity in situations in which the gestational mother is not the biological mother is addressed in this writer's *Contemporary Halakhic Problems,* I (New York, 1977), 106–109; II (New York, 1983), 91–93; and IV (New York, 1995), 237–272.
3. See *supra,* pp. 227–231.
4. See Rema, *Oraḥ Ḥayyim* 656:1.
5. Cf., *Magen Avraham, Oraḥ Ḥayyim* 656:7.
6. See, *inter alia,* Rambam, *Hilkhot Ishut* 15:2 and *Sefer ha-Ḥinnukh, mizvah* 1.
7. Nor, pursuant to the edict of Rabbenu Gershom forbidding divorce other than with consent of the wife, does the husband have the right to divorce his wife on grounds of infertility. Although dispensation in the form of a *hetter me'ah rabbanim* for the husband to enter into a polygamous relationship for purposes of fulfilling his obligation to "be fruitful and multiply" might well be forthcoming, there is ample authority serving to relieve the husband of availing himself of that opportunity. See *Pitḥei*

Teshuvah, Even ha-Ezer 154:27 and *Oẓar ha-Poskim, Even ha-Ezer* 1:26.

8. Cf., however, *Mishneh la-Melekh, Hilkhot Ishut* 15:4, who asserts that the possibility of pregnancy occurring in this manner is a matter of dispute and is both inherently contradicted by other talmudic discussions and normatively rejected in the adoption of the rule imputing bastardy to the child of a married woman whose husband had no access to her for twelve months prior to its birth. See also R. Moshe Shick, *Maharam Shik al Taryag Miẓvot*, no.1, sec. 3. *Mishneh la-Melekh*'s arguments are rebutted by various later authorities. See, for example, R. Yonatan Eibeschutz, *Bnei Ahuvah, Hilkhot Ishut* 15:6 and R. Jacob Ettlinger, *Arukh la-Ner, Yevamot* 12b. See also *Tashbaẓ*, III, no. 263; cf., *Teshuvot Mahari Asad, Yoreh De'ah,* no. 179.
9. Published in J.D. Eisenstein, *Oẓar Midrashim* (New York, 5688), p. 43. That report is quoted by a noted fourteenth-century scholar, R. Jacob Ben Moses Mölln, in the first of the addenda (*likkutim*) to his *Sefer Maharil.* That work is cited, in turn, by numerous later sources.
10. Cf., however, R. David Gans, *Ẓemaḥ David,* in his entry for the year 3448, who challenges the reliability of that report and advances a number of alternative theories regarding the identity of Ben Sira and the age in which he lived. See also R. Solomon ibn Verga, *Shevet Yehudah* (Hanover, 1924), p. 2.
11. See R. Judah Leib Zirelson, *Ma'arkhei Lev,* no. 73; R. Ovadiah Hadaya, *No'am*, I (5718), 130–137, reprinted in *idem, Teshuvot Yaskil Avdi,* V, *Even ha-Ezer*, no. 10; R. Joel Teitelbaum, *Ha-Ma'or,* Av 5724, pp. 3–13; *idem, Teshuvot Divrei Yo'el,* II, nos. 107–110; R. Samuel Aaron Yudelevitz, *No'am,* X (5727), 57–103; and R. Abraham Lurie, *Ha-Posek,* Ḥeshvan-Kislev 5710, pp. 1754–1756.
12. See, for example, R. Shalom Mordecai Schwadron, *Teshuvot Maharsham,* III, no. 268; R. Aaron Walkin, *Teshuvot Zekan Aharon,* II, no. 97; R. Joshua Baumol, *Teshuvot Emek Halakhah,* no. 68; R. Ben Zion Uziel, *Mishpetei Uzi'el, Even ha-Ezer,* I, no. 10; and R. Eliyahu Meir Bloch, *Ha-Pardes,* Sivan 5713, pp. 1–3. For a survey of these and other sources see R. Michal Stern, *Ha-Refu'ah le-Or ha-Halakhah,* vol. I (Jerusalem, 5740), part 2, pp. 56–68. For a comprehensive bibliography of the rabbinic periodical literature devoted to artificial insemination see Nahum Rakover, *Oẓar Mishpat,* I (Jerusalem, 5735), 322–333.
13. However, implanatation of an embryo in the uterus of a host

mother subsequent to fertilization, since it does not involve deposit of semen, is a different matter. Cf., however, Yitzchak Mehlman, "Multi-Fetal Pregnancy Reduction," *Journal of Halachah and Contemporary Society*, no. XXVII (Spring 1994), pp. 43–44, who reports an oral communication by R. Aaron Soloveichik to the effect that, in the latter's opinion, the status of an embryo during the first forty days of gestation is identical to that of the male "seed." Assuming, as Rabbi Soloveichik apparently does, that during that forty-day period the embryo does not have the status of a fetus, the conclusion that it has the status of "seed" is intellectually alluring and indeed almost intuitive: the male seed undergoes a metamorphosis and becomes a fetus; until it actually becomes a fetus it remains "seed." That position, however, is contradicted both by the authorities who apparently maintain that, unlike semen, an embryo may be destroyed during that period with impunity as well as by the conflicting authorities who maintain that destruction of an embryo even in that early stage of gestation constitutes feticide. Thus, to cite one example, unlike Rabbi Soloveichik, R. Yechiel Ya'akov Weinberg, *Seridei Esh*, III, no. 127, places no restriction on termination of pregnancy during the first forty days. Those authorities apparently maintain that, in light of the description of the embryo during that period by the Gemara, *Yevamot* 69b, as "mere water," the sperm loses its status as "seed" upon fusing with the ovum with the result that, according to those authorities, the nascent embryo is neither "seed" nor fetus. However, R. Ya'ir Bacharach, *Teshuvot Ḥavot Ya'ir*, no. 31, and R. Jacob Emden, *She'ilat Ya'aveẓ*, I, no. 43, who maintain that feticide in all stages of pregnancy is prohibited as a form of "destruction of the seed," clearly maintain that the fetus is endowed with the halakhic status of "seed" during the entire period of gestation. It might cogently be argued that, according to those authorities, embryo transfer at any stage of gestation is no different from AID insofar as the issue of adultery is concerned.

14. One authority, *Teshuvot Ma'arkhei Lev*, no. 73, understands the comments of Ramban quite literally in declaring not only that AID constitutes adultery, but that the physician performing the insemination, in effect, acts as an agent of the donor in committing adultery.
15. See Ramban, *Commentary on the Bible*, Leviticus 19:20.
16. See R. Eliezer Waldenberg, *Ẓiẓ Eli'ezer,* IX, no. 51, sec. 4. Cf., R. Moshe Feinstein, *Iggerot Mosheh, Even ha-Ezer*, II, no. 11.

17. See R. Yosef Eliyahu Henkin, *Ha-Ma'or,* Tishri–Ḥeshvan 5725, pp. 9–11, reprinted in *idem, Kol Kitvei ha-Grya Henkin* (New York, 5746), II, 100–101.
18. Rambam, *Sefer ha-Mizvot, mizvot lo-ta'aseh,* no. 350, understands *"lo yiheyeh kadesh"* as a reiteration of the prohibition against homosexual acts.
19. See *supra,* note 11. See also *Zekher Ḥagigah, Ḥagigah* 15a; *Teshuvot Bar Leva'i,* II, no. 1; and R. Eliyahu Meir Bloch, *Ha-Pardes,* Sivan 5713, pp. 1–3. For a discussion of these various sources see *Ha-Refu'ah le-Or ha-Halakhah,* vol. I, part 2, pp. 68–76.
20. See *supra,* pp. 219–224. See also *Ha-Refu'ah le-Or ha-Halakhah,* vol. I, part 2, pp. 36–43.
21. See *Ha-Refu'ah le-Or ha-Halakhah,* I, part 1, pp. 113–119. Cf., however, *Ẓiẓ Eli'ezer,* XIII, no. 102 and the sharp rejoinder of *Iggerot Mosheh, Ḥoshen Mishpat,* II, no. 69, sec. 4.
22. Some few authorities maintain that AID does establish a paternal-filial relationship between the donor and the child born of such a procedure but that, since no sexual act is involved, the donor does not thereby fulfill his obligation with regard to procreation. See R. Jacob Emden, *She'ilat Ya'aveẓ,* II, no. 97, sec. 3; R. Chaim Joseph David Azulai, *Birkei Yosef, Even ha-Ezer* 1:14; *Maharam Shik al Taryag Miẓvot,* no. 1; *Bigdei Yesha,* no. 123; and *Bigdei Shesh, Even ha- Ezer* 1:11.
23. Authorities who espouse the latter view include *Teshuvot Emek Halakhah,* I, no. 60; R. Shlomoh Zalman Auerbach, *No'am,* I, 157; and R. Judah Gershuni, *Or ha-Mizraḥ,* Tishri 5739, pp. 15–22, reprinted in *idem, Kol Ẓofayikh* (Jerusalem, 5740), p. 367.
24. See *Bet Shmu'el, Even ha-Ezer* 1:6. This view is accepted by most authorities including, *inter alia, Tashbaẓ,* III, no. 263; *Teshuvot Bet Ya'akov,* no. 124; *Bnei Ahuvah, Hilkhot Ishut* 15:6; *Teshuvot Ben Ya'akov,* no. 122; *Turei Even, Ḥagigah* 15a; *Arukh la-Ner, Yevamot* 10a; R. Malki'el Zevi Tennenbaum, *Teshuvot Divrei Malki'el,* IV, no. 107; R. Ya'akov Yitzchak Weisz, *Teshuvot Minḥat Yiẓḥak,* I, no. 50; *Ẓiẓ Eli'ezer,* IX, no. 51; and R. Yisra'el Zev Mintzberg, *No'am,* I, 129.
25. See also *Teshuvot Bar Leva'i, Even ha-Ezer,* no. 1; *Mishpetei Uzi'el, Even ha-Ezer,* I, no. 19; R. Menachem Kasher, *No'am,* I, 125–128; *idem, Torah Shelemah,* XVII, 242; and R. Moshe Aryeh Leib Shapiro, *No'am,* I, 138–142. For further sources see *Ha-Refu'ah le-Or ha-Halakhah,* vol. I, part 2, pp. 14–29.
26. See also, R. Shlomoh Goren, *Ha-Ẓofeh,* 7 Adar I, 5744.
27. Cf., however, *Bet Shmu'el, Even ha-Ezer* 13:1, who asserts that

the ban against remarriage of a woman within three months of her divorce or of the death of her husband that is predicated upon the same consideration is rabbinic in nature.

28. See Matter of Baby, 109 N.J. at 422; 537 A.2d at 1240. See also Barbara Cohen, "Surrogate Mothers: Whose Baby Is It?" *American Journal of Law and Medicine*, vol X, no. 3 (Fall 1984), pp. 247–248; and Mark Rust, "Whose Baby Is It? Surrogate Motherhood After Baby M," *American Bar Association Journal*, vol. LXXIII (June 1, 1987), pp. 53–55. A number of states explicitly exempted surrogacy agreements from provisions criminalizing baby-selling. See *infra*, note 34.

    In one case brought by the attorney general of Kentucky to clarify the state's law on surrogacy, the Supreme Court of Kentucky found that surrogate contracts did not violate state baby-selling statutes because the child produced by the arrangement is the natural child of the father. See *Surrogate Parenting Ass'n.* v. *Com. Ex. Rel. Armstrong*, 704 S.W.2d 209 (1986). According to that reasoning, it would then follow that, if the wife is the sole contracting party, the contract would be illegal. Similarly, if the surrogate was impregnated by donor sperm because of the husband's infertility, the contract would be illegal.

29. Thus R. Ben Zion Uziel, *Mishpetei Uzi'el, Even ha-Ezer*, no. 91, writes: "Neither the sons nor the daughters of a person are owned by him in the same way that he owns his property or livestock . . . they are the inheritance of the Lord given to parents in order to receive an education in Torah, *mizvot* and daily life."

30. See also *Osef Piskei Din Rabbaniyim*, ed. Z. Wahrhaftig (Jerusalem, 5710), p. 11 and *Piskei Din shel Batei ha-Din ha-Rabbaniyim be-Yisra'el*, III, 358; XI, 161; and XI, 172–173. See also *Piskei Din shel Batei ha-Din ha-Rabbaniyim be-Yisra'el*, XIII, 337.

31. Hence, when it is obvious that the father will not fulfill that obligation he has no presumptive claim to custody. Indeed, in one case, the Rabbinical District Court of Jerusalem ruled that when the child is educated by teachers rather than by the father and spends the entire day in school with the result that "the father has no time left to teach his son" he has no superior claim to custody. See *Piskei Din shel Batei ha-Din ha-Rabbaniyim be-Yisra'el*, VII, 17.

32. See *Osef Piskei Din Rabbaniyim*, pp. 11 and 32; *Piskei Din shel Batei ha-Din ha-Rabbaniyim be-Yisra'el*, I, 56, 61; I, 66, 75–76; I, 147, 157–158; III, 353, 358–360; XI, 154, 157, 158–159, 161–

162; XI, 172–173 and 366, 368–369; and XIII, 336–337. See also *Mishpetei Uzi'el, Even ha-Ezer*, no. 83, and R. Ovadiah Hadaya, *Teshuvot Yaskil Avdi, III, Even ha-Ezer*, no. 8.

33. For a detailed survey of sources establishing this principle see Eliav Shochetman, "On the Nature of the Rules Governing Custody of Children in Jewish Law," *Jewish Law Annual*, X (1992), 115–117.

34. A significant minority of states have legislation addressing surrogacy agreements. Some simply deny enforcement of all such agreements. See Ariz. Rev. Stat. Ann. § 25-218 (A) (West 1991); D.C.Code Ann. § 16- 402(a) (1997); Ind. Code Ann. §§ 31-20-1-1, 31-20-1-2 (Michie 1997); Mich. Comp. Laws Ann. § 722.855 (West 1993); N.Y. Dom. Rel. Law § 122 (McKinney Supp.1997); N.D. Cent. Code § 14-18-05 (1991); Utah Code Ann. § 76-7-204 (1995). Others expressly deny enforcement only if the surrogate is to be compensated. See Ky. Rev. Stat. Ann. § 199.590(4) (Michie 1995); La. Rev. Stat. Ann.§ 9:2713 (West 1991). Neb. Rev. Stat. § 25-21, 200 (1995); Wash. Rev. Code §§ 26.26.230, 26.26.240 (1996). Some states have simply exempted surrogacy agreements from provisions making it a crime to sell babies. See Ala. Code § 26-10A-34 (1992); Iowa Code § 710.11 (1997); W. Va. Code § 48-4-16(e)(3) (1996). A few states have explicitly made unpaid surrogacy agreements unlawful. See Fla. Stat. ch. 742.15 (1995); Nev. Rev. Stat. § 126.045 (1995); N.H. Rev. Stat. Ann.§ 168-B:16 (1994 & Supp. 1996); Va. Code Ann. §§ 20-159, 20-160(B)(4) (Michie 1995). Florida, New Hampshire and Virginia require that the intended mother be infertile. See Fla. Stat. ch. 742.15(2)(a); N.H. Rev. Stat. Ann. § 168-B:17(II) (1994); Va. Code Ann. § 20-159(B), 20-160(B)(6). Arkansas raises a presumption that a child born to a surrogate mother is the child of the intended parents and not the surrogate. See Ark. Code Ann. § 9-10-201(b), (c) (Michie 1993)

There are few appellate court opinions regarding the enforceability of traditional surrogacy agreements subsequent to the decision of the New Jersey court in the case of Baby M. In *In re Marriage of Moschetta*, 25 Cal. App. 4th 1218 (1994), the court declined to enforce a traditional surrogacy agreement because it was incompatible with California parentage and adoption statutes. More recently, the Supreme Judicial Court of Massachusetts declared surrogate contracts to be unenforceable on the grounds that consent to custody cannot be recognized unless given on or after the fourth day following the child's birth and because payment of money to influence the mother's custody decision renders the agreement as to custody void. See *R. R.* v. *M. H. & Another*, No. SJC-07551, 1998 WL23540 (Mass. Jan. 22, 1998).

35. Indeed, the halakhic provisions set forth herein pertain only in situations in which both parties are Jewish. The halakhic provisions are presented, not as normative prescriptions for a non-Jewish society, but as model for social legislation.
36. Cf., Nehama Leibowitz, *Iyyunim be-Sefer Bereshit* (Jerusalem, 5729), pp. 111–112.

10

Pregnancy Reduction

Women suffering from certain medical problems that prevent them from becoming pregnant because they do not experience normal ovulation can now be treated with fertility drugs that may result in the production of a multiple number of ova. Similarly, women who experience normal ovulation but fail to become pregnant because of other problems such as a blockage of the fallopian tubes may be able to conceive and bear multiple fetuses by means of in vitro fertilization.[1] Since the statistical probability of successful implantation of any single ovum fertilized in this manner is relatively low, fertility specialists treat such women with drugs that cause production of multiple ova. As many as eight or nine ova may be produced in a single cycle, thus enabling the physician to implant a multiple number of fertilized ova and thereby increase the chances for a successful pregnancy. In some instances most or even all of the ova may become implanted in the uterus with the result that a woman who had heretofore been experiencing fertility problems may actually become pregnant with a multiple number of fetuses.

Simultaneous gestation of multiple fetuses may present a serious risk to the life of the mother. Beyond a certain number, there is virtually no likelihood that any of the fetuses will survive to term. Problems resulting in the mortality or morbidity of at least some of the fetuses, including premature birth and the problems attendant thereupon, may occur with as few as four, and perhaps even three, simultaneous pregnancies. To avoid such complications, gynecologists recommend reducing the number of fetuses in the uterus at a relatively early stage of pregnancy. The halakhic discussions of pregnancy reduction are limited to situations in which failure to intervene will result in the certain loss of all of the fetuses. That problem generally arises only in pregnancies involving six or perhaps five fetuses. That, of course, is a medical issue that must be determined upon assessment of all relevant factors.

When the presence of multiple fetuses will result in loss of the life of the mother the status of the fetus is that of a *rodef* or "pursuer" whose "aggression" must be blocked even at the cost of the life of the *rodef*. This is true even when, as in this case, there is no moral turpitude insofar as the *rodef* is concerned since the *rodef* is acting in an entirely involuntary manner. However, a significant question of Jewish law arises in largely theoretical cases in which there is no threat to the life of the mother rising to the level that renders the law of *rodef* applicable but in which failure to intervene will result in the demise of all the fetuses. In such circumstances the question is whether it is permissible to destroy some fetuses in order to save others.

Were the question to be posed with regard to the sacrifice of an already born baby in order to save the life of another person—adult or infant—the answer would be fairly clear. The Mishnah, *Oholot* 7:6, declares that from the moment the major portion of a baby emerges from the birth canal it cannot be killed in order to save the mother. The Palestinian Talmud adds the explanatory comment that mother and child are, in effect, reciprocal *rodfim*, each one threatening the life of the other. In such situations, the proper course of action is passive non-intervention.

The sacrifice of a fetus in order to preserve the life of the mother is sanctioned on the premise that fetal life is inherently inferior to the life of a person already born coupled with the consideration that the fetus is a *rodef* with regard to the life of the mother.[2] That principle is not applicable in situations involving pregnancy reduction in which some fetuses are sacrificed to save others because the lives of the fetuses are, in terms of their halakhic status, equal in quality.[3]

The status of the halakhic prohibition with regard to feticide is a matter of some controversy. Many authorities regard the destruction of the fetus as a form of non-capital homicide while others regard it to be a forbidden form of "wounding," a form of "destruction of the seed" or as a prohibition merely rabbinic in nature.[4] Rabbinic decisors who accept one of the latter positions have no difficulty sanctioning abortion for therapeutic reasons not involving a threat to the life of the mother.[5] R. Chaim David Halevy, in a contribution to *Assia*, no. 47–48 (Kislev 5750),[6] relies upon those permissive views in permitting pregnancy reduction. Similarly, R. Eliezer Waldenberg, in his recently published *Ẓiẓ Eli'ezer*, XX, no. 22, in a manner consistent with his highly controversial position regarding abortion of a Tay-Sachs fetus,[7] cites those views in reaching an identical conclusion. The problem, however, is far more complex for the many authorities who regard feticide as a form of homicide and consequently refuse to sanction abortion other than for the purpose of preserving the life of the mother.[8]

The Mishnah, *Oholot* 7:6, is emphatic in its ruling prohibiting embryotomy once the major portion of the child has been delivered. The inferred presumption is that the sacrifice of one life will assuredly save the other. There is, however, no specific statement of halakhic determination dealing with cases in which non-interference would lead to the loss of both mother and child. Halakhic grounds that may justify an embryotomy under such conditions even subsequent to the commencement of parturition are set forth by R. Israel Lipschutz, the author of *Tiferet Yisra'el*, in his commentary on this Mishnah. One of the issues[9] hinges upon the applicability of a law recorded by Rambam, *Hilkhot Yesodei ha-Torah* 5:5, ". . . if the heathen said to them, 'Give us one of your company and we shall kill him; if not we will kill all of you,' let them all be killed but let them not deliver to [the heathens] a single Jewish soul. But if they specified [the victim] to them and said, 'Give us so and so or we shall kill all of you,' if he had incurred the death penalty as Sheba the son of Bichri, they may deliver him to them . . . but if he had not incurred the death penalty let them all be killed, but let them not deliver a single Jewish soul."

Rambam's ruling is based upon the explication of the narrative of II Samuel 20:4–22 found in the Palestinian Talmud, *Terumot* 8:12. Joab, commander of King David's troops, had pursued Sheba the son of Bichri and besieged him in the town of Abel and demanded that he be delivered to the king's forces. Otherwise Joab threatened to destroy the entire city. From the verse "Sheba the son of Bichri has lifted up his hand against the king, against David" (II Samuel 20:21), Resh Lakish infers that acquiescence with this demand can be sanctioned only in instances in which the victim's life is lawfully forfeit, as was the case with regard to Sheba the son of Bichri who is described as being guilty of *lèse majesté*; in instances in which the victim is innocent, all must suffer death rather than become accomplices to murder. R. Yoḥanan maintains that the question of guilt is irrelevant, but that the crucial element is the singling out of a specific individual. Members of a group have no right to select one of their number arbitrarily and deliver him to death in order to save themselves since the life of each individual is of inestimable value. However, once a specific person has been marked for death in any event, either alone if surrendered by his companions or together with the entire group if they refuse to comply, those who deliver him are not accounted as accessories. Rambam's ruling is in accordance with the opinion of Resh Lakish.[10]

In a medical context, when confronted by the imminent loss of both mother and child, those authorities who require merely that the victim be "specified" would advocate dismemberment of a partially delivered child having no possibility of survival in order to save the mother since they do not require that he necessarily be guilty of a capital offense. However, according to Rambam, the intended victim must be culpable as well. Since a newly-born child is certainly guilty of no crime it may not be sacrificed in order to preserve the life of the mother. Furthermore, this line of reasoning does not apply to the many cases where either the mother or child may be saved through the sacrifice of the other; in such situations the crucial element of "specification" is totally absent.[11]

Teshuvot Panim Me'irot, II, no. 8, discusses the selfsame problems but does not conclude with a definitive ruling. *Panim Me'irot*'s comments are cited by *Tosefot R. Akiva Eger, Oholot* 6:17, no. 17. *Panim Me'irot*'s arguments for permitting the destruction of the child in order to save the mother seem to be predicated upon the consideration that sacrifice of the child will save the mother whereas the child is doomed in any event. Since the death of the child can save the mother but the death of the mother cannot save the child, the child is to be regarded as "specified" for death as was Sheba ben Bichri. Similar views are also advanced in other contexts by *Yad Ramah, Sanhedrin* 72a, and *Maharam Ḥal'avah, Pesaḥim* 25b.

In an article published in *Assia*, vol. 12, nos. 1–2 (Tevet 5749),[12] Rabbi Yitzchak Zilberstein finds tentative support in the comments of *Panim Me'irot* for resolution of the classic lifeboat dilemma as well as for the problem of pregnancy reduction. An overloaded boat will sink and drown all its passengers. If one or more passengers are thrown overboard the remainder will be rescued. May some of the passengers, who will in any event die if no one intervenes, be cast from the boat in order to save at least one of the passengers? May some of the fetuses be eliminated in order that the others develop to term? Citation of *Panim Me'irot* in this context does not at all seem to be apropos. In addressing the parturition situation, *Panim Me'irot* seems to be tracking the reasoning advanced by *Tiferet Yisra'el*, i.e., the child has been "specified" for death whereas the mother has not. That is manifestly not the case with regard to either the lifeboat passengers or the woman pregnant with multiple fetuses. The situation is entirely analogous to the paradigm case, *viz.*, "Give us one of your company and we shall kill him; if not we will kill all of you." *Ḥazon Ish*, *Sanhedrin*, no. 25, as well as R. Shlomoh Zalman Auerbach, as cited by the editor of *Assia* in a footnote appended to Rabbi Zilberstein's article, explicitly rule that it is forbidden to sacrifice one member of an endangered group in order to save the rest.

To be sure, application of the rule "Be killed but do not transgress" to situations in which even the person delivered to death will perish in any event is fraught with conceptual difficulty. The Gemara, *Pesaḥim* 25b, states that the principle "Be killed but do not transgress" as applied to an act of homicide is an *a priori* principle based upon reason alone, i.e., upon the principle "Why do you think that your blood is sweeter than the blood of your fellow?" If so, questions *Kesef Mishneh, Hilkhot Yesodei ha-Torah* 5:5, what is the basis for the extension of the ruling "Be killed but do not transgress" to a situation in which the victim is singled out and the entire group warned that, if the specified individual is not delivered, all will perish. In such cases the dictates of reason would indicate that it is preferable by far to sacrifice a single life rather than to suffer the loss of the entire group. *Kesef Mishneh* concludes that the Sages possessed a tradition extending this principle even to cases in which the *a priori* reason advanced does not apply.[13]

The most authoritative, although somewhat tentative, pronouncement with regard to pregnancy reduction that has appeared thus far is that of R. Shlomoh Zalman Auerbach. Rabbi Auerbach is quoted by Dr. Abraham S. Abraham, *Nishmat Avraham, Ḥoshen Mishpat* 425:2, sec. 22, as having stated that he "is inclined to permit" (*da'ati noteh le-hattir*) pregnancy reduction in appropriate circumstances. Dr. Abraham cites Rabbi Auerbach as having expressed that opinion with regard to "multiple fetuses, e.g., a sextuplet." Unfortunately, further details of Rabbi Auerbach's reasoning are not provided. A similar ruling by R. Mordecai Eliyahu is published in *Teḥumin*, XI (5720), 272–274. Again, a detailed discussion of the considerations involved is unfortunately lacking.

A similar conclusion is reached by Rabbi Zilberstein in his earlier cited article in *Assia* and by Rabbi Joshua Ze'ev Zand in an article appearing in a journal published by the Hebrew Theological College, *Or Shmu'el* (Skokie, 5752).[14] Rabbi Zand carefully cautions that, unless the mother's life is endangered, the procedure can be sanctioned only in situations in which none of the fetuses can otherwise survive, but that the procedure cannot be sanctioned if any of the fetuses can survive even though the surviving fetus is likely to suffer some defect or abnormality. A more detailed discussion was subsequently published by Rabbi Zand in his *Birkat Banim* (Jerusalem, 5744), chap. 12, sec. 41.

Both writers explain that the procedure is permissible because a non-viable fetus, i.e., a fetus that cannot survive for a period of at least thirty days subsequent to birth, is not considered to be a "live" creature for purposes of Jewish law and hence the prohibition against feticide does not apply. Indeed, the Gemara, *Shabbat* 135a, *Yevamot* 80a and *Bava Batra* 20a, compares a non-viable neonate, i.e., a baby that cannot survive for a period of thirty days, to a stone and declares that it cannot be moved on *Shabbat*.[15]

There is yet another conceptual problem that must be confronted in analyzing the basis of a permissive ruling with regard to pregnancy reduction. If feticide is a form of homicide it must be because the fetus has the status of a human being even during gestation. If a neonate that cannot survive does not also enjoy that status it must be because although only a viable fetus enjoys the status of a human being it nevertheless enjoys that status either from conception or from an early period of gestation. Conversely, a non-viable neonate does not enjoy that status in utero. The crucial point is that, although the status of the fetus may not be known until it either survives or perishes, its objective status is determined from the very beginning of its existence.

This gives rise to a dilemma in the contemplation of pregnancy reduction. It is certainly the case that at the moment of intervention all of the fetuses are doomed. Which fetus shall be selected for reduction and which fetus shall be allowed to develop to term depends upon the act of the physician. Assuming there is no prohibition in eliminating a non-viable fetus, choosing between non-viable fetuses presents no halakhic problem. Pregnancy reduction, however, is advocated precisely in order to assure that some fetuses will survive to term. After intervention, the remaining fetuses are viable. It is clear that in performing a medical procedure a physician does not generate life but simply preserves a life already in existence. Accordingly, when pregnancy reduction is an option, each of the fetuses is potentially viable. The physician merely selects which fetus shall live and which shall perish. Assuredly, the surviving fetuses had the status of viable fetuses from the earliest stage of gestation. Choosing between viable fetuses does present a problem in the form of "on what account do you think the blood of one is sweeter than the blood of another? (*mai ḥazit*)." In the act of intervention it becomes determined that the surviving fetus was viable from the moment of conception. Does the principle of *mai ḥazit* operate in precluding a selection of that nature? It is that principle that is codified by Rambam, *Hilkhot Roẓeaḥ* 1:9, in the words "for one dare not set aside one life for [another] life."

In effect, multiple pregnancies of such nature give rise to a paradox: If there is no intervention, the fetuses are all foredoomed and no prohibition attends upon their destruction. The very act of reduction renders some of the fetuses viable and hence would appear to trigger the rule "one dare not set aside one life for [another] life." Hence it would seem that the very act of intervention serves to render such intervention illicit.

The predicament is analogous to the classical paradox presented by Epimenides the Cretan who declared that all Cretans were liars and that all other statements made by Cretans were certainly lies.[16] Accordingly, if the statement "All Cretans are liars," when uttered by a Cretan, is also understood as meaning that Cretans always lie,[17] the following propositions follow from that statement: All Cretans are liars. I am a Cretan. Therefore, I am a liar. But if I am a liar then "All Cretans are liars" is a lie. If that is a lie, then I am telling the truth. If I am telling the truth, then it is true that all Cretans are liars and that I am telling a lie. . . .[18]

It would appear to this writer that, methodologically, proper resolution of the paradox is akin to the methodology employed in resolution of the philosophical paradox presented by the seemingly contradictory principles of divine omniscience and human freedom. The various resolutions of that problem propounded by medieval philosophers serve to confirm both principles in insisting that human will is indeed free but that the Deity has foreknowledge of the choice that men will make.[19] Similarly, it may be argued that the surviving fetuses were created as viable fetuses from the onset of conception. The physician may indeed randomly choose fetuses for elimination but his choice, albeit not preordained, is nevertheless foreknown. Hence, those fetuses that are eliminated were *ab initio* not endowed with viability with the result that their elimination is not prohibited.

This situation is not analogous to that of a physician who aborts a perfectly viable fetus. Such a fetus is perfectly viable save for the act of the abortionist. Divine omniscience is a significant factor only in determining that the fetus was never viable and hence its destruction does not constitute an illicit act. Assuming that feticide is a form of homicide, the elimination of a viable fetus is comparable to the sacrifice of one human being for the preservation of another. Prior knowledge on the part of the Deity is neither a defense nor a justification for engaging in such an act, just as divine omniscience does not serve to exculpate an act of homicide. Pregnancy reduction, on the contrary, is comparable to a situation in which a fetus would perish if not for medical intervention. When rescued, the fetus is regarded as having been viable from conception since such rescue was foreknown to the Deity. When, absent pregnancy reduction, no fetuses can survive, none of the fetuses is viable other than upon an act of rescue. Accordingly, the act of rescue, involving, to be sure, the destruction of other nonviable fetuses, serves to determine that only the preserved fetuses were viable from the moment of conception.[20]

This line of reasoning serves to sanction pregnancy reduction only when it is a virtual certainty that no fetuses will otherwise survive and serves to sanction the elimination of only the minimum number of fetuses necessary in order to make it possible for some fetuses to survive.

NOTES

1. For a discussion of in vitro fertilization from the perspective of Jewish law see J. David Bleich, *Judaism and Healing* (New York, 1981), pp. 92–95.
2. A detailed analysis of this involved concept is presented in J. David Bleich, *Contemporary Halakhic Problems*, I (New York, 1977), pp. 347–354.
3. It is indeed the case that in situations in which the fetuses are not viable solely because there are too many fetuses in a single uterus each fetus is a "pursuer" with regard to each of the other fetuses and hence it might appear that the "law of the pursuer" would permit, and even require, elimination of the "pursuer" in order to preserve a potential victim. However, as is evident from the deliberations of the Palestinian Talmud, *Avodah Zarah* 2:2 and *Sanhedrin* 8:9, in situations in which two individuals are mutual

aggressors the acts of aggression, in effect, cancel each other, and the law of pursuit does not apply. See *Teshuvot Divrei Yissakhar*, no. 168 and *Iggerot Mosheh, Ḥoshen Mishpat*, II, no. 59. Cf., R. Joshua Ze'ev Zand, *Birkat Banim* (Jerusalem, 5754), p. 376.

4. For an analysis and discussion of these various positions see *Contemporary Halakhic Problems*, I, 325–371.
5. See sources cited in *Contemporary Halakhic Problems*, I, 109–115 and 354–356.
6. Reprinted in *Sefer Assia*, VIII (5755), 3–6.
7. See the vigorous rebuttal of R. Moshe Feinstein, *Iggerot Mosheh, Ḥoshen Mishpat*, II, no. 69. See also *Contemporary Halakhic Problems*, I, 112–115.
8. *Teshuvot Aḥi'ezer*, III, no. 72, contends that references to feticide as a form of homicide apply only to a fetus that has "torn itself loose" from the uterus, i.e., during the final stages of labor. According to that view, the fetus is regarded as a separate entity only after the process of parturition has begun whereas in earlier periods of gestation the fetus is regarded as but an organic limb of the mother's body with the result that pregnancy reduction in order to preserve other fetuses presents no halakhic problem. *Teshuvot Torat Ḥesed, Even ha-Ezer*, no. 42, sec. 4, also explains Rambam's ruling in *Hilkhot Roẓe'aḥ* 1:9 in a similar manner. This is apparently the position adopted by R. Aaron Soloveichik as reported by Yitzchak Mehlman, "Multi-Fetal Reduction," *Journal of Halacha and Contemporary Society*, no. XXVII (Spring 1994), pp. 59–62.
9. Other issues discussed by *Tiferet Yisra'el* are analyzed in *Contemporary Halakhic Problems*, I, 359–360.
10. Rosh and Ran, however, both rule in accordance with the opinion of R. Yoḥanan; Rema, *Yoreh De'ah* 157:1, cites both views without offering a definitive ruling.
11. See, however, R. Chaim Sofer, *Teshuvot Maḥaneh Ḥayyim, Ḥoshen Mishpat*, no. 50, who advances a number of considerations that serve to distinguish the "specification" of Sheba ben Bichri from the danger posed by a child in the course of delivery. These considerations are discussed in *Contemporary Halakhic Problems*, I, 358.
12. Reprinted in *Sefer Assia*, VIII (5755), 7–13.
13. For an elucidation of the basis of that tradition see *Teshuvot Aḥi'ezer*, II, no. 16, sec. 5.
14. The various halakhic authorities who permit reduction of multiple embryos are cited by Richard V. Grazi and Joel B.

Wolowelsky, "Multiple Pregnancy Reduction and Disposal of Untransplanted Embryos in Contemporary Jewish Law and Ethics," *American Journal of Obstetrics and Gynecology*, vol. 165, no. 5 (November, 1991), pp. 1268–71, and by Richard V. Grazi, Joel B. Wolowelsky and Raphael Jewelewicz, "Assisted Reproduction in Contemporary Jewish Law and Ethics," *Gynecologic and Obstetric Investigation*, vol. 37, no. 4 (May, 1994), pp. 217–225.

15. It must however be noted that despite these statements of the Gemara, R. Eleazar Fleckles, a disciple of the *Noda bi-Yehudah*, in a cryptic statement appearing in his *Teshuvah me-Ahavah*, I, no. 43, states that one who causes the death of a non-viable neonate incurs the penalty of "death at the hands of heaven." That statement has neither been analyzed nor cited by contemporary scholars.
16. For a discussion of this paradox see Bertrand Russell, *Logic and Knowledge*, Richard C. Marsh, ed. (London, 1956), pp. 59–83, reprinted in Irving M. Copi and James A. Gould, *Comtemporary Readings in Logical Theory* (New York, 1969), pp. 135–153. For references to this paradox in classical sources see Theodore K. Scott, *James Buridan: Sophisms on Meaning and Truth* (New York, 1966), pp. 49–60 and p. 49, note 89.
17. Expressed more generally, the identical paradox is presented by the statement. "This sentence is false." If it is false, then it must be true that "This sentence is true." But if it is true, then the sentence is false. Thus the truth of the sentence implies that it is false, which in turn implies that it is true, which in turn. . . .
18. Russell's Theory of Types designed to resolve paradoxes of this nature is of no avail with regard to the dilemma posed by pregnancy reduction. Russell argued that a proposition concerning a class of propositions is not itself a member of that class. Thus the proposition "All Cretans are liars" is not itself a member of the class of lies ascribed to Cretans. Similarly, the self-referential proposition "This sentence is false" is not really a member of the class of false propositions. However, as expressed by Hans Reichenbach, "Bertrand Russell's Logic," *The Philosophy of Bertrand Russell*, Paul A. Schilpp, ed. (New York, 1963), I, 38, Russell's Theory of Types is merely "an instrument to make language consistent," i.e., a linguistic rule designed to interpret the manner in which language is employed. As such, it offers no solution to a paradox that is ontological in nature.
19. Among the Jewish philosophers who affirm and reconcile both

principles are R. Sa'adia Ga'on, R. Judah Halevi, Rambam and their followers. Ibn Daud excluded human actions from divine foreknowledge while Ralbag denied knowledge of contingent events. Crescas, on the other hand, sacrificed freedom of the will in staunchly championing divine omniscience. For relevant sections from the writings of these philosophers see *With Perfect Faith: The Foundations of Jewish Belief*, ed. J. David Bleich (New York, 1983), pp. 415–594. It must be reiterated that mainstream Jewish thought accepts the veracity of both divine omniscience and human freedom.

20. This argument is developed at some length and in a somewhat different form in *Birkat Banim*, pp. 366–372.

11

Conjoined Twins

I. DESCRIPTION AND HISTORY

A report in the March 25, 1996 issue of *Time* together with a feature article published in the April, 1996 issue of *Life* describing the remarkable case of Abigail and Brittany Hensel have focused attention upon the rare phenomenon of conjoined twins, i.e., congenitally united twins who may also share common anatomical structures. These emotion-laden journalistic accounts, accented by an accompanying complement of photographs, evoke empathy with the plight of the children and their parents.

The Hensel twins have separate necks and heads, separate hearts, gallbladders, stomachs and spinal cords. They have one right kidney but two left kidneys. It is unclear whether they have three or four lungs. They do, however, share a single set of organs below the waist, including intestines, one pair of ovaries, a single uterus, bladder, vagina and urethra. They have separate nervous systems but a common blood stream. Together they have two hands and two feet; the limbs on each side are controlled by the twin whose head is on the corresponding side of the body. A third central but anomalous arm was surgically removed after birth. Despite all indications of separate nervous systems the twins have developed remarkable dexterity in coordinating movement of their separate limbs.

Twins, such as the Hensel sisters, who share an undivided torso and two legs represent an extremely rare example of conjoined twins. The total incidence of all forms of conjoined twins, i.e., twins physically connected to each other by some part of the body but who do not necessarily share common organs, is approximately one in fifty thousand births.[1] Approximately forty percent are stillborn and another thirty-four percent die within twenty-four hours after birth.[2] Oddly, the incidence of female conjoined twins is far higher than that of males.[3]

Conjoined twins are the product of a single ovum that for some unknown reason fails to divide fully into separate twins in the early weeks of gestation.[4] Although the reason for the occurence of this phenomenon has not been established with certainty, most scientists believe that conjoining occurs within the first twenty days after conception when some of the cells within a single fertilized ovum that is in the process of dividing into identical twins fail to separate completely.[5] Although it is estimated that in the United States alone sixty-seven such births occur each year[6] only about five hundred such babies are known to have survived until their first birthday.[7]

The popular term "Siamese twins" used to describe this phenomenon came into use as a description of the conjoined twins Eng and Cheng who were born in Siam in 1811 and widely exhibited by P.T. Barnum. Eng and Cheng each had a full complement of normal limbs and organs but were joined at the sternum by a flexible band of cartilage several inches long. They were discovered by a British merchant in 1824 and after tours of the United States and Europe they adopted the surname Bunker and settled as farmers in North Carolina. At the age of forty-four they married two British sisters aged twenty-six and twenty-eight. The twins maintained their wives in separate households and alternated weekly in visiting each wife. Cheng fathered six children and Eng had five; all of the children were normal and healthy. The brothers lived until 1874 and died within hours of each other.

Eng and Cheng were by no means the first known case of fully developed twins connected by a band of tissue. A description of such an occurrence was published as early as 1752.[8] There are much earlier reports of other forms of conjoining. One report speaks of twins joined back to back who were born in Rome in 1493.[9] Another account relates that twins joined at the forehead by a fusion of the cranial bones were born in 1495 and survived until the age of ten.[10] The "Scottish Brothers" were a curiosity in the Court of James III of Scotland. They survived their royal patron who died in 1488. The King took diligent care in educating them with the result that they became proficient in music, languages and other court accomplishments.[11]

One of the earliest descriptions of conjoined twins concerns the "Biddenden Maids," Mary and Eliza Chulkhurst, born in England in Biddenden, Kent in 1100. They are reported to have been united at the hips and shoulders and to have survived until 1134. The existence of the Biddenden Maids is remembered despite their deaths over 850 years ago because of a curious legacy left by them. The twins bequeathed twenty acres of land to the church wardens of their parish with instructions that the rental income be used to defray the cost of distribution of cakes to all strangers present in Biddenden on Easter Sunday together with gifts of bread and cheese to the poor of the parish. They further directed that their effigies, which readily identified them as conjoined, be imprinted on the cakes.[12] There is an even earlier report of a chronicler who, in 1062, observed female twins joined at the umbilicus and sharing a single lower extremity[13] and also a record of male conjoined twins brought from Armenia to Constantinople for exhibition in the year 945.[14]

Both the father of R. Levi ben Gershon (Ralbag), in his *Sha'ar ha-Shamayim* (Venice, 1547), *ma'amar* 8, and Tobias

Katz, *Ma'aseh Tuvyah* (Venice, 1708), p. 69, quote a narrative attributed to Avicenna regarding female Siamese twins born "in the land of the West." One of the twins wished to marry but the other, for reasons of modesty, sought to prevent her sister from doing so. The twins brought their dispute before a judge. The judge cleverly ordered the recalcitrant sister to rise but she was incapable of following his instruction. The judge then ordered the other twin to rise. She did so with alacrity, dragging her sister into an upright position together with her. Thereupon the judge ruled that, as the dominant twin, she was entitled to make the decision to marry. This brief account concludes with a report that shortly thereafter the subservient twin died of "shame and pain" and that resultant putrefaction of her body caused the other sister to die as well.

The phenomenon of conjoined twins is also reported in the responsa literature.[15] R. Jacob Reischer, in his responsa collection first published in 1709,[16] *Shevut Ya'akov*, I, no. 4, reports the exhibition of fully-formed non-Jewish male twins joined in the cranial area. *Shevut Ya'akov* remarks that "there is nothing new under the sun" (Ecclesiastes 1:9). He notes that the phenomenon is not novel since, according to the Gemara, *Eiruvin* 18a, and, according to one opinion recorded in *Ketubot* 8a, Adam and Eve were created simultaneously as fully formed but conjoined individuals and only later were they separated. *Shevut Ya'akov* further asserts that the talmudic opinion concerning simultaneous creation of Adam and Eve serves to establish that twins united in such a manner are separate persons since Scripture refers to Adam and Eve in their conjoined state in the plural: "Male and female did He create them . . . and He called their name Adam" (Genesis 5:2).

Accordingly, *Shevut Ya'akov* rules that twins conjoined in a like manner must be regarded as separate individuals for all purposes of Jewish law. Nevertheless, he expresses the opinion that such twins should not be permitted to marry since perforce both brothers would be compelled to share a single bed with the wife of either one and also because cohabitation in the presence of a third party is forbidden. The latter consideration, he asserts, would also prevent female twins from marrying a single husband even in Oriental countries not subject to the edict of Rabbenu Gershom in which polygamy is permissible.[17]

In another late seventeenth-century account, R. Jacob Hagiz, *Halakhot Ketanot*, I, no. 245, presents a rather bizarre description of conjoined male twins he reports having seen in Italy. The twins were approximately twenty-five years old. The larger twin appeared to be perfectly normal; the body of the second twin was significantly shorter with the result that his feet did not reach the ground. *Halakhot Ketanot* reports that the shorter twin experienced no sensation. The circulatory systems of the twins seem to have been connected since apparently the smaller twin was parasitically dependent upon the larger. *Halakhot Ketanot* regards the two brothers as separate individuals although he states that the smaller twin should be categorized as a *goses*, i.e., as being moribund.[18]

Even more unfortunate is a situation such as that of the Hensel sisters in which the twins are not only conjoined but lack a full complement of limbs and organs. That anomaly frequently occurs when the twins are conjoined in the anterior thoracic or upper abdominal area. The area of the thoracopagus is the most common site of union in conjoined twins with thoracopagus twins representing appproximately seventy-five percent of all reported cases of conjoined twins.[19] In all described cases of thoracopagus twins the livers have been found to be fused; the hearts are reported as fused in seventy-five percent of such cases.[20]

There are numerous references to two-headed and even three-headed conjoined babies, who may or may not have other dual organs in the upper part of the body, but who have only a single set of organs below the waist.[21] There is also one report of the opposite abnormality—one head and chest but a double abdomen as well as four feet.[22] Apparently, none of the three-headed neonates survived for any significant period of time.[23]

There are a number of fleeting references to the birth of two-headed children in antiquity.[24] However, the oldest detailed description of the birth of dicephalous twins is probably the narrative recorded in the Gemara, *Menaḥot* 37a. A certain Pelemo inquired of R. Judah the Prince, "If a man has two heads, on which one must he place the *tefillin*?" R. Judah considered the question to be both irrelevant and irreverent and accordingly ordered the interlocutor to "go into exile"[25] or suffer excommunication. However, at that very moment, another person appeared and said, "A [firstborn] infant with two heads has been born to me. How much must I give the priest?" An old man[26] came forward and instructed the father to give the priest ten *sela'im*. Since the statutory requirement for redemption of the firstborn is five *sela'im*, the aged respondent in issuing this ruling declared, in effect, that the father was liable for the redemption of each of the two heads.[27] Although the discussion was not recorded until the redaction of the Talmud in the fifth century C.E., it is quite evident that the report refers to an actual incident that took place during the life of R. Judah the Prince who lived in the latter part of the second century C.E.

Tosafot, obviously unaware of extant reports of dicephalous twins born in Europe during the medieval period, remark, "In our world (*ba-olam ha-zeh*) this does not exist," but cite a midrashic narrative[28] relating that Ashmedai, in the presence of King Solomon, brought forth "from under the ground" a person having two heads. That man subsequently married and sired children having two heads like himself as well as children having one head like his wife.[29] When the time came to divide their inheritance, the two-headed children demanded a double portion of the legacy. The case was brought before King Solomon for adjudication. Although not quoted by *Tosafot*, the Midrash further relates the curious information that such beings live in a far-off place in an abyss at a depth of five hundred years' journey below the ground and at an additional distance of five hundred years' journey horizontally, that they live in a world in which the sun rises in the west and sets in the east and that they are descended from Cain.[30]

The inheritance issue cited by *Tosafot* highlights a problem not discussed by the Gemara. The Gemara establishes only that the obligation of payment of the sum of five *sela'im* for redemption of the firstborn is occasioned by the emergence of each head that "opens the womb" of the mother. In the birth of ordinary twins, as Rashi explains, it is "impossible" for both heads to present simultaneously. Hence, although there may be some doubt with regard to which twin emerged first, there can be only one firstborn. However, in the delivery of dicephalous twins, it is entirely possible for both heads to present simultaneously. Accordingly, in instances in which the heads emerge first and both heads are delivered simultaneously, each of the heads "opens the womb."[31] Since Scripture establishes a requirement for redemption in the sum of "five shekels for the skull" (Numbers 3:47) the sum to be presented to the priest is doubled when both heads present simultaneously. Accordingly, the question pertaining to redemption of the firstborn is resolved without reference to whether dicephalous twins are deemed to be two people or one person. That question is, of course, crucial with regard to the issue addressed by *Tosafot*, i.e., establishment of rights of inheritance vis-à-vis other siblings.

Thus, the question of whether dicephalous twins are halakhically regarded as separate individuals or whether they share a single personality is raised by *Tosafot* and identified as a question placed before King Solomon but is left unresolved. However, King Solomon's decision, culled from the same midrashic source quoted by *Tosafot*, is presented by *Shitah Mekubeẓet, ad locum*. According to this midrashic source, Solomon heated water, covered one of the heads and then poured the scalding water on the other head. Both heads screamed in pain. Thereupon Solomon ruled, "It can be deduced that both heads have a single source and [the twins] should be deemed a single person."[32]

This writer's search of works devoted to the history of medical anomalies as well as of current medical literature has failed to uncover a parallel report of dicephalous twins sharing a common nervous system.[33] Quite to the contrary, a number of the sources cited in the literature make it a point to inform the reader that each of the twins was endowed with a unique personality. Thus, in the case of dicephalous twins born in the fourth century during the reign of the Emperor Theodosius, it is reported that "the emotions, affections and appetites were different. One head might be angry while the other laughed, or one feeding while the other was sleeping. At times they quarrelled and occasionally came to blows."[34] The "Scottish Brothers" had no synchronous sensation above the point of union, while below, sensation was common to both.[35] Of Ritta and Christina, born in Sardinia in 1829, we are told that "sensations in the upper extremities were distinct" and that "the nervous systems of the twins had little in common except in the line of union."[36] The dicephalous twins, Maria and Rosa Druin, born in Montreal in 1878, did not experience sensations of hunger and thirst at the same time.[37] Of the present-day Hensel twins *Time* magazine reports: "Tickle Abby on her side anywhere from head to toe, and Britty can't feel it—except along a narrow region on their back where they seem to share sensation. The girls experience separate urges to urinate and sleep."[38]

Unlike Solomon's twins, the dicephalous conjoined twins described in the literature would not both respond to pain stimuli applied to a single head. According to *Shitah Mekubeẓet*, such twins must be deemed to be separate persons, not only for purposes of inheritance, but for all other halakhic purposes as well. Moreover, conjoined twins, each endowed with a full complement of organs, are clearly separate individuals, regardless of whether or not they respond autonomously to pain stimuli. This is evident from the earlier cited responsum of *Halakhot Ketanot*, I, no. 245. In the case described in that responsum, the smaller, parasitic twin is reported to have been incapable of experiencing any sensation. Nevertheless, *Halakhot Ketanot* regards the twins as separate individuals for purposes of inheritance. An early twentieth-century scholar, R. Chaim Eleazar Shapiro, *Ot Ḥayyim ve-Shalom* 27:9, note 13, expresses a similar view, albeit somewhat tentatively, with regard to twins having separate limbs and organs above the waist but who share a single body below the waist. That authority understood the uncertainty expressed by the Gemara as limited to a situation in which the second head was a mere appendage but that situations involving more clearly defined separate bodies were not the subject of the Gemara's discussion. Consequently, the status of such twins is not at all a matter of doubt.

However, halakhic status as separate persons is not an unmitigated blessing. The logical conclusion of such a determination is that twins having separate heads and discrete nervous systems but who share a common torso are halakhically incapable of entering into a licit marital relationship. To be sure, each of the twins, as a separate person, enjoys legal capacity to contract a marriage. But having done so, it would appear that consummation of the marriage would be tantamount to adultery on the part of the non-spousal twin.[39] Since the twins share a single set of genital organs, any sexual act must be considered to be the act of both twins with the result that the twin who is not the marriage partner is engaged in an adulterous relationship with the spouse of his or her twin. Adultery is a far graver transgression than the offenses of reclining in a bed occupied by the wife of another man or violation of the norms of modesty in cohabiting in the presence of a third party, as identified by *Shevut Ya'akov*.

The concept of a person's single set of sexual organs having two distinct, and even contradictory, legal identities is not unknown in the annals of Halakhah. A slave owned in common by two individuals may be emancipated by one of his masters. Thereupon his status is that of a person who is half-slave and half-freeman. The Gemara, *Ḥagigah* 2b, declares that, unless that individual is emancipated by his second master as well, he may cohabit neither with a female slave nor with a free woman. Free men are forbidden to cohabit with slaves and slaves are forbidden to cohabit with persons of legitimate Jewish birth. A person who is half-slave, half-freeman cannot legitimately enter into a marital relationship with any woman since the part of his person that is free is forbidden to cohabit with a slave while the part that is a slave is forbidden to cohabit with a person of legitimate Jewish birth. To be sure, an individual who is half-slave, half-free is a single biological person whose dual personality exists only as a legal construct whereas dicephalous twins are separate biological entities who physically share a single set of sexual organs. Nevertheless, if Halakhah proscribes sexual activity because it regards the partially emancipated slave to be possessed of dual legal personae, the identical result should obtain, *a fortiori*, in instances of shared biological proprietorship of sexual organs. Indeed, even in the absence of the paradigm of the half-slave, half-freeman, it is only logical that shared biological proprietorship of sexual organs also gives rise to dual halakhic identity insofar as legal status of those organs is concerned.

II. THE PHILADELPHIA CASE OF 1977

1. *Background*

Most tragic is the anguishing decision that must be made in the case of dicephalous twins who share a single heart. Unfortunately, until very recently, no thoracopagus twins with conjoined hearts remaining attached survived for longer than nine months.[40] In the absence of surgical intervention, twins sharing a single heart are both doomed, apparently because the heart mass is not strong enough to maintain adequate circulation to both bodies. Although in 1982 it was reported that over fifty pairs of other forms of conjoined twins had been separated surgically,[41] very few attempts have been made to separate dicephalous twins. Separation, which is essentially the amputation of one head, means that one twin must be sacrificed in order to give the other an opportunity to survive.

Early attempts at separation of thoracopagus twins with conjoined hearts met with little or no success and received scant public attention.[42] The first such case to receive widespread attention was a procedure performed at Children's Hospital in Philadelphia in October, 1977 by Dr. C. Everett Koop, who later became Surgeon General of the United States during the Reagan administration.[43] The infant sisters were joined at the chest. An essentially normal four-chamber heart was fused to a stunted two-chamber heart. The connecting wall was only one-tenth of an inch thick and hence far too thin to divide. Even if divided, the two-chamber heart was incapable of supporting life.[44] Separation necessitated sacrificing one twin in order to preserve the life of the other.[45] That factor served to rivet attention upon the procedure.[46]

2. *Rabbi Feinstein's Ruling*

As might be anticipated, the situation posed a serious moral, religious and legal dilemma.[47] The parents of the twins, who resided in Lakewood, New Jersey, were devout Jews and members of a family of rabbinic scholars; the father himself was a rabinical student in his early twenties.[48] The parents sought the sanction of the late R. Moshe Feinstein before consenting to the procedure. Several of the nurses scheduled to assist at the operation were practicing Catholics and sought religious guidance.[49] Although reassurance by a Catholic moralist was forthcoming, three anesthesiologists and two nurses asked not to be put on the case.[50] Dr. Koop himself feared potential homicide charges and sought prospective legal immunity from criminal prosecution. Permission was readily granted by a three-judge panel of the Philadelphia Family Court.[51] Ultimately, the surviving twin died forty-seven days later of causes not related to the surgical procedure. The infant succumbed as a result of contracting hepatitis B from a blood transfusion.[52]

There is no record of a written opinion authored by Rabbi Feinstein. However, various accounts of his decision and of the reasoning upon which it was based have been published in a variety of sources.[53] Rabbi Feinstein is quoted in one source as having relied upon two analogies in resolving the dilemma.[54] The simpler analogy is to the case described in the Palestinian Talmud, *Terumot* 8:10. The *beraita* cited by the Palestinian Talmud declares that, in a situation in which heathens come upon a group of travelers and say to them, "Give us one of your company and we shall kill him; if not, we will kill all of you," the rule is "Let them all be killed but let them not deliver to [the heathens] a single Jewish soul." However, "If the heathens specify one [of the group] such as Sheba the son of Bichri they may deliver him [so that] they not be killed." Invocation of this paradigm assumes that one of the twins has been "designated" for death in the sense that it is doomed in any event and that any attempt to save its life, rather than the life of the other twin, will fail. In such circumstances, it is argued, the twin "designated" for certain death may be sacrificed in order to save the life of the other.[55]

That argument, as cited, fails to take cognizance of the balance of the discussion recorded in the Palestinian Talmud. The Palestinian Talmud adduces a controversy between two Amora'im with regard to explication of the rule formulated in the *beraita*. R. Simeon ben Lakish asserts that designation of a victim justifies delivering him to death only if the victim is indeed deserving of the death penalty as was Sheba the son of Bichri; R. Yoḥanan maintains that designation even without attendant guilt is sufficient. The talmudic discussion centers upon the narrative recorded in II Samuel 20:4–2. Joab, commander of King David's forces, pursued Sheba the son of Bichri and besieged him in the town of Abel. Joab demanded that Sheba the son of Bichri be delivered to the king's troops; otherwise, threatened Joab, he would destroy the entire city. On the basis of the verse "Sheba the son of Bichri has lifted up his hand against the King, against David" (II Samuel 20:21) R. Simeon ben Lakish infers that acquiescence to Joab's demand could be sanctioned only in instances in which the victim's life is lawfully forfeit, as was the case with regard to Sheba the son of Bichri who is described as having been guilty of *lèse majesté*; but in instances in which the victim is innocent all must suffer death rather than become accomplices to murder. R. Yoḥanan maintains that the issue of guilt is irrelevant; the sole relevant element is the singling out of a particular individual. Members of a group have no right to select one of their number for death in order to save their own lives. However, once a specific person has been marked for death, either alone if surrendered by his companions or together with the entire group if they do not comply, those who deliver him are not accounted as assassins. Ran, *Yoma* 82b, and other early authorities rule in accordance with the opinion of R. Yoḥanan; however, Rambam, *Hilkhot Yesodei ha-Torah* 5:5, rules in accordance with the opinion of R. Simeon ben Lakish. Rema, *Yoreh De'ah* 157:1, cites both views without adjudicating between them.

In the case of the conjoined twins, although the twin that is not capable of surviving under any circumstances may well be regarded as "designated" for death,[56] the "designated" twin is clearly innocent of any wrongdoing and cannot be regarded as culpable for the penalty of death. In light of the unresolved controversy between early-day authorities with regard to this matter, a rabbinic decisor would find grave difficulty in sanctioning an overt act designed to extinguish the life of one twin on the basis of this consideration alone.[57]

The second analogy is to a situation involving two men who jump from a burning airplane. The parachute of the second man does not open and, as he falls past the first man, the second seizes the first man's legs. If the parachute cannot support both men, is the first man justified in kicking the second man away in order to save himself?[58] The answer is yes. The reason, however, is not because the second man was "designated" for death,[59] but because the second is a "pursuer" who through his actions will bring about the death of the first.[60] Jewish law regards it not only as permissible, but as mandatory, to eliminate a pursuer when it is necessary to do so in order to preserve the life of a putative victim.[61]

It is precisely because the case of the two men bailing out of an airplane involves the concept of a pursuer that it is not entirely analogous to the case of conjoined twins sharing a single heart. In the case of the burning airplane it is clear which person is the pursuer and which is the victim. However, in the case of conjoined twins, each twin threatens the life of the other. R. Akiva Eger, in his novellae on *Ketubot* 33b, establishes that, in the case of mutual pursuers, the law of pursuit does not apply and hence intervention by a third party is not halakhically justified.

To be sure, there may exist a set of circumstances in which one of the twins may be judged to be a pursuer. If the heart can be shown to belong to one twin exclusively, the second is, in effect, a parasite. The second twin, who has no claim to the heart, is then quite literally a pursuer with regard to the first twin, whereas the first twin, in making use of a heart that is rightfully his, commits no act of aggression against the second twin. Indeed, in the case under consideration, Dr. Koop asserted,[62] and continues to assert, that the four-chambered heart "definitely belongs to one of the twins" exclusively.[63]

It appears to this writer that Dr. Koop's statement that the heart "belonged to one of the twins" is conclusory in nature and not supported by any halakhically relevant evidence. Mere relative proximity to one head rather than to the other does not serve to resolve the issue either scientifically or halakhically.[64] Development and configuration of blood vessels leading to the heart, and from it the other organs, may be extremely significant in determining which of the two twins is potentially viable but does not necessarily determine or reflect "ownership" of the heart. DNA evidence cannot resolve the question of "ownership" of the heart since the twins develop from a single ovum and possess an identical chromosomal structure. Quite to the contrary, since a single heart is the embryological result of failure of certain cells to develop, the single organ, or the portion of the organ that failed to divide, should be presumed to be held in common by both twins. The twins operated on by Dr. Koop had a six-chamber heart; it may be surmised that the additional chambers arose from an incomplete division of the organ. Since the organ remains fused it is difficult to perceive a basis for the assumption that nature gave one child a normal heart and the other a malformed two-chamber heart;[65] prior to actual division of the heart the entire organ would appear to be held in common by both twins.[66] In the case under discussion this assessment is bolstered by the fact that blood passed through a hole between the ventricles where the two fused hearts touched[67] and by the fact that the single six-chamber heart was supplying blood to both infants.

However, if it could be established that, halakhically speaking, the four-chamber heart should be assigned to one of the twins, the resolution of the dilemma from the vantage point of Jewish law would, upon first analysis, appear to be obvious and any analogy is superfluous.[68] It would appear that the twin lacking a heart, if that fact can be established, is a pursuer and hence no further justification is required in order to sanction surgical separation in order to preserve the life of the other twin. The "pursuer" argument, however, requires closer scrutiny.

3. *Objection to Rabbi Feinstein's Ruling*
Indeed, R. Baruch Dov Povarsky, a Rosh Yeshivah at the Ponivezh Yeshivah in Bnei Brak, *Bad Kodesh*, IV, no. 52, s.v. *ve-sham'ati*, states that he heard an oral report to the effect that Rabbi Feinstein had permitted separation of the twins precisely on the grounds that, as a parasite, the second twin was a pursuer. That line of reasoning is, however, subject to an obvious objection. Consequently, Rabbi Povarsky proceeds to question the grounds for Rabbi Feinstein's ruling on the basis of the discussion recorded in the Gemara, *Sanhedrin* 72b.

The Mishnah, *Oholot* 7:6, declares that if a pregnant woman is in "hard travail" the fetus may be destroyed in order to preserve the life of the mother. However, declares the Mishnah, once the head of the fetus has emerged, the fetus may not be harmed "for one life may not be set aside for the sake of [another] life." The Gemara raises an objection to the latter ruling by pointing out that the emerging fetus is, in effect, a pursuer, i.e., in emerging through the birth canal the fetus will cause the mother to perish. The Gemara responds by announcing that the law of pursuit does not apply in such instances because the mother is being "pursued by Heaven." In codifying that rule, Rambam, *Hilkhot Roẓeaḥ* 1:9, rephrases that distinction in an explanatory comment stating that the unborn fetus is not a pursuer for "this is the natural course of the world." The thrust of this modification of the law of pursuit is clear: In situations in which death of the victim is the result of natural, physiological processes, the law of pursuit cannot be invoked to eliminate the threat posed by another party whose "aggression" is limited to natural physiological activities. Such danger is not to be attributed to the other party but to nature or Heaven.[69]

In the case of dicephalous twins, the "parasitic" twin, if it is endowed with independent juridic personhood, is neither a parasite nor an aggressor. Accordingly, argues Rabbi Povarsky, its status is entirely comparable to that of a neonate whose head has already emerged from the birth canal. Since the danger is the product of natural processes, the infant, who upon entering the birth canal is a "person" (*nefesh*) in the full sense of the term, cannot be sacrificed in order to save the mother "for [one] life may not be set aside for the sake of [another] life." The "parasitic twin," argues Rabbi Povarsky, is similarly a full-fledged person in its own right. Since the danger it poses to the other twin is physiological in nature and entirely caused by Heaven, its life cannot be sacrificed in order to save the other twin.[70]

4. *Rabbi Baruch Dov Povarsky's Thesis*

Rabbi Povarsky himself offers an argument totally unrelated to the law of pursuit as justification for sacrificing the twin deemed to be a parasite. That twin, lacking a heart of its own or possessing a two-chambered heart, is dependent upon the other twin for circulation of blood; cut off from the circulatory system of its twin it would succumb in a matter of minutes. A nonviable neonate incapable of survival for a minimum period of thirty days is deemed to be a *nefel*, i.e., it has the halakhic status of an abortus or stillborn infant. Rabbi Povarsky takes note of the fact that the Gemara, *Shabbat* 135a, speaks of a nonviable neonate that has not yet expired as having a status analogous to that of a stone that may not be moved on the Sabbath. Accordingly, since the nonviable neonate is not regarded as a living person, Rabbi Povarsky sees no reason why it may not be sacrificed in order to save the other twin.[71]

In formulating this argument Rabbi Povarsky acknowledges that the twin in question did survive longer than thirty days and that, ostensibly, the twin who was sacrificed would also have survived for a similar period of time; consequently, the twin lacking its own heart should similarly not be deemed to be a *nefel*. Rabbi Povarsky counters that objection by claiming that a neonate who can survive only with the assistance of artificial organs has no independent vitality and hence is to be deemed a *nefel* even if it survives more than thirty days. Taking this line of reasoning one step further, Rabbi Povarsky categorizes the twin drawing upon her sister's circulatory system as lacking independent vitality and hence as analogous to a neonate attached to an artificial heart.

Rabbi Povarsky's basic premise regarding a neonate capable of survival only with the assistance of artificial life support systems is certainly subject to challenge. Rabbinic decisors who have discussed related matters have generally reached the opposite conclusion. A closely related question arises with regard to infants who are placed in incubators either because they are premature or because they suffer from congenital abnormalities. If the baby is a firstborn male and survives in an incubator for a period of thirty days, is the father obligated to fulfill the *mizvah* of redemption of the firstborn? If the baby survives in an incubator more than thirty days but dies some time thereafter without having been removed from the incubator, must the laws of mourning be observed by parents and siblings?

The matter was apparently first addressed in a published responsum by R. Mordecai Winkler, *Teshuvot Levushei Mordekhai, Mahadura Telita'i, Oraḥ Ḥayyim,* no. 14 and no. 35. A premature baby was placed in an incubator and survived for six months. *Levushei Mordekhai* ruled that a child known to be premature retains the status of a *nefel* unless it survives to the age of twenty years.[72] The clear inference to be drawn from his response is that a child who was carried to term but suffers from a condition unrelated to gestational maturity with the result that it survives for thirty days only by virtue of having been placed in an incubator is indeed not regarded as a *nefel*. Thus, R. Akiva Sofer, *Da'at Sofer, Yoreh De'ah*, no. 114, rules unequivocally that mourning practices must be observed upon the death of a neonate who required an incubator but survived only for three months. Similarly, R. Shlomoh Zalman Auerbach is quoted by Dr. Abraham S. Abraham, *Nishmat Avraham*, IV, *Yoreh De'ah* 305:1, as ruling that a baby who has been carried to term but nevertheless requires an incubator must be redeemed in the usual manner.[73]

Unlike *Levushei Mordekhai, Da'at Sofer* apparantly maintains that even a child known to be prematurely born who survives in an incubator for thirty days is no longer a *nefel*. *Da'at Sofer*'s responsum is cited and relied upon by R. Eliezer Waldenberg, *Ẓiẓ Eli'ezer*, IX, no. 28, sec. 8. A contemporary authority, R. Moshe Stern, *Teshuvot Be'er Mosheh*, I, no. 64, rules that a premature infant possessing normal hair and fingernails at birth must be redeemed upon expiration of the statutory thirty-day period even if the baby is still maintained in an incubator. This is also the position of R. Abraham Jaffe-Schlesinger, *Teshuvot Be'er Sarim*, I, no. 75. For purposes of redemption of the firstborn, R. Ya'akov Breisch, *Teshuvot Ḥelkat Ya'akov*, III, no. 109, accepts the position of Rambam who maintains that survival for thirty days is sufficient even if hair and fingernails are not properly formed[74] and, accordingly, rules that a premature baby who survives in an incubator for thirty days must be redeemed. Thus, according to all rabbinic decisors, a baby who is born after a full nine month period of gestation but nevertheless requires an incubator in order to live is not deemed a *nefel* if he survives for a period of thirty days even though he is still maintained in an incubator.[75]

Elsewhere,[76] this writer has discussed the status of a patient whose heart has been removed and who is dependent upon an implanted artificial heart for survival and the considerations pointing to the conclusion that such a person must be considered to be alive for all purposes of Jewish law. If so, there is no reason to distinguish between a child who survives in an incubator and a child who survives with the assistance of an artificial heart. In both cases, if the baby is born at term and survives for thirty days, it should not be deemed a *nefel*. Accordingly, there is no reason to categorize the parasitic twin as a *nefel* on the basis of the fact that it is artificially sustained by the heart of its sibling.[77]

However, the argument advanced by Rabbi Povarsky does acquire cogency if it is maintained that the absence of some organs because of incomplete embryological cell division is tantamount to arrested development of the fetus. For example, a premature baby who succumbs because of incomplete development of its lungs is clearly a *nefel*. Hence, if one of the twins completely lacks lungs because cell division creating two sets of organs failed to occur it, too, might be considered to be gestationally immature and hence a *nefel*. Accordingly, it might be argued that the twin lacking a heart must be regarded as "prematurely" born, i.e., a *nefel*. If so, since the child is known to be "premature" at birth, it has the status of a *nefel* with the result that, according to *Levushei Mordekhai*, survival by "artificial" means for more than thirty days does not remove the child from the category of a *nefel*, as is the case, in his view, with regard to a neonate known to be gestationally premature.

Nevertheless, the argument, whether formulated in this manner or as formulated by Rabbi Povarsky, fails unless it is possible to categorize the twin who is to be sacrificed as a parasite. That, in turn, requires a determination that the heart in its entirety, or at least four of the chambers of the heart, belong to the twin whose life is to be preserved. If, as has been argued earlier, an acceptable demonstration of that fact has not been forthcoming, the heart must be regarded as shared equally by both twins. If the heart belongs to both twins, neither can be regarded as incompletely formed by virtue of the absence of a heart and, hence, neither can be considered a *nefel*.

5. *A Suggested Explanation of Rabbi Feinstein's Ruling*

Although the information presented by the media and in other reports does not intimate this line of reasoning, it seems to this writer that Rabbi Feinstein's ruling may readily be explained in light of his earlier and highly incisive analysis of the concept of "specification." As recorded in the Palestinian Talmud, *Terumot* 8:10, if the heathens designate an individual for execution and threaten to annihilate the entire company if that person is not delivered to them, R. Yoḥanan permits the threatened individuals to turn over the designated victim. Rashi, *Sanhedrin* 72b, s.v. *yaẓa rosho*, explains that, based upon the narrative concerning Sheba ben Bichri, R. Yoḥanan reasons that such an act is permissible because the designated individual is destined to perish in any event, either alone if delivered to those demanding his life or together with the entire company if that demand is not satisfied.

Rabbi Feinstein, *Iggerot Mosheh, Yoreh De'ah*, II, no. 60, *anaf* 2 and *anaf* 3, raises a serious question: It is indeed the case that the designated victim will surely die. However, if he is delivered to those intent upon putting him to death, he will be killed immediately, but, if he is not delivered to them, he will survive for at least a brief period of time until the evildoers carry out the execution of the entire company. Certainly in the paradigm involving the handing over of Sheba ben Bichri to Joab the death of Sheba ben Bichri would have been delayed at least until the siege of the city had accomplished its objective. Since hastening the death of even a moribund patient is a capital crime, queries *Iggerot Mosheh*, how could R. Yoḥanan sanction an act whose effect was to hasten the demise of a designated victim?

Iggerot Mosheh explains that the general rule is that if each of two individuals threatens the life of the other the law of pursuit does not apply. In cases of mutual pursuers bystanders dare not intervene because there is no reason to prefer one over the other in light of the presumption that both lives are equally "sweet."[78] The Gemara, *Sanhedrin* 74a, establishes the rule that a person may not take the life of another even in order to save his own life on the basis of the *a priori* principle "How do you know that your life is sweeter than the life of your fellow?" However, argues *Iggerot Mosheh*, when one of the two individuals is engaged in an act of pursuit that is qualitatively greater than that engaged in by the second pursuer, the objection in the form of "How do you know that the life of one is sweeter than the life of the other?" is removed. To be sure, in the case discussed by the Palestinian Talmud, the putative victim is entirely innocent and is not at all engaged in an overt act of aggression. Nevertheless, the very existence of the designated victim poses a threat to others and hence he is adjudged to be a "pursuer."[79]

The situation depicted in the Palestinian Talmud, then, involves two pursuers: the victim who endangers those who continue to harbor him and the others who seek to deliver the designated victim to the heathens and who thereby themselves become the victim's pursuers. However, the nature of their pursuit is quite different from the "pursuit" of the designated victim. The victim, by virtue of his continued existence and presence among the members of the group, threatens the normal longevity anticipation of those surrounding him; the others, in delivering the victim, jeopardize only the brief period of time (*ḥayyei sha'ah*) that the victim's life would have been prolonged until he is actually seized by those making the threat. Thus, argues *Iggerot Mosheh*, R. Yoḥanan reasons that, although both parties are pursuers, the victim poses a threat to the others that is qualitatively greater than their threat to him. Elimination of the designated victim rather than allowing the others to be put to death results in a net gain in the qualitative category of life preserved, *viz.*, normal longevity anticipation as opposed to ephemeral prolongation of life.

In support of this thesis *Iggerot Mosheh* adduces a discussion of the Palestinian Talmud, *Shabbat* 14:14. That discussion focuses upon whether the law of pursuit is applicable in instances in which the pursuer is a minor. In a tentative attempt to demonstrate that a minor, by virtue of his lack of legal capacity, is not culpable as a pursuer, the Palestinian Talmud cites the statement of the Mishnah, *Oholot* 7:6, "If the major portion [of the fetus] has emerged he may not be touched for [one] life may not be set aside on behalf of another." In effect, the Palestinian Talmud regards the emerging fetus as a pursuer as indeed does R. Ḥisda in a similar query reported in the Babylonian Talmud, *Sanhedrin* 72b. However, unlike the Gemara, *Sanhedrin* 72b, the Palestinian Talmud rebuts that contention with the declaration that, in the situation to which reference is made in *Oholot*, "You do not know who is killing whom," i.e., mother and child are mutual pursuers. *Korban ha-Edah* and *Pnei Mosheh*, in their commentaries *ad locum*, amplify that comment in explaining that, since each is endangering the other, it is not possible to make a determination that the child is pursuing the mother or, vice versa, that the mother is pursuing the child. Accordingly, there are no grounds for intervention.

Iggerot Mosheh further asserts that, in light of the comments of the Palestinian Talmud, the distinction drawn by the Gemara, *Sanhedrin* 72b, *viz.*, that in the case of the women in hard travail "it is Heaven that pursues her," must be understood in an identical manner, i.e., as an assertion that, since nature causes mother and child to become locked in mutual pursuit of one another, they must be regarded as mutual pursuers with the result that the law of pursuit becomes inoperative.

Rambam, *Hilkhot Roẓeaḥ* 1:9, invokes the law of pursuit in justifying the sacrifice of a fetus in order to save the life of the mother despite the fact that later, during actual parturition, intervention is forbidden. The difficulty is obvious: If the law of pursuit does not apply during partrution because "it is Heaven that pursues her" or, as paraphrased by Rambam, because "such is the nature of the world,"[80] how can the law of pursuit be invoked to justify elimination of the fetus while it is still in the mother's womb? Resolution of that difficulty has been the subject of concerted attention over a span of centuries.[81]

For *Iggerot Mosheh*, the resolution of that difficulty is simple. Mother and fetus, as well as mother and child, are indeed mutual aggressors. Qualitatively, the aggression of the mother vis-à-vis the child and the aggression of the child vis-à-vis the mother are identical; hence the resultant rule is nonintervention. However, the aggression of the mother vis-à-vis her unborn fetus is not qualitatively identical to that of the fetus against the mother. Homicide is a capital offense whereas feticide is not; hence, the threat against the mother is qualitatively more serious than the threat to the fetus. Accordingly, since the fetus is engaged in a qualitatively greater act of aggression, there is an objective reason to eliminate the fetus that renders nugatory the consideration "How do you know that the life of one is sweeter than the life of the other?"

Iggerot Mosheh further maintains that R. Simeon ben Lakish, who disagrees with R. Yoḥanan in maintaining that the specified victim may not be delivered to death even though he has been marked for death by the heathens and is destined to die in any event, does not challenge the basic thesis concerning relative degrees of pursuit. R. Simeon ben Lakish, argues *Iggerot Mosheh*, maintains that a person cannot be deemed to be a pursuer simply because evildoers arbitrarily and capriciously seek his death and will cause others to perish in order to kill their intended victim as well. In effect, R. Simeon ben Lakish contends that the only pursuers are the heathens; the individual designated by them, who is entirely passive, is not a pursuer but a victim. Only when the individual identified for execution is culpable of the death penalty does R. Simeon ben Lakish agree that he may be delivered to the heathens, i.e., only when he has committed an overt act that gave rise to the danger is he regarded as a pursuer. Consistent with that view, *Iggerot Mosheh* cites *Taz*, *Yoreh De'ah* 157:8, in insisting that the act for which the heathens seek to punish the designated victim need not necessarily constitute a capital offense in Jewish law, but that any act sufficient to give offense to the heathens renders the individual a pursuer.

The case of a fetus threatening its mother in "hard travail" is significantly different from the case of an individual whom the heathens demand be delivered to them in that it is not simply the existence of the fetus that threatens the life of the mother but rather the activity of the fetus as it attempts to force its way through the birth canal that constitutes the source of danger. That activity is, of course, both natural and nonvolitional; however, as both the Palestinian Talmud and the Gemara, *Sanhedrin* 72b, conclude, the law of pursuit applies even to an unintentional pursuer.

Iggerot Mosheh's thesis is readily applicable to the case of dicephalous twins. At the time that Rabbi Feinstein's ruling was issued, medical experience indicated that, if not separated, conjoined twins sharing a single heart could survive for a maximum of nine months.[82] Moreover, in the particular case addressed by Rabbi Feinstein, the twins were experiencing heart failure and, had they not been separated, they both would have expired in a relatively short period of time.[83] In the case of dicephalous twins, there is medical evidence indicating that, generally speaking, it is the left twin that has a chance for survival; the indications are that the right twin will not survive even if assigned a full complement of organs.[84] In the case under discussion, it is clear that only one twin had a chance for survival. For unexplained reasons, the right twin usually has complex cardiovascular anomalies that are not amenable to surgical correction.[85] In the conjoined state, the twins are certainly mutual aggressors. The right twin unintentionally threatens the normal longevity anticipation of the left twin. The right twin, however, because of its congenital anomalies, cannot survive for a period of more than twelve months. Such an individual, it may well be argued, must be regarded as a *treifah*.[86] As is the case with regard to feticide, murder of a *treifah* is not a capital offense. Accordingly, although both are pursuers, the right twin is engaged in an act of pursuit that is qualitatively of greater magnitude than the pursuit in which the left twin is engaged. Hence, according to *Iggerot Mosheh*'s analysis, the right twin may, and indeed must, be eliminated in order to preserve the life of the left twin.[87]

Thus, Rabbi Feinstein's ruling with regard to the separation of dicephalous twins is not only consistent with his earlier published responsum[88] but was logically compelled by the thesis developed therein. However, disagreement with any element in his analysis of the discussion of the Palestinian Talmud, including the rationale underlying R. Simeon ben Lakish's disagreement with R. Yoḥanan with regard to the sufficiency of specification alone, would in all likelihood result in a different conclusion regarding separation of dicephalous twins.[89]

NOTES

1. Estimates based upon imperfect reporting vary between 1/30,000 and 1/100,000 births. Most writers accept 1/50,000 as a likely approximation. See Larry D. Edmonds and Peter M. Layde, "Conjoined Twins in the United States, 1970–1977," *Teratology*, vol. 25, no. 3 (June 1982), pp. 302 and 305; R. Patel, K. Fox *et al.*, "Cardiovascular Anomalies in Thoracopagus Twins and the Importance of Preoperative Cardiac Evaluation," *British Heart Journal*, vol. 39, no. 11 (November 1977), p. 1254; James W. Hanson, "Incidence of Conjoined Twinning," *Lancet*, vol. 2, no. 7947 (December 20, 1975), p. 1257; A.F. Guttmacher and B.L. Nichols, "Teratology of Conjoined Twins," *Conjoined Twins: Birth Defects Original Article Series*, vol. III, no. 1 (April 19, 1967), p. 6; Edith L. Potter and John M. Craig, *The Pathology of the Fetus and the Infant*, 3rd ed. (Chicago, 1995), pp. 220–221; and R. Mark Hoyle, "Surgical Separation of Conjoined Twins," *Surgery, Gynecology and Obstetrics*, vol. 170 (June 1990), p. 549. Hoyle reports that for some unexplained reason the incidence of conjoined twins in Africa is one in 14,000.
2. See Edmonds and Layde, p. 302. Cf., Hoyle, p. 549, who reports that approximately 60% are stillborn.
3. The figures given range from 76% higher, as given by Edmonds and Layde, p. 302, to 70–95% higher, as given by William D. Edwards, Donald K. Hagel *et al.*, "Conjoined Thoracopagus Twins," *Circulation*, vol. 56, no. 3 (September 1977), p. 494.
4. Strangely, although conjoined twins presumably are uniovular

they are not always entirely identical. See Ian Aird, "The Conjoined Twins of Kano," *British Medical Journal*, vol. 1, no. 4866 (April 10, 1954), p. 833.

5. See Aird, p. 831; E. Graeme Robertson, "Craniopagus Parietalis," *Archives of Neurology and Psychiatry*, vol. 70, no. 2 (August 1953), pp. 198–199; Miguel Marin-Padilla, Alvin J. Chin and Teresa M. Marin-Padilla, "Cardiovascular Abnormalities in Thoracopagus Twins," *Teratology*, vol. 23, no. 1 (February 1981), pp. 101 and 106; A.A. Zimmermann, "Embryologic and Anatomic Considerations of Conjoined Twins," *Conjoined Twins: Birth Defects Original Article Series*, pp. 18–21; and *Pathology of the Fetus and the Infant*, pp. 221–222.
6. Edmonds and Layde, p. 305. *Time*, p. 60 gives the figure as 40 per year.
7. *Life*, p. 51.
8. See George M. Gould and Walter L. Pyle, *Anomalies and Curiosities of Medicine* (New York, 1896), p. 168.
9. *Ibid.*, p. 168.
10. *Ibid.*, p. 173.
11. *Ibid.*, p. 184.
12. For a description of other conjoined twins who achieved renown over the centuries see *Anomalies and Curiosities*, pp. 167–189; and A.F. Guttmacher, "Bibliographical Notes on Some Famous Conjoined Twins," *Conjoined Twins: Birth Defects Original Article Series*, pp. 10–17.
13. *Anomalies and Curiosities*, p. 184.
14. *Ibid.*, p. 172
15. See also *Sefer Yuḥasin ha-Shalem*, ed. Herschell Filipowski (London, 1857), pp. 249–250, who describes a case of dicephalous twins and astonishingly reports that one died three years before the other.

A medical work of purported Maimonidean authorship, *Pirkei Mosheh* (Vilna, 5648), chap. 24, contains a report of a rash of dicephalous births attributed to what apparently was an eclipse of the sun. R. Chaim Joseph David Azulai, *Maḥazik Berakhah, Yoreh De'ah* 13:5, quotes from a work of R. Isaiah di Trani: "I heard from Jews who saw a woman with two backs, two spines, two heads, four eyes and four hands . . . but from the waist down there was a single body. She was about twenty years old and they were escorting her to the king dressed in beautiful clothes. I also heard from non-Jews that they had seen a man with two backs and two spines from the waist and above but from the waist down there was a single body."

16. The date of this observation is given as Channukah 5498 (1737–38). The date is clearly a typographical error since the *editio princeps* of *Shevut Ya'akov* is dated 5470.
17. *Shevut Ya'akov*'s comment that such polygamous marriage is prohibited solely because of the stricture against cohabitation in the presence of a third party is quite remarkable. The marriage of two living sisters to one male constitutes a biblical offense and hence is biblically forbidden in all locales. This objection is raised by R. Joseph Saul Nathanson in a note appended to his letter of approbation to R. Jacob Reischer's *Teshuvot Shevut Ya'akov*. Rabbi Nathanson advances the equally remarkable position that (1) each of the twins in question must be regarded as a *treifah* and (2) since the prohibition against marrying two sisters does not apply to marrying the sister of a deceased wife, it is not applicable to a sister of a *treifah*. Although, as will be shown later, a baby born with two heads is indeed a *treifah* that is so because of the principle that duplicate organs are both regarded as absent (*yeter ke-natul dami*). That principle does not apply when there exist two complete, albeit, conjoined bodies. Rabbi Nathanson asserts that some other form of *treifut* was present in the case described by *Shevut Ya'akov*. He cites the tentative view of R. Chaim Alefandri, *Teshuvot Maggid me-Reshit*, *Yoreh De'ah*, no. 2, to the effect that a man may marry the sister of his wife who is a *treifah*. That quite novel view is rejected by *Pitḥei Teshuvah*, *Even ha-Ezer* 15:11; R. Chaim Joseph David Azulai in *Birkei Yosef*, *Even ha-Ezer* 15:4; and R. Yitzchak Schmelkes, *Teshuvot Bet Yiẓḥak, Yoreh De'ah*, no. 62, sec. 18. See also R. Joseph Totzanovsky, *Pardes Yosef, Parashat Bereshit*, sec. 27.

    It is of interest to note that *Bet Yiẓḥak* asserts that *Shevut Ya'akov*'s hypothetical case involved non-Jewish twins who might convert to Judaism but to whom the biblical prohibition against marrying two sisters would not apply. [Nevertheless, such a marriage is normally prohibited by rabbinic law as recorded in *Shulḥan Arukh, Yoreh De'ah* 269:5. For a possible reason that such a marriage may not be forbidden in the case of conjoined twins, see R. Eliyahu Posek, *Koret ha-Brit, Naḥal Brit* 262:10.] *Pardes Yosef* cites one scholar who questions whether conjoined twins can undergo a valid conversion since, in immersion in the *mikveh*, each twin represents an interposition or *ḥaẓiẓah* to the other. It seems to this writer that there is no problem of *ḥaẓiẓah* in the immersion of conjoined twins. The Gemara, *Yevamot* 78a, indicates that a fetus may be converted together with its mother. The Gemara declares that the mother's body does not constitute a *ḥaẓiẓah* between the waters of the *mikveh* and the child because "that is its natural growth." The same principle should apply to conjoined twins.

18. Indeed, *Halakhot Ketanot* suggests that the blessing *Barukh dayyan ha-emet* may perhaps be recited even though the twin has not yet died since it is already a *goses*. It is remarkable that *Halakhot Ketanot* adds that the second twin should be circumcised. Since it is forbidden to so much as move a limb of a moribund patient, there is no question that circumcision dare not be performed on a *goses*.
19. Marin-Padilla *et al*., p. 101, and Edwards *et al*., p. 494.
20. *Loc. cit.*
21. The statements in *Time*, p. 62, that there are "only three or four cases on record" and in *Life*, p. 51, that "no more than four sets of surviving twins in recorded history have shared an undivided torso and two legs" are inaccurate.
22. Aird, p. 832.
23. See *Anomalies and Curiosities*, p. 167.
24. Livy, Book XLI, 21, 12; *Scriptores Historiae Augustae*, Antoninus Pius, IX, 3; and Ammianus Marcellinus, XIX, 12, 19, are cited by Prof. Saul Lieberman, "Tanna Heikha Ka'i," *Koveẓ Mada'i le-Zekher Mosheh Shor*, ed. Louis Ginzberg and Abraham Weiss, (New York, 1945), p.185. Lieberman includes the *Annals* of Tacitus, Book XII, 64, in this list. That text, however, reads *biformis hominum* or "hermaphrodite" rather than "biceps." See the Loeb Classics Series edition of Tacitus, trans. by John Jackson (Cambridge, 1937), III, 409. *Chronique de Michel le Syrien*, ed. J.B. Chabot (Paris, 1901), II, 2–3, relates that a child with two chests and two heads was born in Emmaus, Palestine at approximately the beginning of the fifth century during the reign of Flavius Honorius. See Daniel Sperber, *Magic and Folklore in Rabbinic Literature* (Ramat Gan, 1994), p. 14. Aristotle, *De Generatione Animalium*, IV,3,30, describes "monstrosities" that are "spoken of" as being formed with "extra heads."
25. *Seder ha-Dorot, Tanna'im ve-Amora'im*, s.v. *Pelemo*, cites a statement of the *Zohar* indicating that Cain was exiled to a place known as "Arka," a locale in which everyone was born with two heads. *Seder ha-Dorot* explains R. Judah's retort as indicating that Pelemo should go into exile to the same place to which

Cain was exiled and that in that place he might appropriately pose his question but that elsewhere the question is frivolous and the intelocutor is deserving of excommunication. See also *Zohar, Parashat Va-Yeẓei*, p. 157a, and *Zohar*, introduction, p. 9b. The latter source speaks of descendants of Cain possessing two heads. Cf., R. Chaim Eleazar Shapiro, *Ot Ḥayyim ve-Shalom* 27:9, note 13. See also *Zohar, Hashmattot, Bereishit*, pp. 253b–254a.

26. The term *ha-hu saba* occurs numerous times in the Gemara. For a complete list of those occurrences see R. Joshua L. Maimon, *Sinai*, vol. 19, no. 1–6 (Nisan-Elul 5756), p. 15. The references are not to a single anonymous person since they occur in contexts that span many centuries. *Tosafot*, *Ḥullin* 6a, cite the opinion that this individual is the prophet Elijah, but demonstrate that, in at least one of its occurences, the reference cannot be to Elijah. *Teshuvot ha-Ge'onim*, ed. Isaac Harkavy (Berlin, 5646), no. 23, also rebuts the opinion that the reference is to the prophet Elijah. See also R. Chaim Joseph David Azulai, *Petaḥ Einayim, Shabbat* 34a.

27. *Teshuvot Ḥatam Sofer, Yoreh De'ah*, no. 294, states that, according to Rashi's understanding of the ensuing talmudic discussion, the Gemara concludes that a neonate with two heads is a *treifah* incapable of survival for more than a period of twelve months and, accordingly, the response of the "old man" serves to establish an ancillary principle to the effect that a *treifah* requires redemption. *Ḥatam Sofer* further explains that *Tosafot* also understand the Gemara as concluding a child with two heads is a *treifah* but that, according to *Tosafot*'s understanding of that discussion, other *treifot* do not require redemption; the obligation to redeem a two-headed child constitutes an exception to the general rule that a *treifah* need not be redeemed and is based upon an explicit biblical verse. A similar analysis of *Tosafot*'s position is presented by R. Abraham Isaiah Karelitz, *Ḥazon Ish, Menaḥot* 42:4. *Ot Ḥayyim ve-Shalom* 27:9, note 13, similarly regards a two-headed person to be a *treifah*. This is also the view of R. Joseph Saul Nathanson as cited *supra*, note 17. Cf. also, *Teshuvot Bet Yiẓḥak, Yoreh De'ah*, no. 62, sec. 17. However, R. Chaim Soloveitchik, *Ḥiddushei ha-Graḥ al ha-Shas, Menaḥot* 37a, and R. Shlomoh Zalman Auerbach, cited by Abraham S. Abraham, *Nishmat Avraham, Yoreh De'ah* 305:12, note 3, regard the Gemara as adopting, as its final position, the view that a two-headed child is not a *treifah*. Cf., R. Jacob Emden, *Migdal*

Oz, Birkhot Horai 1:30 and 3:18. Cf. also, the analysis offered by *Ḥazon Ish* in his own name. *Ḥazon Ish* asserts that at no time did the Gemara consider a two-headed person to be a *treifah*. His argument is apparently that, although the principle is that duplicate organs are both regarded as non-existent (*yeter ke-natul dami*), a person without a head is a cadaver, but not a *treifah*; hence, there is no basis for assuming that a person with duplicate heads is a *treifah*. Similarly, *Avnei Nezer, Yoreh De'ah*, no. 399, offers two analyses of the discussion in *Menaḥot* according to which the Gemara concludes that a two-headed person is not a *treifah*.

28. This midrashic narrative is published in *Bet ha-Midrash*, ed. Adolph Jellinek, 3rd edition (Jerusalem, 5727), IV, 151–152 as well as in *Yalkut Sippurim u-Midrashim*, ed, Zev Wolf Greenwald, vol. II (Warsaw, 5683), pp. 115–116 and *Oẓar Midrashim*, ed. J.D. Eisenstein (New York, 5675), II, 533–534. Some scholars have erroneously assumed that the abbreviation *mem resh* appended to *Tosafot* stands for Midrash Rabbah. Cf., *Magic and Folklore in Rabbininc Literature*, p. 13, note 1. Those letters represent the words *mi-pi rabbi* or, as Urbach prefers, *me-divrei rabbi*. The identical abbreviation appears in numerous instances in *Tosafot*'s commentary on *Menaḥot* 25b–37a, including no less than six occurrences on the same page on which this midrashic narrative is cited, in conjunction with halakhic comments that are certainly not based on midrashic references. Cf., Ephraim E. Urbach, *Ba'alei ha-Tosafot* (Jerusalem, 5740), II, 663. For a comparison with other similar narratives see R. Judah L. Slotnick, "Anashim Ba'alei Shnei Roshim," *Sinai*, vol. 9, no. 4 (Tishri 5706), pp. 19–25.

29. The Midrash relates that this person amassed a phenomenal fortune and became the father of six normal children and of one two-headed child. A variant version in which no reference is made to Ashmedai or to other worlds and which speaks of only two children is recorded in *Sefer ha-Ma'asiyot (The Exempla of the Rabbis)*, ed. Moses Gaster (New York, 1968), p. 74.

30. See *Zohar*, introduction, p. 9b and cf., sources cited *supra*, note 25. *Zohar, Parashat Va-Yikra*, pp. 9b–10a, states that just as there are seven firmaments above, there are seven earths below. Between each of these earths, which include the Garden of Eden and Gehinnom, is a firmament dividing them from one another. The creatures inhabiting the earths are also different, some with two faces, some with four, and some with one. See also

Tikkunei Zohar, tikkun 64 and cf., *Zohar, Parashat Yitro*, p. 80a.

31. In breach births the obligation of redemption is established on the basis of the delivery of the major portion of the body. Since dicephalous twins share a common trunk, if the twins present in the breach position, only the standard five *sela'im* would be required for redemption.
32. R. Chaim Eleazar Shapiro, *Ot Ḥayyim ve-Shalom* 27:9, note 13, reports that, as a child, he saw dicephalous male twins sharing one set of organs below the waist who had been brought to Vienna from London. That authority completely ignores the comments of *Shitah Mekubeẓet*, presumably because of the principle that halakhic matters are not subject to determination on the basis of aggadic statements. Nevertheless, he rules that each twin must don *tefillin* both on his head and on his left arm. Rabbi Shapiro regards the matter as having been left unresolved by the Gemara but applies the principle *safek de-oraita le-ḥumra*, i.e., in matters pertaining to biblical law a doubtful issue must be adjudicated stringently.

    Ot Ḥayyim ve-Shalom also asserts, but with some hesitation, that the question left unresolved by the Gemara is limited to a situation in which the sole duplicated organ is the head. However, twins possessing dual sets of organs above the waist, but a single body below the waist, he regards as two persons whose status is not the subject of the Gemara's unresolved question. It seems to this writer that twins having two complete sets of limbs, even though they share a liver and heart, are certainly separate individuals and that, in such a case, *Ot Ḥayyim ve-Shalom* would not have expressed any qualms in making such a determination.
33. There is, however, one report of a fusion of two heads in which "every movement and every act of the natural face was simultaneously repeated by the supernumerary face in a perfectly consensual manner, i.e., when the natural mouth sucked, the second mouth sucked; when the natural face cried, yawned, or sneezed, the second face did likewise; and the eyes of the two heads moved in unison." If this account is accurate, it may reflect the existence of a common nervous system. See *Anomalies and Curiosities*, p. 187.
34. *Ibid.*, p. 184.
35. *Loc. cit.*
36. *Ibid.*, p. 185.
37. *Ibid.*, p. 186.

38. *Time*, p. 64. However, despite their independently experienced sensations, a physician at Johns Hopkins Medical Center has stated, "Given the fact that they have shared organs, it's almost impossible for there not to be some overlapping in their autonomic nervous systems." See *Life*, p. 56.
39. There is a report of dicephalous twins, born in Switzerland in 1530 who had a single wife with whom they were said to have lived in harmony. See *Anomalies and Curiosities*, p. 184. Even more curious is the case of Rosalie and Josepha Blazek, pygopagus twins born in Bohemia in 1878, and joined posteriorly by a single very broad sacrum, by the lower lumbar region and by the ilia, who are said to have married one man. Rosalie, the only conjoined twin to have borne a child, gave birth to a normal son on April 17, 1910, some time before her marriage. See Guttmacher and Nichols, pp. 14–15.
40. George J. Annas, "Siamese Twins: Killing One to Save the Other," *Hastings Center Report*, vol. 27, no. 2 (April, 1987), p. 27. See, however, *People*, August 5, 1991, pp. 43–44, for a report of conjoined twins sharing a heart who survived until the age of seven. See also, *People*, July 3, 1989, p. 1.
41. E.S. Golladay, G. Doyne Williams *et al.*, "Dicephalus Dipus Conjoined Twins: A Surgical Separation and Review of Previously Reported Cases," *Journal of Pediatric Surgery*, vol. 17, no. 3 (June, 1982), p. 259. It is commonly assumed that the earliest attempt at surgical correction was made by Dr. Farius of Basle in 1689. The first successful separation of conjoined twins was performed in 1912 at the Military Families Hospital in Portsmouth, England. See Aird, p. 832; and E.W. Jenkins, T.R. Watson and W.T. Mosenthal, "Surgery in Conjoined Twins," *American Medical Association Archives of Surgery*, vol. 76, no. 1, (January, 1958), p. 35. There is, however, a report of an earlier separation in 1866 as a result of which one of the babies died after three days but the other survived. See *Anomalies and Curiosities*, p. 173. There is also an account of an attempt to separate female conjoined twins who were born in Italy in 1700. These twins died as the result of the surgeon's attempt to separate them. See *ibid.*, p. 178.

Recently, a remarkable case involved the separation of Lin and Win Htut at the Hospital for Sick Children in Toronto. The twins, born in Burma, shared a liver but each had its own gallbladder and bioducts. They shared a large intestine and rectum, bladder and penis. Each had his own quite normal heart, lungs, spleen, pancreas, stomach, small intestine, testes, spinal column, a single kidney and one normal leg. They shared a joint bladder with a vertical dividing wall, making two almost complete and separable bladders. In separating the twins, the surgeons severed the liver, leaving half to each twin complete with its gallbladder and bioducts. The twins each had one leg and each was to be fitted with a second artificial leg. The male genitalia were assigned to one child and artificial external female genital organs were surgically crafted. In effect, the second twin underwent a sex-change procedure. See Joan Hollobon, "Making Individuals of Siamese Twins," *Globe and Mail*, August 6, 1984, p. M7. For the halakhic implications of sex-change surgery see this writer's *Contemporary Halakhic Problems*, I (New York, 1977), 100–105.

42. See Norman J. Johnson and James E. Doherty, "Simultaneous Electrocardiagrams in Thoracopagus Twins," *American Heart Journal*, vol. 53, no. 1 (January 1957), pp. 150–156; and W. Riker and H. Traisman, "Conjoined Twins: Report of Three Cases," *Illinois Medical Journal*, vol. 126, no. 4 (October 1964), pp. 450–454.
43. See Donald C. Drake, "The Twins Decision: One Must Die So One Can Live," *Philadelphia Inquirer*, Oct. 16, 1977, p. 1A and pp. 14A–15A. This article also appears in *Nursing Forum*, vol. 16, no. 3–4 (Fall 1997), pp. 228–249.
44. Shortly after the attempted separation of the Philadelphia twins, conjoined thoracopagus twin sisters with a shared atrial myocardium were successfully separated in Salt Lake City, Utah. That procedure was accomplished with survival of both twins because it is possible that joined atria without joined ventricular myocardium may be divided with survival of both patients. In that case, one twin had hypoplastic right heart syndrome and was dependent on the other twin for oxygenation of her blood. An aortopulmonary shunt to increase her pulmonary blood flow was created. In addition, the prognosis of that twin was compromised by donation of skin to provide sufficient tissue for closure of the incision in the chest and abdominal wall of the other twin. Approximately one week after surgery, the twin affected by those complications suffered hepatic and renal failure. Death was attributed to severe cardiac and hepatic failure. See David Synhorst, Michael Matlak *et al.*, "Separation of Conjoined Thoracopagus Twins Joined at the Right Atria," *American Journal of Cardiology*, vol. 43, no. 3 (March 1979), pp. 662–

665. It should be noted that compromising the life of one twin in order to preserve the other represents a halakhic problem similar to that involved in the sacrifice of one twin in order to save the other.

45. A second, almost identical procedure was undertaken at the same hospital some ten years later in early 1987. The surgeon, Dr. James O'Neill Jr., did not seek a court order granting legal immunity in advance. The hospital's attorneys did, however, ask the District Attorney to sign a letter indicating that the procedure would not result in an attempt to prosecute for homicide. Unfortunately, neither twin survived. See Annas, p. 28.

A more recent case involved the Lakeberg twins, Amy and Angela. The twins, born in Loyola University Medical Center in Chicago, were born with a fused liver and a six-chamber heart with a hole in one chamber and blood from the lungs entering the wrong side. Physicians at Loyola estimated that there was less than a 1% chance that even one baby could survive separation and therefore counselled non-intervention. However, surgery was performed by Dr. James O'Neill Jr. at Children's Hospital in Philadelphia. In that case as well, one twin, Amy, was sacrificed in order to save the other. Angela survived the surgery but ten months later died suddenly as the result of a blockage in a blood vessel leading from the heart to the lungs. See *Newsweek*, August 23, 1993, p. 44; *Time*, August 30, 1993, pp. 43–44; and *Time*, June 27, 1994, pp. 61–62. That case engendered discussion by ethicists regarding the propriety of the expenditure of the large sums of money involved in treatment of the infant. See *Time*, August 30, 1993, p. 44 and June 27, 1994, p. 27; John J. Paris, "Ethical Issues in Separation of the Lakeberg Siamese Twins," *Journal of Perinatology*, vol. 13, no. 6 (November-December 1993), pp. 423–424; Brian M. Foley, "Siamese Twins Spark Debates Over Ethics and Rationing Health Care Resources," *Health Span*, vol. 10, no. 8 (September 1993), p. 2; Charles J. Dougherty, "A Life and Death Decision: The Lakeberg Twins," *Health Progress*, vol. 74, no. 9 (Summer 1995), pp. 16, 30–31; Kevin O'Rourke, "Separating the Lakeberg Twins: Ethical Issues," *Health Care Ethics USA*, vol. 2, no. 1 (1994), pp. 1–3; Charles J. Dougherty, "Joining in Life and Death: On Separating the Lakeberg Twins," *Bioethics Forum*, vol. 11, no. 1, (Spring 1995), pp. 9–16; and David C. Thomasna *et al.*, "The Ethics of Caring for Conjoined Twins: The Lakeberg Twins," *Hastings Center Report*, vol. 26, no. 4 (July-August 1996), pp. 4–11.

46. There were reports of at least two earlier attempts to save one conjoined twin by sacrificing the other. Karl Leiter, "Ein Craniapagus Parietalis Vivens," *Zentralblatt für Gynäkologie*, vol. 56, no. 27 (July 2, 1932), pp. 1644–1651, describes a case involving craniopagus conjoined twins who shared brain tissue. The brain of one child was removed, thereby causing its death. In that case, there was no compelling medical reason to prefer one twin over the other. After the separation both infants died. It is of interest to note that it was presumed that German law would regard killing one twin to save the other as homicide. However, unlike the position of the Philadelphia Family Court, it was decided that the twins were not two human beings but one monster from which a normal human being might be formed. See Robertson, p. 205. A second earlier attempt to save one twin closely resembled the case of the Philadelphia twins. Separation of twins born with a six-chamber heart was undertaken in Switzerland during the summer prior to Dr. Koop's endeavor. In that case the chest cavity appeared to have been closed too tightly to allow the six-chamber heart assigned to one twin to beat properly. The rescued twin died shortly after surgery. See *Philadelphia Inquirer*, p. 14-A, col. 3. Another reported case also involved craniopagus twins in whom the presence of a common sagittal sinus necessitated the sacrifice of one child. See Aird, p. 832. However, an examination of the original account of the procedure performed does not at all give the impression that the surgeons intended to sacrifice one of the infants. See Herbert J. Grossman, Oscar Sugar *et al.*, "Surgical Separation in Craniopagus," *Journal of the American Medical Association*, vol. 153, no. 3 (September 19, 1953), pp. 201–207.
47. At approximately the same time, dicephalous twins possessing two hearts were born at Children's Hospital in Little Rock, Arkansas. In that case, it became apparant that the twins could not be successfully separated with the survival of both. The County Prosecuting Attorney, with the concurrence of the State Attorney, concluded that surgical separation was legally justified and that no criminal prosecution would be sought. The surgery was performed on October 1, but the surviving twin expired on November 17th. See Golladay *et al.*, pp. 259–260.
48. *Philadelphia Inquirer*, p. 14-A., col. 1.
49. See Francis X. Meehan, "The Siamese Twin Operation and Contemporary Catholic Medical Ethics," *Linacre Quarterly*, vol. 45, no. 2 (May 1978), pp. 157–164. For a contradictory con-

clusion regarding the propriety of such a procedure from the vantage point of Catholic moral theology see C.K. Pepper, "Ethical and Moral Considerations in the Separation of Conjoined Twins," *Conjoined Twins: Birth Defects Original Article Series*, p. 133, as well as Annas, p. 28.

50. *Philadelphia Inquirer*, p. 14-A., col. 6.
51. *Philadelphia Inquirer*, p. 15-A, cols. 1–2; Annas, pp. 27–28.
52. *Legal Intelligencer*, p. 1.
53. Meehan, pp. 158–159; Annas, pp. 27–28; Joseph F. Kattner, "OK to Kill Twin to Save Other, Scholars Say," *Legal Intelligencer*, March 25, 1985, pp. 1 and 22; Rabbi Moshe D. Tendler, "Ke-she-Doḥin Nefesh Mipnei Nefesh," *Le-Torah ve-Hora'ah: Sefer Zikaron* (New York, 5749), pp. 114–122, reprinted in *idem, Responsa of Rav Moshe Feinstein*, I (Hoboken, N.J., 1996), pp. 209–213; and *idem*, "Unpublished Responsum: 'So One May Live,'" *ibid.*, pp. 125–133. The latter is not at all a responsum but an attempted reconstruction of the reasoning underlying Rabbi Feinstein's ruling. Rabbi Tendler carefully prefaces his analysis of Rambam's ruling in *Hilkhot Roẓeaḥ* 1:9, upon which he asserts Rabbi Feinstein based his reasoning, with the phrase "in my humble opinion" (*le-aniyut da'ati*). A different analysis of Rambam's statement based upon a published responsum of Rabbi Feinstein will be presented later in this discussion.
54. Annas, p. 27. See also *Philadelphia Inquirer*, p. 14-A, cols. 5–6.
55. See *Philadelphia Inquirer*, p. 14-A, col. 6; and Annas, p. 27.
56. Cf., R. Chaim Sofer, *Teshuvot Maḥaneh Ḥayyim, Ḥoshen Mishpat*, no. 50, who argues that "designation" is a factor only when it is within the power of the person specified for death to remove the danger to others by turning himself over to those demanding his life. It is not a factor, asserts *Maḥaneh Ḥayyim*, when the danger arises because the victim is "pursued by Heaven," i.e., a natural process totally independent of human volition. In the former case, argues *Maḥaneh Ḥayyim*, the individual is regarded as a *rodef* because he has the option of delivering himself to those seeking his death; in the case of the child emerging from the birth canal, there is no such option. In addition, *Maḥaneh Ḥayyim* asserts that "designation" is a factor only in situations involving an act of homicide since delivery of the designated victim serves to diminish the total number of instances of homicide. However, when death will result from natural causes, the rule in all cases, he maintains, is, in effect, "Better two deaths than one murder."

57. See *Teshuvot Panim Me'irot,* III, no. 8; R. Akiva Eger, *Tosefot R. Akiva Eger, Ohohot* 7:6, no. 16; and *infra,* note 70. The argument that one of the twins should be regarded as "designated" for death since that twin would certainly die in any event and that "designation" is sufficient grounds to sacrifice one person in order to save another was apparently suggested to Rabbi Feinstein and rejected by him. See *Responsa of Rav Moshe Feinstein,* p. 131.
58. See Annas, p. 27; and *Philadelphia Inquirer,* p. 14-A, col. 5.
59. That rationale is erroneously given in the sources cited *supra,* note 53.
60. A variant version of this analogy depicts a mountain climber who has fallen and is dangling from a rope attached to a friend. The friend cannot hold the weight of the fallen mountain climber and hence both climbers will imminently fall to their death. The person to whom the rope is attached may cut the rope even though it will lead to his partner's death. See Meehan, pp. 158–159; and *Philadelphia Inquirer,* p. 15-A, col. 2. Here, too, the person dangling from the rope is clearly a "pursuer" whose act causes the death of the person to whom the rope is attached.
61. See Rambam, *Hilkhot Roẓeaḥ* 1:9.
62. *Legal Intelligencer,* p. 22.
63. Personal communication, dated April 8, 1996, addressed to this writer.
64. See Leon M. Gerlis, Jeong-Wook Seo, Siew Yen Ho, and Je G. Chi, "Morphology of the Cardiovascular System in Conjoined Twins: Spatial and Sequential Segmental Arrangements in 36 Cases," *Teratology,* vo. 47, no. 2 (February 1993), p. 103.
65. Gerlis *et al.*, p. 103, emphasizes that even conjoined twins having two well-developed hearts should be described as having "shared hearts" rather than separate individual hearts. See also *ibid.*, p. 107.
66. It may indeed be cogently argued that King Solomon's use of scalding water as a test to determine whether both heads respond to a single pain stimulus was, in actuality, an attempt to determine whether or not the two heads share a common nervous system. If so, separate identity is predicated upon an independent nervous system. Accordingly, it might well be argued that "ownership" of individual organs is to be determined on the basis of control by, or association with, a particular nervous system. Consequently, it has occurred to this writer that it might

be possible to show that the heart, or an individual chamber of the heart, is controlled by the nervous system of one twin rather than by the nervous system of the other. There is, however, no indication that Dr. Koop performed the neurological tests necessary to make that determination. Moreover, on the basis of information provided by neonatologists consulted by this writer, there may well exist significant neurological crossover with the result that such tests would be rendered meaningless.

67. See *Philadelphia Inquirer*, p. 14-A, col. 3.

68. There may be an indication that Rabbi Feinstein did not regard the four-chamber heart as the "exclusive property" of one twin. It is reported that, in the midst of his deliberations, Rabbi Feinstein sought reassurance that it would be medically futile to assign the heart to the other twin. See *Philadelphia Inquirer*, p. 14-A, col. 4. He apparently was not prepared to sanction the sacrifice of one twin if the choice was an arbitrary one. The query would certainly have been inappropriate if the decision was predicated upon the concept of "ownership" of the heart.

69. This principle, to be sure, renders somewhat inconsistent Rambam's invocation of the law of pursuit, *Hilkhot Roẓeaḥ* 1:9, in justifying elimination of the fetus in order to preserve the life of the mother. That inconsistency will be addressed later in this discusion.

70. Rabbi Povarsky, however, fails to take cognizance of one highly significant difference between the case of dicephalous twins and the paradigmatic case of a pregnant woman in hard travail. The ruling of the Mishnah, *Oholot* 7:6, forbidding the sacrifice of a neonate whose head has already emerged from the uterus in order to save the mother can readily be understood as limited to circumstances in which the choice is between survival of the mother and survival of the child. The medical hazard described by the Mishnah is apparently death as the result of hemorrhaging. Termination of labor by performance of an embryotomy serves to eliminate that risk at the cost of the life of the fetus. Allowing labor to continue will cause bleeding to continue unabated but is likely to result in a live birth. A situation in which non-intervention will result in the certain loss of both mother and child with the sole option being sacrifice of the already doomed child in order to preserve the life of the mother is not explicitly discussed in the Mishnah. The question of the permissibility of killing the infant in order to save the mother when failure to do so would result in the loss of both is posed by *Te-*

shuvot Panim Me'irot, III, no. 8, whose comments are, in turn, cited by R. Akiva Eger, *Oholot* 7:6, no. 16. The comments of both *Panim Me'irot* and R. Akiva Eger seem to indicate that the issue hinges upon whether specification alone without attendant culpability is sufficient to warrant sacrifice of the one specified in order to save the other when, otherwise, both would die. Nevertheless, since both authorities declare that the matter requires further investigation, overt intervention cannot be sanctioned in such cases. For additional considerations present in the case of hard travail but of no direct relevance to the dilemma posed by conjoined twins see *Tiferet Yisra'el, Oholot, Bo'az* 7:10 and additional sources cited in *Contemporary Halakhic Problems*, I, 359–360.

71. Rabbi Povarsky's conclusion regarding the state of a *nefel* seems to be unexceptionable. Nevertheless, attention should be drawn to the puzzling statement of R. Eleazar Fleckles, *Teshuvah me-Ahavah*, I, no. 53, who declares that hastening the death of a *nefel* constitutes an infraction punishable by death at the hands of Heaven. *Teshuvah me-Ahavah* cites no source for that statement. Moreover, that assertion seems to contradict the position of the Gemara recorded in *Shabbat* 135a equating a *nefel* with a stone. The penalty of death at the hands of Heaven must, perforce, reflect the fact that a *nefel* is considered to be endowed with human life of a nature analogous to that of a *treifah* whose life, in terms of normative Halakhah, cannot be sacrificed in order to preserve the life of another person. For a discussion of that issue see *Contemporary Halakhic Problems*, IV (New York, 1955), 333, note 42. Cf., *Teshuvot Radvaz*, I, no. 695, who declares emphatically that hastening the death of a nonviable fetus does not entail even "doubtful homicide," but yet, for reasons that he does not explain, adds the comment "nevertheless, we restrain [people] so that they not hasten its death by means of an overt act."

72. See *Yevamot* 80a and *Tosafot, ad locum*, s.v. *ve-ha*.

73. In the case of a premature child maintained in an incubator, unlike other decisors, Rabbi Auerbach requires a waiting period of thirty days after the infant is removed from the incubator. He does not require any delay in the case of a baby carried to term who is maintained in an incubator for thiry days. See *Nishmat Avraham*, IV, *Yoreh De'ah* 305:11, note 1; and R. Neriyah Gotel, *Or ha-Mizraḥ*, Tevet 5749, p. 122, note 8. See also R. Yitzchak Zilberstein and R. Moshe Rothschild, *Torat ha-Yole-*

det 57:5, note 8; and *Nishmat Avraham, Yoreh De'ah* 374:8, note 1. This is also the opinion of R. Shmu'el ha-Levi Woszner, as cited by R. Gedaliah Oberlander, *Pidyon ha-Ben ke-Hilkhato* (Jerusalem, 5753), 3:31, note 67, with regard to a child who cannot survive outside of an incubator. A similar view is expressed more recently by Rabbi Woszner himself in an article appearing in *Kovez̤ Or Torah*, vol. 1, no. 1 (Tishri 5756), in which he expresses the view that every neonate placed in an incubator should be pressumed to be in this category. Rabbi Auerbach's view is disputed by R. Joseph Shalom Eliashiv, as reported in the same sources as well as by *Teshuvot Ḥelkat Ya'akov*, III, no. 109; *Teshuvot Be'er Mosheh*, I, no. 64; *Teshuvot Be'er Sarim*, I, no. 75; and *She'arim Mez̤uyanim be-Halakhah* 164:10, note 20. R. Ovadiah Yosef is cited in *Yalkut Yosef*, VII, chap. 8, sec. 5, note 6, as ruling that such a child requires redemption but, in light of the rule that, with regard to the laws of mourning, doubtful matters are adjudicated permissively, laws of mourning need not be observed.

74. See also R. Abraham Isaac Glick, *Teshuvot Yad Yiz̤ḥak*, II, no. 67, who rendered a similar decision with regard to observance of the laws of mourning. Cf., however, the analysis of Rambam's position presented in *Teshuvot Ḥatam Sofer, Even ha-Ezer*, II, no. 69, s.v. *ve-amnam*. *Ḥatam Sofer* maintains that, an infant born prematurely must be redeemed only after nine months have elapsed from the time of conception plus another thirty days.

75. See also R. Shlomoh Zalman Braun, *She'arim Mez̤uyanim be-Halakhah*, IV, 164:10, note 20; R. Joseph Shalom Eliashiv, cited by R. Yitzchak Zilberstein, *Assia*, no. 38 (Elul 5744), p. 34 and in *Torat ha-Yoledet* 57:5, note 8; Abraham S. Abraham, *Lev Avraham*, I (Jersualem, 5737), 32:5; *Nishmat Avraham, Yoreh De'ah*, 305:11, note 2; and *Nishmat Avraham*, IV, *Yoreh De'ah*, 305:11, note 1; R. Eliezer Waldenberg, *Z̤iz̤ Eli'ezer*, IX, no. 28, sec. 8; R. Jacob David Weisberg, *Oz̤ar Pidyon ha-Ben* (Jerusalem, 5754), 3:10–11 and *ibid.*, notes 31–32; and *Pidyon ha-Ben ke-Hilkhato* 3:31, notes 63–67.

Oz̤ar Pidyon ha-Ben 3:10, cites and rejects a minority view that does not sanction the redemption of even a baby carried to term so long as it requires an incubator. *Oz̤ar Pidyon ha-Ben, ibid.*, note 30, ascribes this view to the interlocutor in *Teshuvot Ḥelkat Ya'akov*, III, no. 109, and to sources cited by Rabbi Gotel, *Or ha-Mizraḥ*, p. 122. In actuality, the interlocutor quoted by *Teshuvot Ḥelkat Ya'akov* refers explicitly to a premature infant. Rabbi Gotel similarly cites the opinion of R. Shlomoh Zalman Auerbach that was pronounced only with regard to a premature infant. Rabbi Auerbach explicitly ruled that a baby carried to term must be redeemed on the thirty-first day even if it is still maintained in an incubator. See *Nishmat Avraham*, IV, *Yoreh De'ah* 305:11, note 1. See also *Pidyon ha-Ben ke-Hilkhato* 3:31, note 67.

76. *Contemporary Halakhic Problems*, III (New York, 1989), 160–193.
77. Indeed, such a neonate is more closely analogous to the situation of a child born without a stomach who survives for more than thirty days because he is sustained by means of artificial nutrition. R. Ya'akov Yitzchak Weisz, *Teshuvot Minḥat Yiẓḥak*, IX, no. 120, and R. Joseph Shalom Eliashiv, cited by *Nishmat Avraham*, IV, *Yoreh De'ah* 305:11, note 1, ruled that the child is not a *nefel* but a *treifah*, and, accordingly, laws of mourning must be observed. Rabbi Auerbach is quoted by *Nishmat Avraham* as being of the opinion that since, in the the absence of medical treatment, the infant would not have survived for a period of thirty days, it must be regarded as a *nefel*. Rabbi Auerbach apparantly distinguished between an incubator, which merely provides warmth and oxygen, and artificial nutrition which is necessary because of the absence of natural organs of digestion. The opposing view cogently regards a baby carried to term but lacking a vital organ who survives for thirty days as no different from a baby born with a perforation of that organ who survives for thirty days, i.e, as a *treifah* rather than a *nefel*. Such an infant is a *treifah* rather than a *nefel* even if it requires medical treatment in order to survive for thirty days.
78. See also *Ḥiddushei R. Akiva Eger, Ketubot* 33b.
79. *Iggerot Mosheh*'s categorization of Sheba ben Bichri as a pursuer is not novel; *Tiferet Yisra'el, Oholot, Bo'az* 7:10, similarly categorizes Sheba the son of Bichri as a pursuer. See also *Teshuvot Maḥaneh Ḥayyim, Ḥoshen Mishpat*, no. 50.
80. As earlier noted, Rambam's ruling concludes with the explanatory statement that the child cannot be sacrificed in order to save the life of the mother because "such is the nature of the world." Rambam clearly does not intend to ignore, much less to reject, the talmudic formulation "it is Heaven that pursues her." Thus, it is clear that Rambam seeks to clarify that the import of the talmudic dictum "it is Heaven that pursues her" is that the reason that the child is not deemed to be a pursuer is

because the danger is the result of nonvolitional physiological processes subject only to providence. In light of the talmudic basis of Rambam's statement, an interpretation of his statement as a reference to an ordinary versus a statistically rare threat to the life of the mother is not supportable. Frequency of occurence is entirely irrelevant to the meaning of Rambam's phrase "such is the nature of the world." Cf., *Le-Torah ve-Hora'ah*, p. 116; *Responsa of Rav Moshe Feinstein*, p. 211 and pp. 130–131.

81. For a discussion of rabbinic literature focusing upon that difficulty, see *Contemporary Halakhic Problems*, I, 347–349.
82. There is indeed a question with regard to the halakhic credibility of this type of evidence. See *Contemporary Halakhic Problems*, I, 360.
83. Personal communication, dated June 19, 1996, by Dr. C. Everett Koop addressed to this writer. This point is noted simply to confirm the existence of a cardiac anomaly that would render at least one of the twins a *treifah*. See Rambam, *Hilkhot Roẓeaḥ* 2:8, discussed *infra*, note 86. Whether, according to Rambam, human *treifut* is defined objectively, i.e., as an anomaly or trauma that generally results in death, or relatively, i.e., as an anomaly or trauma that will cause the affected person to die within a period of twelve months, is a matter of some doubt. See *Iggerot Mosheh, Ḥoshen Mishpat*, II, no. 73, sec. 4, and *Encyclopedia Talmudit*, vol. XXI (Jerusalem, 5753), p. 5, note 55.
84. In the case addressed by Rabbi Feinstein, Dr. Koop has stated that "it would have been impossible to separate the children and assign the heart to the child that was sacrificed." Personal communication, dated June 19, 1996, addressed to this writer.
85. See Golladay *et al.*, p. 263, and Gerlis *et al.*, p. 95.
86. The assumption that an infant lacking a heart or possessing a congenitally malformed heart is a *treifah* requires clarification. An obvious source for that position is the eighteenth-century ruling of R. Yonatan Eibeschutz in a celebrated controversy between himself and R. Zevi Ashkenazi.

A young woman eviscerated, soaked and salted a chicken, but failed to find a heart. She consulted R. Zevi Ashkenazi who, as recorded in his *Teshuvot Ḥakham Ẓevi*, nos. 74, 76 and 77, ruled that the animal was kosher. *Ḥakham Ẓevi* reasoned that, since it is impossible for any creature to survive without a heart for even a brief period of time, it must be assumed that the chicken, which had thrived and developed in a normal manner, must indeed have been endowed with a heart. The absence of a heart, declared *Ḥakham Ẓevi*, must assuredly be attributed to the predatory nature of a cat which must have been in close proximity. Not content with simply ruling with regard to the case presented to him, *Ḥakham Ẓevi* further announced that "even if witnesses will come and testify that they saw with open eyes that nothing was removed from the body of the chicken, it is certain that their testimony is false for it is contrary to reality." In sharp disagreement, R. Yonatan Eibeschutz, *Kereti u-Peleti* 40:4, declared that the testimony of credible witnesses cannot be dismissed peremptorily but rather "it must be assumed that there was some piece [of tissue] which does not appear as a heart but which is designed to fulfill the functions of the heart, but yet the chicken is *treifah* since it is not a normal heart." Thus, *Kereti u-Peleti* clearly regards an animal born with an anomalous heart to be a *treifah* because it lacks a normal heart.

However, *Ḥazon Ish, Yoreh De'ah* 4:14, takes issue with *Kereti u-Peleti* in arguing that the chicken thus described is indeed kosher. *Ḥazon Ish* argues that, although removal of the heart does indeed render the animal a *treifah*, there is no source for a ruling that an anomaly of the heart similarly renders the animal a *treifah*. Moreover, there is no indication that *Kereti u-Peleti* would regard a six-chamber heart in the same light as a mere piece of tissue that fulfills the functions of a heart.

The dispute between *Ḥazon Ish* and *Kereti u-Peleti* occurs in the context of the status of an animal. Rambam, *Hilkhot Roẓeaḥ* 2:8, asserts that the talmudic enumeration of the various *treifot* is exhaustive. However, insofar as human *treifot* are concerned, Rambam asserts that, in every era, the particular anomalies or traumas that render a human being a *treifah* are to be assessed in accordance with the medical knowledge of the day. Thus Rambam rules that a human being is not to be considered a *treifah* (and his murderer must be executed) unless "it is known with certainty that this [person] is a *treifah* and the physicians declare that this wound has no cure in a human being or he will die as a result of it unless something else kills him [sooner]." See also *Ḥazon Ish, Hilkhot Ishut* 27:3. Rambam's categorical statement regarding medical assessment of human *treifot* indicates both that a wound or anomaly that would render an animal a *treifah* does not necessarily render a human being a *treifah* and also that a wound that will cause death in man renders a human being a *treifah* even though, with regard to animals, it is not one of the enumerated *treifot*.

There are indeed many early authorities who disagree with Rambam's position and maintain that the determination of status as a *treifah* in humans is no different from determination of that status in animals. For a list of those authorities see *Encyclopedia Talmudit*, XXI, 4–7, and, in particular, *ibid.*, p.4, note 40. See also *Nishmat Avraham, Yoreh De'ah* 29:1, note 1. Nevertheless, Rambam's position together with the view expressed by *Kereti u-Peleti* with regard to anomalies of the heart might provide a rabbinic decisor with ample grounds for a determination that a child born with such a cardiac anomaly is a *treifah.*

87. To be sure, according to some analyses of the discussion of the Gemara, *Menaḥot* 37a, a child born with two heads is a *treifah.* See *supra*, note 27. Accordingly, it might be argued that each of the twins has the status of a *treifah* and hence they are, qualitatively speaking, equal pursuers of one another. However, such a conclusion is not necessarily correct. *Tosafot* indicate that a child possessing two heads is a *treifah* because of the principle that duplicate organs are both halakhically regarded as non-existent (*yeter ke-natul dami*); hence, the halakhic status of the child is that of a headless person. In context, the Gemara does not explicitly address the question of whether dicephalous twins are one person or two individuals. It appears to this writer that it may be argued that the Gemara seeks to assert that a two-headed individual has the status of a *treifah* only with regard to an individual who has the status of a single person, i.e., according to the analysis of the *Shitah Mekubeẓet*, if each head feels the pain of the other. However, if the twins are two separate individuals, i.e., they respond to pain stimuli separately and independently, there is no reason to assume the Gemara asserts that both are *treifot.* [Pelemo's query, "If a man has two heads, on which one must he place the *tefillin*?" is also best understood as applying to an individual regarded as one person. If the two-headed individual is regarded as two separate people, it stands to reason that each is obligated to don *tefillin*.] Since each is an independent entity, one twin possessess a full complement of organs but the second head is not an intrinsic part of its body and hence is not a duplicate organ. The second twin may perhaps be a *treifah* by virtue of the fact that it lacks other organs but nevertheless remains liable for redemption. Cf., *Ot Ḥayyim ve-Shalom* 28:9, note 13. On the other hand, one may argue that, if the twins are separate individuals, neither is a *treifah* since each possesses all vital organs, albeit in commom with the other

twin. Alternatively, Rabbi Feinstein may well have agreed with the scholars who understood the Gemara's final position to be that a two-headed individual is not at all a *treifah*; if so, the problem is entirely dispelled.

It should be noted that, according to those authorites who do not accept the position of Rambam discussed *supra*, note 86, if the twins are two separate individuals and the twin lacking independent organs is regarded to be a *treifah*, as argued by *Ot Ḥayyim ve-Shalom*, and assuming that the other twin is not a *treifah*, it would follow that, according to Rabbi Feinstein's analysis, the twin lacking independent organs should be sacrificed in order to save the other twin. The problem, then, would be identification of the twin to whom those vital organs belong. However, as argued earlier contra the view of *Ot Ḥayyim ve-Shalom*, it is not at all clear that either twin must be a *treifah* since all vital organs are present, albeit shared in common. In any event, Rabbi Feinstein's ruling may have been predicated upon acceptance of the view that a two-headed person is not a *treifah* or upon Rambam's position regarding human *treifut* as explained *supra*, note 86.

88. This responsum was written by Rabbi Feinstein in 1935 while he resided in the U.S.S.R. and addresses the totally different, but halakhically related, question of whether, in order to preserve the sanctity of other synagogues in the city, the sanctity of one synagogue may be violated by turning it over to Communist authorities who would use it for improper purposes.
89. See the exchange between Professor Zev Low and this writer in *Tradition*, vol. 31, no. 4 (Summer 1997), pp. 80–82.

12

The Cases of Baby Jane Doe and Baby Fae

I. LIFE AS A PARAMOUNT VALUE

"We hold these truths to be self-evident, that all men are endowed by their Creator with certain unalienable rights, that among these are life, liberty and the pursuit of happiness." In these words of the opening section of the Declaration of Independence, the Founding Fathers of this country borrowed and adapted a Lockean concept of natural law. But neither the source nor the particular formulation is of singular importance. What is significant is the express acknowledgment both of the right to life and of its inalienability. Of even greater moment is the acknowledgment "[t]hat to secure these rights, governments are instituted among men." Herein lies a forthright declaration to the effect that society, through its governmental institutions, bears the responsibility for protecting and safeguarding that inalienable right.

This paper was originally delivered at a conference on "The Handicapped Newborn in American Society" sponsored by Fordham University in March 1985.

Even at the time of its formulation in 1776, the doctrine enunciated in the Declaration of Independence was hardly novel in the annals of legal theory. The *parens patriae* doctrine has long been a cardinal principle of common law. Although cast in language of governmental right rather than duty and not necessarily predicated upon natural law theory, this principle embodies the propositions that (1) society has an interest in the preservation of the life of each of its members and (2) this societal prerogative takes precedence over the principle of personal autonomy.

Nowhere in the vast corpus of common law is there so much as a hint of an assertion that the quality of any particular life serves either to diminish an individual's inalienable right to that life or to mitigate society's legitimate interest in its preservation. It was not until 1976 in the decision handed down in *In re Karen Quinlan*[1] that the Supreme Court of the State of New Jersey, in an attempt to balance the conflicting principles of state interest and personal autonomy, declared the State's interest to be less than absolute. The Court expressly affirmed the primacy of the State's interest in "the preservation and sanctity of human life" but qualified that interest in stating:

> We think that the State's interest . . . weakens and the individual's right to privacy grows as the depth of bodily invasion increases and the prognosis dims. Ultimately there comes a point at which the individual's right overcomes the State interest.[2]

Whatever the merits of that decision, or the lack thereof, this assertion of a mitigation of the State's interest in the preservation of human life, limited as it is to patients in a persistent non-cognitive, vegetative state, is certainly irrelevant to questions pertaining to the treatment of neonates suffering from congenital anomalies. Nor does it automatically follow that there exists a right to withhold treatment from even a comatose minor. This is best illustrated by the example of two cases decided on the same day by the Court of Appeals of the State of New York. In the well-known Brother Fox case the Court was perfectly willing to allow life-support systems to be disconnected from a patient in a state of irreversible coma in accordance with the previously announced desire of the patient.[3] The Court, however, in a companion opinion announced the very same day in *In the Matter of Storer*[4] was not prepared to honor the wishes of a parent and to permit the withholding of treatment from a mentally retarded patient whose status in the eyes of the law is comparable to that of a minor.

The latter decision was entirely consistent with well established common law principles. To be sure, parents are entitled to make decisions regarding the health, education and welfare of their offspring. Courts are ordinarily reluctant to interfere with familial decision making if for no other reason than that parenting is best left to parents. However, in a fundamental legal sense, parents are merely the surrogates of the State. Invoking the *parens patriae* doctrine, the State may remove the parents from the decision-making process when it finds that the parents fail to act in accordance with the best interests of the child—or of the State.

Recognition of the inalienable nature of the right to life has traditionally found expression in statutes which forbid abrogation of the right to life not only by others but by oneself as well. Thus, not only is murder proscribed upon pain of criminal sanction, but consensual murder and suicide are forbidden as well. The lack of capacity on the part of a person voluntarily to forego his right to life is in clear conflict with the notion of liberty or personal autonomy which was also expressly regarded by our founding fathers as an inalienable right. The common law tradition clearly manifests a hierarchical ranking of values. The phrase "life, liberty and the pursuit of happiness" was crafted with a precision which reflects that ranking. The earlier cited decision of the New York Court of

Appeals acknowledges that although, as an operative legal principle, preservation of life is tempered, at least at times, by respect for personal autonomy, nevertheless, the inherent presumption that life constitutes the paramount value remains. Hence the right to life, even when it can be waived, can be waived only by an autonomous individual who is fully capable of exercising an informed and reasoned waiver of that right. Accordingly, when parents fail to act in a manner designed to preserve the life of their child, the State, in its role as the ultimate guarantor of the rights of the individual member of society, will intervene.

These principles were affirmed, in form if not in substance, in the judicial decision in the case of Baby Jane Doe.[5] This highly publicized Long Island case involved a child born with spina bifida. The Appellate Division, in affirming the parents' right to refuse surgery for the purpose of closing the baby's spinal column, in no way denied its obligation to assure that the child would receive life-sustaining treatment. Nor did the Court recognize a superior right of parental autonomy. It stated only that, when alternative procedures are available, the decision with regard to the choice of therapy lies with the parents, as indeed it should when such choice is made in a responsible manner. In the case of Baby Jane Doe, the Court ruled that, in withholding permission for the recommended surgical procedure, the parents were not renouncing medical care but were, in effect, choosing an alternative mode of treatment, *viz.*, antibiotics coupled with palliative treatment.

Whether or not this constitutes an accurate categorization of their decision is an entirely different matter. There is no gainsaying the fact that the child did survive despite failure to close the spinal column. Nevertheless, a neurologist might well respond that, medically, such "therapy" is analogous to the treatment of cancer by means of administration of aspirin. Clearly, such treatment would be irresponsible despite the fact that some cancer patients do experience spontaneous remission. Nevertheless, insofar as the decision itself is concerned, the form in which it is couched reflects recognition of the basic principle to be applied even while employing sophistic reasoning in its misapplication. As de la Rochefoucauld wrote, "Hypocrisy is the homage which vice pays to virtue."[6]

II. MAXIMIZING LIFE-QUANTA

This is not to say that the parents of Baby Jane Doe made a morally incorrect decision. On the contrary, their decision, objectively speaking, may have been entirely valid regardless of whether or not they themselves were motivated by considerations endowed with moral validity. The morally legitimate motive for declining surgical intervention in the case of Baby Jane Doe is related to the hazards associated with the surgical procedure required to close the spinal column and not to the question of the severity of the handicap with which Baby Jane must live or the quality of life she may anticipate. The gravity of the hazard posed by the required surgical procedure depends, of course, upon many physiological factors and will certainly not be identical for all patients. Indeed, in many neonates afflicted with spina bifida, the risks associated with surgery may be minimal. Nevertheless, when such risks are significant the moral issues assume an entirely different guise.

A moral system which recognizes preservation of life as a paramount value must come to grips with the stark fact that life is fraught with situations in which risks must be confronted and assessed. Most decisions to perform even the most ordinary and mundane acts involve an assumption of some risk. At times, the risks of intervention are as great, or even greater, than those of inaction. A vaccine against a dread disease may be defective and cause the very disease against which it is designed to provide protection. Although exercise is of demonstrated efficacy in the prevention of obesity, physical exertion may well precipitate a heart attack. For reasons which are quite obvious, assumption of such risks presents no moral dilemma. Statistically, the danger of contracting disease through contagion is far greater than the risk of possible harm resulting from inoculation with material drawn from a defective batch of vaccine. Obesity has caused far more fatal heart attacks than has strenuous exercise. Indeed, in situations in which these statistical considerations do not pertain, the approbation of society is withheld. For that reason we require FDA approval of all drugs and recommend that no one embark upon a regimen of strenuous exercise without first undergoing a thorough physical examination.

There are, of course, innumerable occasions in which risks are assumed even though no such "balancing act" is involved. A motor vehicle is a lethal weapon. Yet we condone the recreational use of passenger cars with no more hesitation than accompanies our endorsement of the emergency use of ambulances. Even as innocuous an activity as crossing the street is not devoid of hazard. Although such risks are statistically significant, we do not feel that we are engaged in weighty decision making every time we hail a cab or go for a stroll in the park. The risks involved in such situations are regarded as minimal and hence as falling below the threshold of moral significance. The Sages of the Talmud dismissed such risks with the citation of a biblical passage, "The Lord preserveth the simple" (Psalms 116:6). In context, this dictum counsels, in effect, that such dangers are best ignored. One almost gets the feeling that we are being advised that exaggerated concern for a minimal danger may constitute a greater hazard than the danger itself. Certainly, exaggerated fear, even when the danger is to some extent real, can breed neuroses and worse.

But there are situations in which the moral dilemma is very real. A patient is afflicted with terminal disease. The only treatment available requires administration of a potent drug which, if successful, will remove all traces of disease and, in terms of longevity anticipation, restore the patient to the *status quo ante.*

However, the drug is highly toxic and in a statistically predictable proportion of patients the drug itself will foreshorten life. Is it morally legitimate for the patient to assume the risks inherent in such therapy? After all, a brief span of human life is endowed with moral value of the highest order. May a patient, in effect, enter into a gamble in which he stakes a limited, but certain, life span against a longer, but uncertain, life expectancy?

Our intuitive feeling that such risks, when reasonable and prudent, are morally acceptable is confirmed by moralists and theologians. Virtually all major surgery poses an issue of this nature and no responsible voice has been raised decrying surgery as an immoral practice of medicine.

But is the assumption of such risks morally mandated or is the assumption of such risks merely morally acceptable? Not every act which falls within the broad zones of moral acceptability is *ipso facto* morally mandated. In cases such as these there are competing life-claims each of which is compelling: preservation of a quantum of life-certain versus acquisition of a greater quantum of life-doubtful.

Perhaps a moral agent might be required to construct a risk-benefit equation. Let us assume that, in the absence of treatment, the patient is endowed with a life-certain longevity anticipation of one week. Let us further assume that the proposed treatment has a predictable success rate of ten percent, with success defined as survival for a period of ten weeks, but that failure will result in immediate death. If the goal is maximization of human life-quanta there is no risk-benefit advantage in treatment over non-treatment or vice versa. By way of illustration, let us assume that there are two groups of patients each of which is composed of 100 such patients and that one group is treated while the other group is left untreated. The 100 untreated patients will each survive for a period of one week. For the untreated group as a whole the aggregate longevity anticipation is 100 human life-weeks. Of the members of the second group, i.e. the recipients of the proposed hazardous therapy, ninety will expire immediately and ten will survive for a period of ten weeks. For this group as well, the aggregate longevity anticipation is 100 human life-weeks. Thus it is readily apparent that, in terms of maximization of human life-quanta, the risk-benefit advantage of treatment is exactly equal to that of non-treatment. Let us posit a third group of patients, identical with the first two groups in every respect save that the predictable success rate, defined as survival for a period of ten weeks, is only five percent. For this group, the beneficial yield of treatment is reduced to 50 human life-weeks as opposed to an aggregate of 100 human life-weeks to be anticipated if treatment is withheld. Since, for members of this group, the risk-benefit yield is negative, treatment is clearly a poor gamble. Assume a fourth group for whom the success rate, as success has previously been defined, is predicted to be 20%. For that group the anticipated aggregate longevity is 200 human life-weeks and, accordingly, if the goal is the maximization of human life-quanta, there is strong reason to recommend that treatment be initiated.

Consider a game of chance in which the stakes are $10 and the return to a winner is $100. If odds of winning are less than one in ten, the gambler is a fool; if the odds of winning are greater than 1 in 10, the gambler is a smart business man. Intuitively, one would discourage the first gambler and encourage the second and one would do so with full conviction. Yet who could, with equal conviction, give such advice to a patient gambling with his life? Of course, medicine remains an art and is not yet an exact science. Survival odds and quanta of life-expectancy cannot be calculated with a precision remotely comparable to that with which slot machines can be calibrated. But more fundamentally, the gambler does not gamble with a single $10 bill. With one chance in nine of winning $100 on a $10 wager the gambler need only play repeatedly and his ultimate gain is, mathematically, a virtual certainty. If the odds of winning are less than one chance in ten the gambler's loss over repeated plays is equally certain. But suppose that the rules provide for only one chance to play. A one in five chance of winning $100 may constitute a very attractive wager, but not if the $10 is immediately needed for some other urgent purpose. A wager which provides one chance in twenty of winning $100 may be a poor investment, but not if there is nothing that one can buy with a $10 bill and a great deal that one can buy with $100.

Were humans blessed with the proverbial nine lives of the cat the comparison would be entirely apt. But each person has only one life, only one $10 bill, and only one chance to play. Under such circumstances there is no determinant risk-benefit ratio which serves as an objective point of demarcation between prudence and foolhardiness. The net result is that, when confronted by such a decision, there is no morally absolute right or wrong. The *desideratum* is enhancement of life quanta. But in any individual situation it is impossible to determine which choice will yield maximum enhancement. Hence, in such circumstances, the decision to treat and the decision not to treat are, morally speaking, equally acceptable.

Thus, in the case of Baby Jane Doe, assuming—and the assumption may well be an unreasonable one—that the infant's general clinical profile was such that surgical intervention itself posed a significant risk of foreshortening her life, the parents' decision not to permit surgery would have been well within the bounds of moral acceptability.

III. EVALUATING AND BALANCING RISKS

It is well established that parents are entitled to make decisions with regard to the health, education and welfare of their children. There are at least three sound reasons why parents ought to be accorded that prerogative: (1) The nature of the parental bond is such that parents can be trusted more so than others to act selflessly and in the best interests of the child. (2) The intimate nature of the parental relationship renders parents more knowledgeable that others insofar as the unique needs and aspirations of a child is concerned. (3) Considerations of physical proximity as well as of economy of time and resources render decision making by parents more efficient than any other readily available alternative. Of course, when, either through malfeasance or nonfeasance, parents are grossly remiss in fulfilling such functions, society has the moral right and obligation to discharge the parents from their decision-making role and to assign that function to some other agent or agency.

There are, however, medical situations in which individuals are powerless to make meaningful decisions unilaterally either for themselves or for their children. A choice between available alternative medical therapies requires an informed decision but all too frequently the patient—or parent—lacks the knowledge and medical sophistication for meaningful decision-making. Quite naturally, the tendency is to rely upon the expert advice of medical practitioners. That advice is, however, not always disinterested and altruistic. Indeed, given the nature of the human condition, it cannot be. Consciously or unconsciously, considerations and concerns having nothing at all to do with the welfare of the patient must intrude and color the advice proffered by medical practitioners. As a class, defective newborns are probably most likely to be adversely affected by the deficiencies of the medical decision-making process.

The celebrated case of Baby Fae[7] involving a cross-species heart transplant represents a striking example of this problem. The decision to implant a baboon heart in the chest of Baby Fae presents a number of moral issues:

1. Should surgical intervention of any type have been attempted? Baby Fae suffered from hypoplastic left heart syndrome, a congenital anomaly that certainly would have caused her to die. But how long could she have been expected to live absent any type of surgical intervention? If it is accepted that

maximization of life-expectancy is the primary goal of such therapy then no procedure can be considered ethical unless there exists a reasonable and realistic anticipation that life-expectancy will be maximized be means of such therapy. When reasonable anticipation of a cure exists, but the statistical probability of success in affecting such a cure is low, we are confronted by the previously discussed quandary attendant upon all hazardous procedures. However, in considering a procedure which offers no realistic benefit to the patient insofar as longevity enhancement is concerned (or, for that matter, insofar as enhancement of quality of life is concerned) the sole justification for initiation of such therapy is its experimental value. The question of whether or not a mentally competent adult patient may ethically consent to a procedure which offers him no therapeutic benefit but which may well foreshorten his life is an entirely different moral problem and is fully deserving of analysis in terms of the issues it presents. Yet, even if such procedures were to be regarded as morally acceptable, no one would argue that assumption of such risk is morally mandated because of the potential utilitarian value of hazardous experimental procedures to society in general. Hence, no one would countenance initiation of such procedures other than upon the informed consent of the person placed at risk.

Granted that parents are empowered to make decisions with regard to the health and welfare of their children, such authority is vested in parents upon the presumption that parents will exercise their discretion in the best interests of the child as those best interests are perceived by the child's parents. Parents have no moral right to predicate such decisions upon any other consideration—not even upon consideration of the greater benefit which may accrue to society. A course of action which, because of moral constraints, cannot be involuntarily imposed upon an individual does not become moral because some party—no matter how closely related—grants vicarious consent.

There is no doubt whatsoever that recognition of the limits of vicarious consent would seriously limit scientific research. It must be candidly recognized and acknowledged that the therapeutic imperative and the experimental imperative are not one and the same. Absent informed consent—which in the case of an infant is an impossibility—advancement of the cause of science, or the interests of children in general, does not constitute justification for placing a child at risk. *Primum non nocere* remains the first commandment governing the physician-patient relationship. The sole justification for subjecting any child to a hazardous procedure is the potential for advancing the cause of *that* child.

2. Assuming that surgical intervention did present a reasonable possibility of benefit to Baby Fae, it surely is the case that, given a choice of procedures, either the procedure offering the optimum risk-benefit ratio or the procedure posing the least hazard to the child should have been pursued. It is, however, reliably reported that doctors at Loma Linda University Medical Center made no effort to obtain a human heart for transplantation. Certainly, the ethics committee which approved the cross-species transplant made no such stipulation. The surgeon, Dr. Leonard Bailey, had performed numerous cross-species transplants in animals over a period of seven years. In Dr. Bailey's own studies the longest animal survival was 165 days.[8] Although Baby Fae survived for 20 days, the longest previous human survival with a heart zenograft was three and one half days.[9] While implantation of a baboon heart was assuredly more useful to the cause of science, there is no doubt that a human heart transplant would have been more beneficial to Baby Fae.

3. Transplantation of a human heart or a cross-species transplant are not the sole options available in the treatment of infants suffering from hypoplastic left heart syndrome. Surgeons at Boston Children's Hospital have developed a two-stage operation for correction of this anomaly.[10] At least the first stage has been performed on approximately 100 children.

Since 40% of the children treated in this way have died, the procedure must certainly be regarded as hazardous in nature. But, by the same token, 60% have survived and that survival rate is far higher than the most optimistic survival rate presently projected for the recipients of zenografts.

No one has imputed, or should impute, venal motives to the physicians associated with the Loma Linda Medical Center. But as physicians and as dedicated medical researchers the decisions and recommendations of those individuals are necessarily colored by two factors: (1) their dedication to the cause of science which, by virtue of its very nature, conflicts with the cause of the patient; (2) their expertise in cross-species transplantation is not matched by similar expertise in either human heart transplantation or in surgical correction of the anomaly presented in cases of hypoplastic left heart syndrome. Since they have not been trained in the surgical procedure developed at Boston Children's Hospital and since Loma Linda lacks approval for human cadaver heart transplantation, the surgeons who recommended a zenograft could hardly be expected to make an unbiased recommendation based solely upon the best interests of the patient. Ignoring the perfectly natural and human inclination for success and glory attendant upon the development of a novel and dramatic procedure, there exists a perfectly understandable inclination to believe sincerely that one's own product is superior to that of one's competitor.

IV. DISPASSIONATE DECISION MAKING

The determination that a proposed procedure is therapeutic (i.e., of potential benefit to the patient) rather than experimental is not always obvious. Determination of the existence of a favorable risk-benefit ratio is often even more difficult. If the attending physician's opinion cannot be regarded as unbiased, to whom shall the patient turn for dispassionate evaluation?

How can one guarantee the right of infants and minors to a decision based solely upon their best interests?

Over a century ago Jewish medical ethics developed a *modus operandi* for dealing with this problem. The specific question involved a patient afflicted with an illness which, if left untreated, would have been fatal. A potentially curative drug was available but there existed a danger that it might cause the immediate demise of the patient. A leading rabbinic decisor was consulted with regard to the proper course of action. He counseled that the risk be evaluated by a number of expert medical practitioners and that subsequent to eliciting multiple medical opinions the view of the majority be followed "upon the acquiescence of 'the wise man' of the town."[11] What role did the "wise man" play in the decision-making process? Although he may have been sagacious, he clearly was not a physician. Perforce he must have relied upon the medical advice of local doctors. Nevertheless, his function was not at all redundant. His role was to assess the reliability and impartiality of the medical advice conveyed and to detect any possible personal or professional bias on the part of the medical consultants. The primary qualification of the "wise man" was that he had neither a personal nor a professional involvement with either the patient or the treatment and hence he could remain detached and dispassionate.

One might suppose that, under present conditions, such a role might be filled by a hospital's ethics committee. Unfortunately, due to the manner in which such committees are constituted, this cannot be the case. The requirement for ethics committee approval of all experimental procedures involving human subjects does place certain meaningful restraints upon potentially unethical procedures. But in a case such as that of Baby Fae there is no greater assurance that the ethics committee will arrive at a decision in a disinterested manner than there is that the surgeon will do so. Procedures such as a zenograft are team efforts; success redounds to the glory and benefit of the institution and of all persons associated with it. Although there is community representation on hospital ethics committees, the overwhelming majority of the members of such committees are members of the institution's own medical and administrative staff. Self-interest can be avoided only if the ethics committee is composed of persons with no ties either to the medical facilities whose procedures are subject to review or to sister and hence "rival" institutions. Of course, the decisions of such a committee can be ethically meaningful only if its members are both knowledgeable of, and committed to, the fundamental principles of ethics which should govern all decision making. But it is imperative that society provide effective ombudsmen to protect the rights and interests of those who cannot possibly protect themselves.

NOTES

1. *In re Karen Quinlan*, 70 N.J. 10, 355 A.2d 647 (1976).
2. *Id. at* 41, 355 A.2d at 664.
3. *Eichner* v. *Dillon,* 52 N.Y.2d 363, 420 N.E.2d 64, 438 N.Y.S.2d 266 (1981).
4. *Eichner* v. *Dillon,* 52 N.Y.2d 363, 420 N.E.2d 64, 438 N.Y.S.2d 266 (1981).
5. *Weber* v. *Stony Brook Hospital,* 95 A.D.2d 587, 467 N.Y.S.2d 685 (App. Div. 2d Dep't 1983), *aff'd* 60 N.Y.2d 208, 456 N.E.2d 1186, 469 N.Y.S.2d 63 (1983).
6. *Maxims*, no. 218.
7. See Leonard L. Bailey, Sandra L. Nehlsen-Cannarella *et al.*, "Baboon-to-Human Cardiac Xenotransplantation in a Neonate," *Journal of the American Medical Association,* vol. 254, no 23 (December 20, 1985), 3321–3329.
8. "The Case of Baby Fae"(Editorial), *Journal of the American Medical Association,* vol. 254, no. 23, p. 3358.
9. See Council on Scientific Affairs, "Zenografts: Review of the Literature and Current Status," *Journal of the American Medical Association,* vol. 254, no. 23, p. 3355.
10. See William I. Norwood, Peter Lang, *et al.*, "Experience with

Operations for Hypoplastic Left Heart Syndrome," *Journal of Thoracic and Cardiovascular Surgery*, vol. 82, no. 4 (October 1981), pp. 511–519; and William Lang and Dolly D. Hanson, "Physiologic Repair of Aortic Atresia-Hypoplastic Left Heart Syndrome," *New England Journal of Medicine*, vol. 308, no. 1 (January 6, 1983), pp. 23–26.

11. R. Jacob Reischer, *Teshuvot Shevut Ya'akov,* III, no.75.

Index of Biblical and Talmudic Sources

BIBLE

MISHNAH AND TALMUD

General Index

C